EXPLORATIONS IN MICROBIOLOGY

EXPLORATIONS IN MICROBIOLOGY

BARBARA K. HUDSON, MT (ASCP), CLS
Montana State University

LINDA SHERWOOD, PhD
Montana State University

Prentice Hall, Upper Saddle River, New Jersey 07458

Acquisition Editor: *Linda Schreiber*
Executive Editor: *David Kendric Brake*
Editorial Director: *Tim Bozik*
Editor-in-Chief: *Paul Corey*
Assistant Vice President of Production and Manufacturing: *David W. Riccardi*
Production Editor: *James Buckley*
Special Projects Manager: *Barbara A. Murray*
Executive Marketing Manager: *Kelly McDonald*
Marketing Assistant: *David Stack*
Manufacturing Buyer: *Ben Smith*
Manufacturing Manager: *Trudy Pisciotti*
Creative Director: *Paula Maylahn*
Supplement Cover Manager: *Paul Gourhan*
Cover Designer: *Liz Nemeth*
Cover Photo: Courtesy of *Center for Biofilm Engineering, Montana State University–Bozeman*

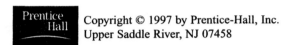

Copyright © 1997 by Prentice-Hall, Inc.
Upper Saddle River, NJ 07458

Library of Congress Cataloging-in-Publication Data

Hudson, Barbara K.
    Explorations in microbiology / Barbara K. Hudson, Linda Sherwood.
      p. cm.
    Includes bibliographical references.
    ISBN 0-13-533589-2
    1. Microbiology—Laboratory manuals. I. Sherwood, Linda.
  II. Title.
  QR63.H83 1997   96-54258
  579'.078—dc21   CIP

ISBN 0-13-533589-2

Prentice-Hall International (UK) Limited, *London*
Prentice-Hall of Australia Pty. Limited, *Sydney*
Prentice-Hall Canada Inc., *Toronto*
Prentice-Hall Hispanoamericana, S.A., *Mexico*
Prentice-Hall of India Private Limited, *New Delhi*
Prentice-Hall of Japan, Inc., *Tokyo*
Editora Prentice-Hall do Brasil, Ltda., *Rio de Janeiro*

Printed in the United States of America

10 9 8 7 6 5 4

CONTENTS

PREFACE

TO THE STUDENTS

Microbiology is a diverse and exciting science. Aspects of many other scientific disciplines—chemistry, biology, genetics, engineering, and mathematics—are incorporated into the exploration and exploitation of microorganisms. Microbiology is also a rapidly changing field. Therefore, not only will you need to learn the skills and major concepts of the day, but you must also be able to adapt to new technologies and theories as they develop. The learning you do now is just the beginning of a process that will continue throughout your career.

All research on learning indicates that you will gain a deeper understanding of microbiology and retain it longer if you are actively involved in the learning process. Active learning entails gathering information (either through experimentation or from written or electronic resources), analyzing information, critical thinking, and problem solving. Studies also indicate you will learn better if you feel the material has immediacy and relevancy to your life. We have written a laboratory manual that we hope will engage you, motivate you, and help you develop learning skills that will be used throughout your career. This manual differs from others in a variety of ways, some of which are listed below. Perhaps the most noticeable difference is that you are often asked to provide more direction for your own learning, while your instructor steps back and acts as a facilitator. As you will see, many exercises require you to design and use your own experimental protocols and then analyze the results. We have used this approach because it allows you to strengthen your critical thinking and problem-solving skills.

There are many other features of *Explorations in Microbiology* that make this manual unique:

- Virtually all exercises begin with a scenario designed to pique your interest in the topic being discussed, establish the relevance of the technique or concept, and serve as a basis for class discussion.
- Each exercise contains up-to-date background information that further establishes the relevance of the exercise.
- Most exercises end with questions that encourage you to reflect on your experience with the exercise. They also allow you to integrate and use concepts and skills learned in the exercise. Some of the questions may require examination of the topic or related topics in more detail by seeking information from sources outside the laboratory or the manual.
- Many exercises are discovery-based, which means that previously learned content and skills are used to design an experiment, conduct the procedure(s), analyze the results, and report the findings. This experience will enable you to develop a deeper understanding of the major concepts covered in the exercise.
- The outcomes of many of the exercises can be described in the form of a research article in a scientific journal. Other exercises lend themselves to being written as reports that follow the format used by microbiologists who work in a clinical setting.
- Most exercises require you to work with a partner or in a group. Working together with classmates not only facilitates your mastery of the material (because what you don't know, your partner may), but also teaches you important communication skills that will benefit you in any career you choose.

It is our hope that by doing these exercises and learning the concepts and skills necessary to study microorganisms, you will gain an appreciation of the diversity of microbes and understand how much we know, and perhaps more important, do not know about them. With this in mind, we have included exercises from many topic areas, including a look at how procaryotic and eucaryotic microorganisms are isolated and classified; how they grow and reproduce; how they are studied at a genetic level, their roles in ecosystems; how they produce disease; how the body defends itself against them; and how microbes are exploited.

We wish to gratefully acknowledge the support of colleagues and our families during the development of this manual. Most importantly, we wish to thank our husbands, Tom Hudson and John Sherwood, for their patience and help. In addition, the following people provided expertise and assistance in developing this manual:

Calvin Abernathy   *Jim Cutler*
Donald M. Anderson   *Todd Damrow*
Mary Bateson   *Peggy Dirckx*
Cliff Bond   *Ken Emerson*
Sue Broadaway   *JoAnn Fenn*
Frank Caccavo   *Tom Foubert*
Kari Cargill   *Gil Geesey*
John Carlsten   *Pati Glee*
Barbara Cooksey   *Karen Kelsey*
Keith Cooksey   *Beth MacConnell*

Bonnie Maidak   *Carol Sharrock*
Tim McDermott   *Robert Sharrock*
Gordon McFeters   *John Sherwood*
Tom McMahon   *Dan Siemsen*
Terry Mudder   *Vance Thurston*
Steve Nold   *Ken Todd*
Barry Pyle   *David Ward*
Neils Ramsing   *Robin Williams*
Kathy Sandoval-Billings

We also thank three reviewers who gave us insightful and meaningful comments that guided our thinking: John Lennox, Galen Renwick, and Linda Kimble. Last but not least, we greatly acknowledge the support and guidance we have received from Linda Schreiber at Prentice-Hall, who was willing to take the risk of developing this different kind of laboratory manual.

Barbara Hudson
Linda Sherwood

LABORATORY SAFETY

A safe laboratory requires that you make a conscious effort to follow guidelines developed to prevent infection by the microorganisms being studied. This manual does not recommend the use of any highly virulent human or plant pathogens. However, *any organism* that is ingested or injected into the body has the potential of being pathogenic. This is particularly true in immunocompromised humans. The human immune system can be compromised in several different ways, including immunosuppressive drugs, surgery, stress, wounds or cuts, or lowered resistance due to another disease.

In addition to microorganisms, you may handle potentially dangerous chemicals, use open flames, and handle sharp objects. Throughout the manual are **caution** warnings in bold print that should be strictly observed.

The following guidelines are meant to help you establish safe laboratory practices to use in these exercises and in any laboratory work you do in the future:

1. Do not eat, drink, smoke, or apply cosmetics in the laboratory. Keep your fingers, pencils, and other materials away from your face and mouth.
2. To avoid taking any organisms out of the laboratory on your clothing, always wear a buttoned lab coat. When removing your laboratory coat at the end of the laboratory period, turn it inside out, fold it over, and store it in the locker provided. At the end of the term, bring a plastic bag to the last laboratory period, place your laboratory coat in it before removing it from the work area, and transfer it directly to a washing machine. Washing the laboratory coat in detergent will adequately kill microbial contaminants.
3. Before each laboratory period, swab your bench space with a sponge and the antimicrobial solution provided. Do the same after completing each period. Leave your work area in a neat and clean condition because sloppiness can lead to laboratory accidents.
4. Although some papers and pencils are necessary to record laboratory observations, keep as few items as possible on the bench top. Do not lay a Petri plate or test tube on your notebook and risk contaminating your notebook. Put your books, backpacks, and coats in a safe area, like a locker, and out of the way. It is important to avoid clutter and possible laboratory accidents.
5. If you do have a spill of any kind, flood the area immediately with a disinfectant, cover it with paper towels, and wait at least 5 minutes. Then clean up the spill thoroughly with other paper towels and discard them in an autoclave bag.
6. If you accidently stab or contaminate yourself, immediately flood the area with alcohol, allow the alcohol to evaporate, and wash the area with a skin antiseptic. Do not get alcohol in your eyes. Report all laboratory accidents to the instructor immediately.
7. Discard contaminated items by placing all used Pasteur pipets, applicator sticks, slides, and swabs in appropriately labeled containers. Also, put contaminated glass plates and tubes in properly labeled containers. Autoclave bags will be provided for disposal of all plastic plates, tubes, and disposable contaminated items.
8. Do not mouth pipet. Learn how to use a pipet pump. When dispensing liquid from a pipet, hold the pipet tip below the lip of the receiving vessel to avoid creating aerosols.
9. To sterilize inoculating loops and needles, hold them almost vertically in the flame until they are red hot, but be careful not to burn your fingers. You may also sterilize the loops and needles in an electric incinerator. When using an incinerator,

do not leave the loop in the incinerator and return to it after several minutes; it will become hot throughout, even in the handle, and cause a burn. Resterilize your loop or needle immediately after use and before placing it on the bench.

10. When using a Bunsen burner, place it on the bench away from your notebook, microscope, or coat sleeves. It is advisable to share a burner with a bench partner and turn it off when not in use.

Fire extinguishers should be readily available. Have your instructor provide you with the locations of the fire extinguishers and the first aid kit and eye wash station, if they are available in your laboratory.

11. For the sake of your health and the health of your friends, family, and other students, wash your hands with a skin antiseptic before leaving the laboratory.

LABORATORY SAFETY

RULES AND REGULATIONS

After you have carefully read the following rules and are sure that you understand them, sign this sheet and return it to your instructor.

1. Do not eat, drink, smoke, or apply cosmetics in the laboratory. Keep your fingers, pencils, and other materials away from your face and mouth.

2. To avoid taking any organisms out of the laboratory on your clothing, always wear a buttoned laboratory coat. When removing your laboratory coat at the end of the laboratory period, turn it inside out, fold it over, and store it in the locker provided. At the end of the term, bring a plastic bag to the last laboratory period and place your laboratory coat in it before removing it from the work area. Then, transfer it directly to a washing machine. Washing the laboratory coat in detergent will adequately kill microbial contaminants.

3. Before each laboratory period, swab your bench space with a sponge and the antimicrobial solution provided. Do the same after completing each period. Leave your work area in a neat and clean condition because sloppiness can lead to laboratory accidents.

4. Although some papers and pencils are necessary to record laboratory observations, keep as few items as possible on the bench top. Do not lay a Petri plate or test tube on your notebook and risk contaminating your notebook. Put your books, backpacks, and coats in a safe area, such as a locker, and out of the way. It is important to avoid clutter and possible laboratory accidents.

5. If you do have a spill of any kind, flood the area immediately with a disinfectant, cover it with paper towels, and wait at least 5 minutes. Then clean up the spill thoroughly with other paper towels and discard them in an autoclave bag.

6. If you accidently stab or contaminate yourself, immediately flood the area with alcohol, allow the alcohol to evaporate, and wash the area with a skin antiseptic. Do not get alcohol in your eyes. Report all laboratory accidents to the instructor immediately.

7. Discard contaminated items by placing all used Pasteur pipets, applicator sticks, slides, and swabs in appropriately labeled containers. Also, put contaminated glass plates and tubes in properly labeled containers. Autoclave bags should be provided for disposal of all plastic plates, tubes, and disposable contaminated items.

8. Do not mouth pipet. Learn how to use a pipet pump. When dispensing liquid from a pipet, hold the pipet tip below the lip of the receiving vessel to avoid creating aerosols.

9. To sterilize inoculating loops and needles, hold them almost vertically in the flame until they are red hot, but be careful not to burn your fingers. You may also sterilize in an electric incinerator. When using an

incinerator, do not leave the loop in the incinerator and return to it after several minutes; it will become hot throughout, even in the handle, and cause a burn. Resterilize your loop or needle immediately after use and before placing it on the bench.

10. When using a Bunsen burner, place it on the bench away from your notebook, microscope, or coat sleeves. It is advisable to share a burner with a bench partner and turn it off when not in use. Fire extinguishers should be readily available. Have your instructor provide you with the locations of the fire extinguishers and the first aid kit and eye wash station, if they are available in your laboratory.

11. For the sake of your health and the health of your friends, family, and other students, wash your hands with a skin antiseptic before leaving the laboratory.

I have read the above rules and regulations and understand their meaning.

_____

(Signature)

SECTION I

GETTING STARTED

Microbes are, by definition, only seen with the aid of a microscope. Therefore, it is easy for the beginner to assume that artful use of the microscope is the only skill to be mastered in a microbiology laboratory. In this section, you will learn that microscopic examination is just one of the tools used in studying microbes. Many other techniques, especially those used to culture microbes, are required to get started as a microbiologist.

TERMINOLOGY

Microbiology is undergoing a major shift in microbial taxonomy. This has resulted in confusing use of terms when referring to different groups of microorganisms. Throughout this laboratory manual, we will use the following terminology.

Eucarya: all eucaryotic organisms.

Archaea: those procaryotes distinguished from other procaryotes based on 16S rRNA sequence and other criteria.

Bacteria: those procaryotes not considered to be Archaea.

bacteria: all procaryotic microorganisms.

EXERCISE 1

GROWING MICROBES ON SOLID SURFACES

Imagine that you are a young student at the University of Berlin. The year is 1882 and you have just learned of an extraordinary German physician who has a fine laboratory at the Imperial Health Office in Berlin. His name is Robert Koch. You are fascinated by the stories of his work on the anthrax microbe and how he proved it causes anthrax. You boldly introduce yourself to him one day and engage him in a conversation about a new way of viewing microbes under the microscope. The "hanging drop," as he calls it, is made using the fluid from the eye of an ox and a piece of glass with a depression in it. The drop of fluid containing the microbe is placed on another piece of glass, inverted, and suspended over the well in the other glass. Koch explains how important it is to study microbes isolated from each other. You are enthralled with this unassuming man and ask him many questions. He invites you back to his laboratory the next day and you notice some of his assistants cutting potatoes and placing the slices on clean glass plates beneath bell jars. The jars protect the potatoes from airborne contaminants. Some of the potatoes have droplets on them. One of the assistants describes how Koch discovered the droplets by accident and later determined that each droplet was composed of one kind of microbe. Some droplets had spherical microbes, others looked like sticks (rods), and still others looked like corkscrews. However, since they were growing on solid surfaces, the different microbes could not move. In other words, they could be studied separately! Koch's work so fascinates you that you ask him if you can work in his laboratory. He hesitates, but admits another pair of hands might help answer some of the new questions he has about the droplets. He is particularly troubled by the cum-

bersome nature of using potatoes to grow microbes, and that some won't grow on potatoes at all.

Over the year, you help Koch design a way to use meat extracts mixed with gelatine. This mixture is then poured over sheets of plate glass to create a solid growth medium. The medium is kept under a bell jar and inoculated with microbes by stroking it with a needle. However, the gelatine has limitations: it melts when incubated at 37°C, the optimum temperature for growth of pathogenic bacteria. Furthermore, some bacteria digest the gelatine, creating soup on the plates. Then one day the wife of another of Koch's assistants, Frannie Hess, suggests using agar. Agar is a substance extracted from seaweed, which has been used as a jam additive for many years. It must be heated to 100°C to melt, but once liquid, it remains a fluid until it reaches 45°C, when it solidifies again. You immediately try the agar and soon learn that its peculiar melting and gelling points, its poor nutritional value, and its lack of inhibitory substances make it an ideal substance for solidifying media.

You eventually become a physician, but still visit occasionally with Koch and his colleagues. In 1887, you learn of a major new contribution by Koch's assistant. His name is Julius Petri. Many microbe hunters had been struggling with the unwieldy nature of the large bell jars. Petri suggested a simpler container for solid growth media—a round plate with an overlapping lid. It permitted a much clearer view of the droplets and, when incubated inverted, both contamination and condensation were eliminated. The dishes (soon called Petri plates) were much less bulky and could be stacked on top of each other in the incubator. They were an immediate success. Now that these two problems were solved, the study of microbes would escalate over the years. Little did you know that the use of agar and the development of the Petri plate would revolutionize the study of microbes for centuries to come!

BACKGROUND INFORMATION

As Koch learned more than one hundred years ago, it is important to study microorganisms isolated from one another. He also recognized that one **colony** (what he called a distinct droplet) arises when one invisible cell divides into millions of cells, which pile up and form the visible colony. Subsequent studies of microbes showed that different microbes had characteristic colony types which could be used to differentiate them. **Figure 1.1** shows some examples of the variety of colony types. Microbiologists use colony morphology to initially describe an organism before confirming its identity.

Koch's laboratory eventually used **agar** to solidify media and it is still used today. Agar is a polysaccharide obtained from red algae. It has poor nutritional value and only a few specialized marine bacteria digest it. This makes it an excellent gelling agent. It is usually used at a concentration of 1.5% and added to

nutrients to isolate a variety of microorganisms. A concentration of agar more than 1.8% gives a harder medium but provides less water for growth, while a concentration of less than 1.0% will not completely solidify a medium.

To study microorganisms in pure culture, a sterile environment—one in which all life is absent—is needed. Exercise 4 will explain and demonstrate how media are prepared to achieve sterility. Our task here is to maintain a sterile environment while preparing agar plates so that unwanted organisms are not introduced. This is called practicing **aseptic technique.** There are several of these techniques, all of which are simple manipulations done to minimize contamination. The first aseptic technique you will learn is how to pour liquid nutrient agar into a sterile Petri plate. If done properly, you should maintain a sterile environment within the dish.

The type of medium you will pour is called **nutrient agar.** It contains beef extract and proteins known as peptones, which allow for the cultivation of organisms that are not fastidious; that is, they have relatively simple nutritional requirements. In future laboratory exercises you will learn

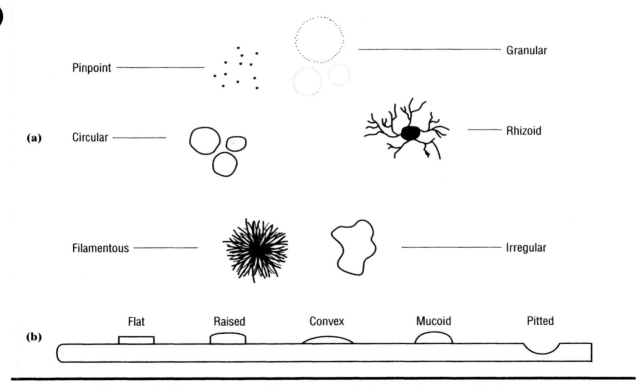

Figure 1.1 Forms of bacterial colony growth: (a) top view and (b) side view.

about other media that contain a variety of nutrients and dyes to select for and differentiate certain types of microbes.

PURPOSE

* To learn how to pour nutrient agar plates and practice aseptic technique
* To detect microorganisms in the air
* To observe microorganisms growing as distinct colonies on exposed plates

THE EXERCISE

MATERIALS:

50 ml of sterile nutrient agar in bottle or flask
Bunsen burner
50°C water bath
37°C incubator
Petri plates

PROCEDURE:

Day 1

Part A: Pouring Nutrient Agar Plates

1. Place two sterile Petri plates, lid side up, in front of you. CAUTION: **Do not open the lids until you have read the entire procedure.**
2. Light a Bunsen burner.
3. Obtain a bottle of sterile nutrient agar from the 50°C water bath and gently swirl it several times to insure a homogenous mixture.
4. Remove the cap of the bottle (**Figure 1.2a**).
5. Lightly pass the lip of the bottle through the open flame (**Figure 1.2b**). The lip of the bottle should already be sterile because it was autoclaved, but passing it through the flame eliminates any dust or contaminants you may have introduced while unscrewing the cap.
6. Pour approximately one-half of the agar into a plate (**Figure 1.2c**). Do not remove the Petri dish lid entirely, but tilt it slightly so that the lid shields the agar from airborne contaminants. Swirl the plate gently so the agar covers the entire bottom of the plate.
7. After one plate is poured, reflame the lip as before and pour the second plate using the same procedure.
8. Allow the plates to sit undisturbed for 15 to 20 minutes on a flat surface.
9. After the medium has solidified, invert each plate and label it with a felt-tipped marker or wax

(a)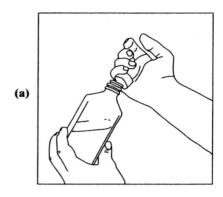

(b)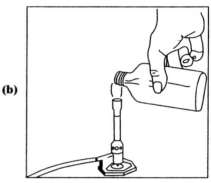

(c)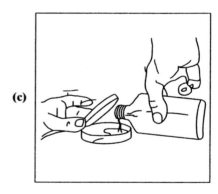

Figure 1.2   Pouring a nutrient agar plate: (a) removing the bottle cap, (b) flaming the lip, and (c) pouring the agar.

pencil. Each plate should have your name, date, and type of medium.

Part B: Testing Your Aseptic Technique

1. Choose a partner. One of you will incubate your plates at 37°C and the other will incubate his plates at room temperature (~25°C).

2. Label one plate "uninoculated" and do not open it. The uninoculated plate tests whether you have accidentally introduced contaminants into the plate when pouring the nutrient agar into it.
3. After the plates are sufficiently cooled, hardened, and dried, expose one plate to the air for one hour. Label this plate "exposed." This plate will allow you to observe colony morphology of different microorganisms. Freshly poured plates have a very moist surface. It is best to wait several hours before the plates are exposed because too much moisture causes the colonies to run together. The plates can be left on the bench top until the next day before being exposed. The plates can also be taped closed and taken home to be exposed to your air at home the next day. If the plates are taken home, they should be brought back to the laboratory to be incubated with the other sterile plate, either at 37°C or room temperature.

Day 2

1. Examine your plates. Observe any colony types that may be growing on your plates. It is important to note the colony differences in color, size, shape and texture. Some of you may see "fuzzy" colonies, which are probably molds growing from spores floating in the air. If your plates do not show many different colony types, observe other plates which may have a greater variety of organisms.
2. Record your observations in the RESULTS section.

REFERENCES

Brock, T.D. *Milestones in Microbiology.* Washington, DC: American Society for Microbiology, 1975.

Collard, P.J. *The Development of Microbiology.* Cambridge: Cambridge University Press, 1976.

De Kruif, P. *Microbe Hunters.* New York: Harcourt Brace Publishers, 1966.

RESULTS

Your Plates: Incubation Temperature _____

Uninoculated Plate	Description of Colonies
Exposed Plate	**Description of Colonies**

Partner's Plates: Incubation Temperature _____

Uninoculated Plate	Description of Colonies
Exposed Plate	**Description of Colonies**

REFLECTIONS

1. Did the uninoculated plates have any growth? If so, speculate why.

2. Was there more, less, or the same amount of growth on the exposed plates when incubated at two different temperatures?

3. Why did some early scientists such as Koch and Pasteur always incubate their plates at 37°C?

4. Is there any uncontrolled variable in this experiment that casts doubt on the validity of comparing the plates incubated at different temperatures?

5. Are the microbes growing on your plates fastidious?

EXERCISE 2

WET MOUNTS AND MICROSCOPY— A MICROBIOLOGY LEGACY

In Exercise 1 you learned how we grow and study microorganisms with the unaided eye. However, microbes were first observed using crude lenses. In this exercise we will begin to view microorganisms, their structures and habits with the aid of an important microbiological tool, the microscope.

Historically, the origins of microbiology can be traced to the development of the microscope. It makes sense that before we could attribute disease, alcohol production, or the decay of organic matter to microorganisms, we had to first see these tiny creatures. In order to see them, lenses had to be developed. It wasn't until Zacharias Janssen, a Dutch spectacle-maker, and Englishman Robert Hooke developed the microscope, that cells and microorganisms were first observed. Hooke not only observed these very small organisms, but also published a book in 1665 called Micrographie, in which he described how a microscope is used. Hooke's book awakened the rest of Europe to the world of microscopic creatures.

In the 1670s another Dutchman, Anton van Leeuwenhoek, began grinding his own pieces of glass into fine lenses, some of which could magnify up to 200 times. For the next fifty years, van Leeuwenhoek used the lenses and communicated his observations of "animalcules" from specimens he obtained from his teeth, feces and many other sources. He eventually constructed 550 single-lens microscopes, but he was very suspicious and would not share them with others. Therefore, microorganisms were only viewed as nature's curiosity until new technology led to the construction of more

efficient microscopes in the late 1800s. It was then that an association between microorganisms and disease was made. Little did early microbiologists know that technology would eventually take us inside these microbes through the use of electron microscopes.

Specimens observed by van Leeuwenhoek and others were immersed in rainwater. The specimens were placed on platforms, and later on pieces of glass, so they could be viewed mingling in water. Such preparations are now termed "wet mounts" and this technique, which is still used today, is said to have been the origin of the first observations of microorganisms and the beginning of microbiology.

BACKGROUND INFORMATION

The most common microscope in use today is called the **compound bright-field microscope.** A compound microscope uses two or more lenses to achieve much greater magnification than possible with a simple microscope like those van Leeuwenhoek built. In a compound microscope, one lens is positioned relatively close to the object being viewed and is called the **objective lens.** The second lens is close to the eye and is called the **ocular lens** or eyepiece. The objective lens magnifies the specimen being examined, creating an image within the tube that holds the lenses. The ocular lens magnifies that image. If the object is magnified 10-fold by the objective lens and that image is magnified 10-fold by the ocular lens, then the total magnification is 100-fold, or 100×. Thus, the total magnification of a compound microscope is the product of the magnification by the objective lens and the magnification by the ocular lens (objective magnification × ocular magnification = total magnification). Using different combinations of objective and ocular lenses allows us greater flexibility in viewing objects of different sizes.

Although compound microscopes are quite powerful, they are limited. The maximum useful magnification is 2,000×. The reason magnification beyond 2,000× is not useful is that the images created are fuzzy and blurred. Blurred images are formed when the magnifying power of the microscope exceeds its **resolving power.** Resolving power is the ability of the microscope to distinguish between two objects that are close together. One way to think of resolving power is to consider the headlights of a car approaching from a distance. They are not resolved as separate images until the car draws closer and we are able to see the headlights as two separate lights. The resolving power of a microscope is determined by a number of parameters, one of which is the wavelength of the light used to illuminate the specimen. The shorter the wavelength of light, the better the resolution. However, if the wavelength of light is too short, we can no longer see it. Therefore, the resolving power of a light microscope is limited by the shortest wavelength of visible light, which is approximately 400 nanometers.

To summarize the optical system of the microscope, it can be said that the magnification of an object increases the size of the object, whereas the resolving power separates the details of the object. Without both magnification and resolution, you would either see nothing, or it would be a big blur. See Appendix A for more on the physics of how lenses, magnifying glasses, and microscopes work.

Two other important parts of the microscope are the **light source** (illuminator) and the **condenser.** A centered light source is critical when viewing an object. The condenser lens system, located between the light source and object, focuses or condenses the parallel light rays on the object. The condenser can move up and down to affect this focus. It can also be adjusted, using the diaphragm lever or knob, to give sufficient light for the object being viewed. Too much light will compromise the image quality more than too little. Too little light reduces color quality but improves resolution or sharpness of the image. A good rule to remember is that the higher the magnification and resolving power of the lenses, the more light is needed to view the object.

Another feature of most microscopes is that they are **parfocal.** That is, when objectives are rotated to change the magnification, very little adjustment of the focus knobs is necessary to bring the object into focus.

Figure 2.1 is a labeled picture of a compound microscope. The basic components of microscopes are the same but they may be configured differently, depending upon the brand. Become familiar with your microscope before proceeding with viewing the wet mounts.

Microbiologists observe microorganisms most often after they have been stained. However, staining usually requires heat fixation, which kills and often shrinks the specimen. By preparing **wet mounts,** living organisms can be observed. Viewing live microbes allows you to observe motility and accurately measure their size. The microbes you will view are eucaryotic algae, protozoa and yeast, and procaryotic bacteria. Algae and protozoa are relatively easy to view at low and intermediate magnifications. Algae contain photosynthetic pigments and can be green, red, or brown. Protozoa are usually colorless and are characterized by rapid movement from cilia (rows of short hair-like appendages) and flagella (one or more long hair-like appendages), or by slower amoeboid motion (slow cytoplasmic flow into the projections of the cell membrane). Yeast are small spheres and most bacteria are very tiny rods and spheres with very low contrast. By suspending the microbes in a drop of liquid on a glass slide and putting a coverslip on the drop, features like color, size, shape, and motility can be observed. Your task in this laboratory exercise is to learn to use a microscope. However, this is also an opportunity for you to observe microbial diversity. Use your microscope to note the defining characteristics of the microorganisms you see.

PURPOSE

- To learn the use of a compound bright-field microscope
- To learn some of the physics of microscopy
- To observe microbes in a wet preparation

THE EXERCISE

MATERIALS:

Microscopes
Cover slips
Inoculating loop
Bunsen burner
Hay infusion
Nutrient agar plates of *E. coli*
Slides
Pasteur pipets
Inoculating needle
Pond water
Overnight broth culture of *S. cerevisiae*
Optional: rumen fluid, hanging drop slide and
    petroleum jelly

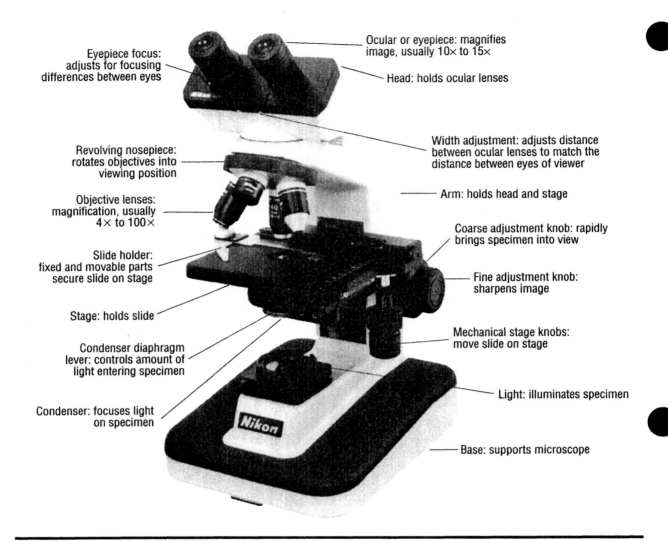

Eyepiece focus: adjusts for focusing differences between eyes

Ocular or eyepiece: magnifies image, usually 10× to 15×

Head: holds ocular lenses

Revolving nosepiece: rotates objectives into viewing position

Width adjustment: adjusts distance between ocular lenses to match the distance between eyes of viewer

Arm: holds head and stage

Objective lenses: magnification, usually 4× to 100×

Coarse adjustment knob: rapidly brings specimen into view

Slide holder: fixed and movable parts secure slide on stage

Fine adjustment knob: sharpens image

Stage: holds slide

Mechanical stage knobs: move slide on stage

Condenser diaphragm lever: controls amount of light entering specimen

Light: illuminates specimen

Condenser: focuses light on specimen

Base: supports microscope

Figure 2.1 A compound microscope. (Photograph courtesy of Nikon, Inc. Instrument Group.)

Care of the Microscope

1. Always carry the microscope with one hand on the arm and the other hand under the base.
2. Use lens paper to clean the ocular and objective lenses before each use. Do not use tissue or other paper, as they will scratch the lenses.
3. If lenses are still dirty after cleaning with lens paper, a dilute solution of methanol (50% methanol: 50% water) can be used with the lens paper to help clean the glass surfaces.
4. Never rotate any objective lens through oil except the oil immersion lens. Oil will seep into non–oil-immersion lenses and ruin them. If you accidentally get oil on any other lenses, wipe them immediately with lens paper.
5. After your observations are complete, remove all slides, clean all surfaces and each lens thoroughly with lens paper. Also center the mechanical stage.
6. Rotate the low-power objective lens into position, wrap the cord around the base of the microscope, and store the microscope, with a cover, if one is available.

Use of the Microscope

1. Plug in the light source and adjust the light so that adequate light flows through the condenser.
2. If you have a binocular microscope, look through the ocular lenes and adjust the width between them so that you are using both eyes to see the object. **Note:** This is an important step, so take your time and adjust the ocular lenses back and forth so that both eyes are comfortable looking through the eyepieces.
3. If you have an eyepiece focus, adjust for eye differences at this time. Your instructor will explain how to do this.
4. Check the location of the condenser. It should be all the way up and directly under the stage opening.
5. Rotate the lowest power objective lens into place and move the stage as close to the objective lens as possible.
6. Look through the ocular lens(es) and slowly bring the object into focus by rotating the coarse adjustment knob.
7. When you find the object, sharpen the image with the fine adjustment knob. **Note:** To practice focusing on an object, you may want to try viewing a wax pencil mark on a glass slide.
8. When the object is clear on low power, move the objective lens to high power (often called high dry lens). If the microscope is parfocal or nearly so, focusing should only require a slight rotation of the fine adjustment knob.
9. Place a drop of oil on the slide or coverslip and slowly rotate the oil immersion lens into position. Adjust the focus by using the fine adjustment knob only. You may have to adjust the light intensity. **Note:** The oil immersion lens is used only when viewing details of larger objects or smaller organisms such as bacteria or yeast.

PROCEDURE

Part A: Wet Mount of Pond Water or Hay Infusion

1. With a pipet, place one or two drops of liquid in the middle of the glass slide (**Figure 2.2**).
2. Place a coverslip over the liquid by gently lowering it as illustrated (**Figure 2.3**). Start at one side of the coverslip and lower the coverslip at an angle to the slide. Try to avoid introducing air bubbles.
3. Observe the microorganisms on low power and then on high power for greater detail. You

should see a variety of protozoa and algae. They will vary in size and can be viewed easily under these magnifications. If you have trouble seeing the organisms, adjust the condenser diaphragm lever to decrease or increase the amount of light passing through the specimen. If you see very small microorganisms, they may be bacteria.

4. Record your observations in the RESULTS section.

Part B: Wet Mount of S. cerevisiae

1. Prepare a wet mount of the broth culture of *S. cerevisiae* using the procedure in Part A (steps 1 and 2).
2. Observe the yeast under low power, high power, and oil immersion. Note its size and shape.
3. Record your observations in the RESULTS section.

Part C: Wet Mount of E. coli

1. Prepare a wet mount of *E. coli* from the nutrient agar plate. This can be done by sterilizing your loop, allowing it to cool, and emulsifying a small portion of a colony in a drop of water.
2. Place a coverslip on the drop as in Part A (step 2) (**Figure 2.3**).
3. Observe this microorganism under low power, high power, and oil immersion. Be persistent in trying to observe *E. coli* as it is not always easy to see bacteria in suspension. This is one of the reasons we stain them. Note their shape, size, and motility.
4. Record your observations in the RESULTS section.

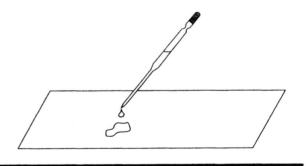

Figure 2.2 Adding liquid to a slide.

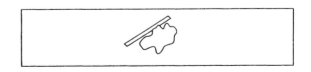

Figure 2.3 Placing coverslip at an angle over the liquid.

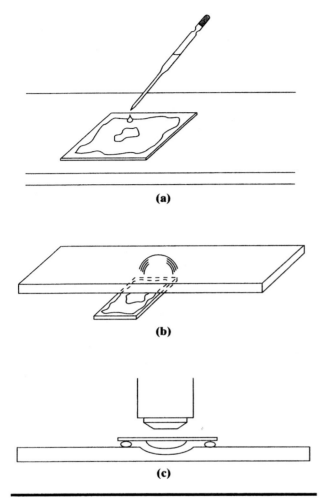

Figure 2.4 Preparation of the hanging drop slide: (a) adding a drop of water to the slide, (b) inverting the slide, and (c) observing the slide.

Optional:

Part D: Hanging Drop Slide

1. Obtain a hanging drop slide, a coverslip, and a toothpick with a small amount of petroleum jelly on the tip. **Note:** Hanging drop slides are made to suspend a fluid sample within an airtight seal so that the sample does not dry out before viewing. The motility of strictly aerobic organisms can be observed for only a brief period of time because the bacteria cease moving once the oxygen is depleted.

2. Apply the petroleum jelly around the edges of the coverslip. Add a drop of the pond water or hay infusion to the center of the coverslip (**Figure 2.4a**).

3. Invert the hanging drop slide over the coverslip so that the drop fits into the depression and the petroleum jelly forms a complete seal between the coverslip and the slide (**Figure 2.4b**).

4. Turn the hanging drop slide over and examine with the low-power objective lens (**Figure 2.4c**). **Note:** Drawing a line on one side of the coverslip before adding the liquid may help you focus on the organisms. The line is in the same plane as the microorganisms.

5. Record your observations in the RESULTS section.

REFERENCES

Alcamo, E.I. *Fundamentals of Microbiology*, 4th ed. Redwood City, CA: Benjamin/Cummings Publishing, 1994.

Collard, P. J. *The Development of Microbiology*. Cambridge: Cambridge University Press, 1976.

Gerhardt, P., et al. *Methods for General and Molecular Bacteriology*. Washington, DC: American Society for Microbiology, 1994.

RESULTS

Draw and describe as many diverse forms of microorganisms as you can from each specimen.

Also record the objective used to view the specimen.

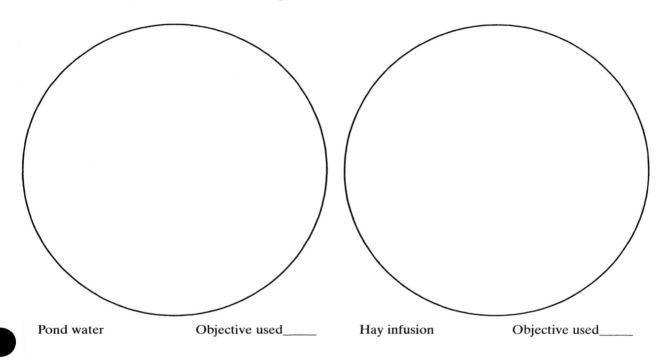

Pond water   Objective used____   Hay infusion   Objective used____

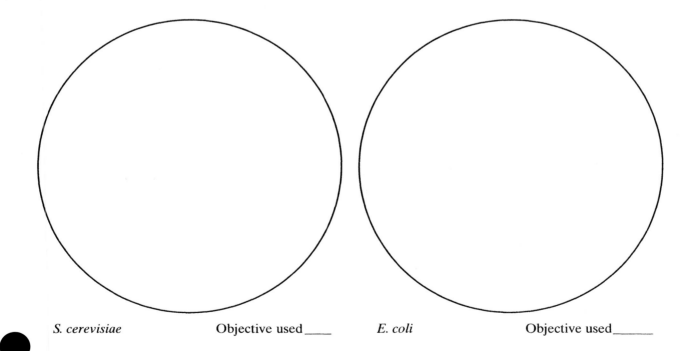

S. cerevisiae   Objective used____   *E. coli*   Objective used____

REFLECTIONS

1. The protozoa, algae, and *S. cerevisiae* are eucaryotes; *E. coli* is a procaryote. Based on your observations, what generalizations can you make about eucaryotic and procaryotic cells?

2. The bacteria and yeast you observed are approximately 2 to 10 micrometers in length and diameter. Based on these known sizes, estimate the average size of some of the protozoa and algae you observed.

3. A student missed the laboratory period where use of the microscope was demonstrated. The instructor asked the student to read the description in the laboratory manual and then proceed to examine bacterial cells with the oil immersion lens. The student skimmed the directions and began. After about 15 minutes of struggling, the student gave up in despair without seeing anything. Below is a detailed description of what the student did. How many mistakes did the student make and why didn't the student see anything?
   a. Plugged in the microscope and turned the light source to maximum intensity.
   b. Made a wet mount and placed it on the stage with the low-power objective lens in position.
   c. Tried to focus with the coarse adjustment knob, but decided the bacteria were too small and needed to be seen with the high-power objective lens.
   d. Rotated the high-power objective lens into position, but saw that the lens would likely touch the slide, so lowered the stage so that the objective lens rotated freely.
   e. Tried to focus with the coarse adjustment knob, but still saw nothing.
   f. Decided to switch to the oil immersion lens, but still saw nothing.

4. Look at the objectives on your microscope. What can you say about the diameter of each lens and its relationship to the magnifying power of the objective?

STREAKING PLATES FOR ISOLATED COLONIES

In Exercise 1 you learned the importance of creating and maintaining a sterile environment for microorganisms. You also learned the importance of observing isolated microorganisms. In this exercise you will learn a technique for isolating colonies by streaking samples containing bacteria on a solid medium.

Sandy was a technician who worked in a clinical laboratory in a large hospital. Her primary job was to inoculate plates with specimens received from different units in the hospital. One afternoon, 15 minutes before her work day ended, she received five specimens—one throat swab, two urine samples, a swab from an infected surgical lesion, and a spinal fluid. She quickly labeled the appropriate media and slides. As she did, her mind wandered to the baseball game her son was playing that evening. With quick, robot-like motions, she began to inoculate the plates and streak them for isolated colonies. She placed the plates in an incubator and quickly left for the game.

The next day, Sarah, a clinical laboratory scientist, retrieved the plates and observed each set of cultures. When she saw the plates from the surgical lesion she immediately realized there was a problem. Two or perhaps three distinct colony types were on each plate, but none were isolated from one another. There was also heavy growth of each colony type in each

quadrant of the plates. Sarah would not be able to identify the bacteria until she isolated each one again on another medium. This meant another 24 hours before identification and antibiotic susceptibility testing could be performed. A delay would leave the patient untreated or with potentially ineffective treatment for another 24 hours. Suddenly, the telephone rang and a physician asked for the culture results of the surgical lesion.

BACKGROUND INFORMATION

Nowhere is the isolation of colonies for identification purposes so important as in the clinical microbiology laboratory. This is clearly demonstrated by the story above. The standard tool used to aseptically transfer bacteria from one specimen or medium to another is an inoculating loop. An **inoculating loop** can also be used to spread the cells over the entire surface of the medium. The procedure of spreading cells over a medium to grow discrete colonies is called the **streak plate method.** This method involves taking a portion of a colony, a loopful of broth, or other material which may contain microorganisms, and spreading the inoculum across sections of the plate using a standard streaking pattern (**Figure 3.3**). Between each streaking phase, the loop is heat sterilized (flamed) to kill any remaining organisms. This results in fewer and fewer cells being moved across the surface of the agar until eventually single cells are deposited far enough apart so that when they grow they pro-

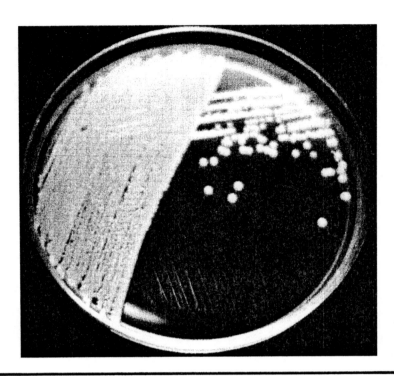

Figure 3.1 An agar plate with isolated colonies.

duce single isolated colonies (**Figure 3.1**). In other words, you have diluted the organism over a solid surface. Once in isolation, a colony can be characterized and the microbe identified by additional testing procedures. If only one type of microbe (one colony type) is isolated on a plate, the plate is said to be a **pure culture** of the microbe.

The aseptic techniques practiced in this laboratory involve heat sterilization of the loop, and manipulating media and inocula without contaminating them with unwanted microorganisms. Removal of the cap from a tube and holding the cap in the hand while inserting a sterile loop into the tube will be demonstrated and practiced in this exercise. Ideally, you should obtain isolated colonies from an inoculum containing a mixture of bacteria. All of these aseptic practices are important techniques used daily in research and clinical microbiology laboratories.

PURPOSE

- To learn the importance of flame sterilization when isolating colonies
- To learn the technique of streaking a plate to isolate colonies

THE EXERCISE

MATERIALS:

Nutrient agar plates
Inoculating loop
Bunsen burner
Overnight broth culture of *Staphylococcus epidermidis* and *Micrococcus luteus*
30°C incubator

PROCEDURE:

Day 1

1. Obtain three nutrient agar plates.
2. Light a Bunsen burner.
3. Label the bottom of the first plate "unflamed loop." **Note:** The plate should also be labeled with your name, date, and medium.
4. Streak the plate using the three-phase pattern above but with *no* inoculum and *no flaming* of the loop throughout the procedure.
5. Label the bottom of the second plate "flamed loop." **Note:** This plate is also labeled with your name, date, and medium.
6. Streak the plate using the three-phase pattern but flame the loop between each of the sections. The loop still has no inoculum.

Aseptic Transfer of Inoculum

Transferring a loopful of culture from a tube to a plate is a technique that requires thoughtful manipulations to avoid contamination. **Figure 3.2** illustrates one technique that many microbiologists use to maintain the sterility of the cap and tube while entering the tube. Remember, placing the cap on the bench top will contaminate the cap. Also, tilting the tube at a slight angle will keep fewer particles (and other microbes) from entering the tube. Follow these three steps when transferring inoculum:

1. Insert the loop and entire wire into the hottest part of the flame until it glows red (**Figure 3.2a**). Hold the handle like a pencil and insert the loop into the flame at an angle to avoid being burned. Allow the loop to cool without waving it in the air.
2. Remove the cap while holding the loop (**Figure 3.2b**).
3. Insert the loop into the inoculum while holding the cap with two small fingers (**Figure 3.2c**). As soon as the loop is removed, replace the cap.

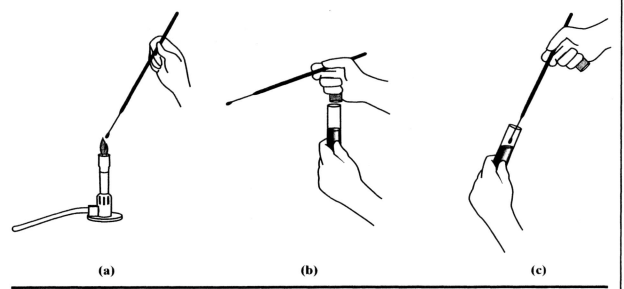

(a)	**(b)**	**(c)**

Figure 3.2 Proper aseptic transfer of inoculum: (a) flaming the loop, (b) removing the cap, and (c) inserting the loop into broth.

7. Label the third plate with *S. epidermidis* and *M. luteus*. Be sure to include your name, date, and medium as well.
8. Flame your loop and allow it to cool.
9. Aseptically obtain a loopful of broth containing *S. epidermidis* and *M. luteus*.
10. Inoculate and streak the plate using the three-phase pattern which includes flaming the loop between each section.
11. Invert the plates and incubate them at 30°C for 2 to 3 days.

Day 2

Observe the plates and record your results in the RESULTS section. *S. epidermidis* will appear as mucoid, white- or cream-colored colonies within 24 hours after inoculation. *M. luteus* will appear as small, mucoid, yellow colonies after 24 to 48 hours of incubation. The two are easily differentiated because of their color and size differences.

Optional:

Your instructor may request a laboratory report for this experiment. This report should be written just like journal articles in leading scientific journals. Refer to Appendix B for instructions on writing a laboratory report and guidelines for better writing.

Streaking a Plate for Isolated Colonies

The following is a description of how to streak a plate using the three-phase pattern. Each of the plates used in this exercise will be streaked for isolation using this method. Four phase patterns are used by some microbiologists and your instructor may choose to illustrate this method.

1. The inoculum is placed on the plate using a swab, pipet, or inoculating loop.
2. Sterilize a loop and allow it to cool.
3. Streak the inoculum lightly over one-third of the plate (**Figure 3.3a**). Use numerous sweeps of the loop and be careful not to gouge the agar.
4. Reflame the loop and allow it to cool.
5. Turn the plate 90 degrees and lightly sweep through a small portion of the original streaked area. Move the inoculum with several strokes to the second portion of the agar surface (**Figure 3.3b**). Care should be taken not to reenter the first streaked area more than three or four times and never reenter the area after exiting the last time.
6. Reflame the loop and allow it to cool.
7. Turn the plate another 90 degrees and streak the final third of the plate as in Step 5 above (**Figure 3.3c**). Isolated colonies should be obtained in the third section of the plate.

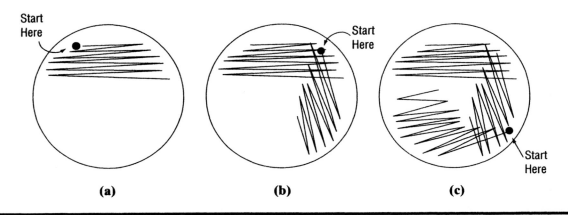

(a)   **(b)**   **(c)**

Figure 3.3   Procedure for streaking a plate: (a) first streak, (b) second streak, and (c) third streak.

RESULTS

Observe your plates and record the results here, noting the amount and type of growth.

Plate 1 (unflamed loop; no inoculum)

Plate 2 (flamed loop; no inoculum)

Plate 3 (*S. epidermidis* and *M. luteus*; properly flamed loop)

REFLECTIONS

1. Were there colonies growing on the "flamed" and "unflamed" plates? If so, please explain why.

2. Did you obtain isolated colonies in the third area of streaking on plate 3? If not, suggest why this may have happened.

3. What mistakes might Sandy have made when streaking the surgical lesion specimen for isolated colonies?

4. Infected surgical lesions are often examples of nosocomial infections. What is a nosocomial infection? Why are nosocomial infections so dangerous?

KILLING
MICROBES

In Exercise 1 you learned about solid growth media and how a sterile medium is poured into a Petri dish without introducing contaminants. But how was the sterile medium prepared? In this exercise, you will learn about how microbes are killed or their growth otherwise controlled so that sterile materials and sanitized work areas can be prepared.

6:30 A.M.—The operating room (OR) staff begins preparation of the room for the first surgery of the day—an emergency appendectomy to be performed on an 11-year-old boy. The instruments required for the surgery are obtained from a supply room containing sterile supplies. They were sterilized by autoclaving after being wrapped in disposable surgical drapes. They will be kept wrapped until the surgery begins.

7:00 A.M.—The surgeon, anesthesiologist, and OR nurse arrive and begin their preparations. They scrub from fingertips to elbows for 10 minutes using antibacterial cleanser, then suit up in clean surgical scrubs. They will cover these areas with sterile gowns and gloves. They will also wear masks and protective eye wear.

7:30 A.M.—The patient arrives and the appendectomy proceeds routinely.

9:00 A.M.—The OR staff arrives to disinfect the room for the next scheduled surgery. All hard surfaces are cleaned and then disinfected with alcohol. Used disposable materials are removed. Those that have been contaminated with blood will be incinerated. The instruments used are removed. They will be washed in disinfectant, machine washed, then wrapped and autoclaved again for future use.

10:00 A.M.—The next surgery begins. An HIV-positive woman is having an emergency caesarean section and delivers a baby girl.

11:45 A.M.—The housekeeping staff washes all hard surfaces, but this time disinfects with bleach. This routine continues throughout the day.

7:00 P.M.—The eighth and last surgery of the day has just been completed. The housekeeping staff soon arrives for terminal cleaning, the last and most thorough cleaning of the day. The walls and all hard surfaces are cleaned with disinfectant cleanser. The floor is flooded with cleanser and wet vacuumed. The room is now ready for tomorrow's surgeries.

BACKGROUND INFORMATION

A microbiology teaching laboratory does not have the same need for disinfection and sterilization as a hospital operating room, but you will use many of the same techniques for controlling microbial contamination in this laboratory excercise. Furthermore, the principles underlying these techniques are used in other settings, including the food industry, drinking water treatment facilities, and sewage treatment plants. The business of killing microbes, or at least decreasing their numbers, is an important one.

A number of terms are commonly used to refer to procedures and agents used to kill microbes (see the box). The term **sterile** refers to materials that are free of all viable microorganisms. Sterile surgical instruments are an obvious necessity in an operating room. Sterile tubes, swabs, and other materials are likewise a necessity in microbiology laboratories to avoid inadvertent introduction of unwanted microbes into growth media and cultures. But not all materials found in an operating room need to be sterile; some can be disinfected. **Disinfection** refers specifically to the killing or removal of disease-causing microbes. A

Terminology

Scientists use a variety of terms when describing antimicrobial agents. Unfortunately, these are not always used or defined in the same way by all scientists. We are using the terms for chemical control agents in the following way:

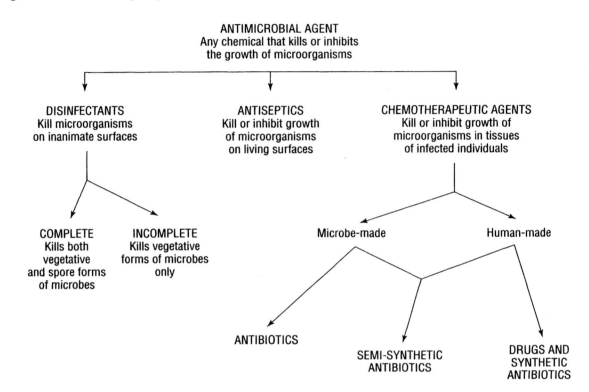

ANTIMICROBIAL AGENT
Any chemical that kills or inhibits
the growth of microorganisms

DISINFECTANTS
Kill microorganisms
on inanimate surfaces

ANTISEPTICS
Kill or inhibit growth
of microorganisms
on living surfaces

CHEMOTHERAPEUTIC AGENTS
Kill or inhibit growth of
microorganisms in tissues
of infected individuals

COMPLETE
Kills both
vegetative
and spore forms
of microbes

INCOMPLETE
Kills vegetative
forms of microbes
only

Microbe-made

Human-made

ANTIBIOTICS

SEMI-SYNTHETIC
ANTIBIOTICS

DRUGS AND
SYNTHETIC
ANTIBIOTICS

All of the above agents can be classified as being either **-static** (e.g., bacteriostatic, meaning it inhibits the growth of bacteria) or **-cidal** (e.g., bactericidal, meaning it kills bacteria). Although disinfectants are -cidal agents, disinfected surfaces are not necessarily sterile because disinfection is often incomplete. That is, the disinfectant only kills vegetative forms of microorganisms.

disinfected surface is not necessarily sterile. Another procedure, **sanitization,** is important in a laboratory setting and in public places. A sanitized surface is one where the number of microbes has been significantly lowered. In a laboratory setting, sanitization is used to decrease the possibility of contaminating sterile media and instruments. In a public restroom, sanitization helps prevent the spread of disease-causing microbes among people using the restroom.

Two methods are commonly used to kill microbes. The first is heat, either dry or moist. Our focus in this exercise will be on moist heat. Moist heat is thought to kill by denaturing proteins and nucleic acids. An important piece of equipment used to kill microbes

with moist heat is an **autoclave.** It is used in both hospitals and laboratories. An autoclave (**Figure 4.1**) is essentially a large pressure cooker. It envelops materials in steam under conditions of increased pressure (fifteen pounds), at which the temperature reaches 121°C. The second common method of killing microbes is the use of chemical agents such as phenolic compounds (e.g., hexachlorophene), alcohols, and halogens (e.g., bleach). Chemical agents are called **disinfectants** if they are used to disinfect inanimate objects. They are called **antiseptics** if used to disinfect living surfaces (e.g., skin).

This exercise consists of two parts: A and B. In Part A, you will determine the effectiveness of

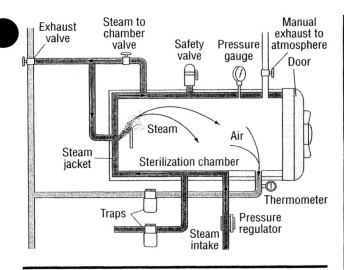

Figure 4.1 The internal workings of an autoclave.

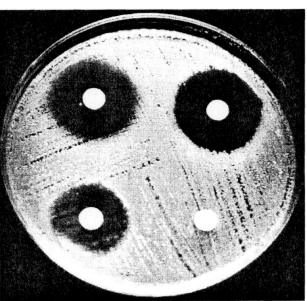

Figure 4.2 Mueller-Hinton agar plate inoculated with *E. coli*. (Note zones of inhibition—the clear zones—around disks saturated with antimicrobial agent.)

boiling and autoclaving for killing the bacterium *Bacillus cereus*. Members of the genus *Bacillus* are Gram-positive rods (see Exercise 6) which form endospores (see Exercise 14). They are common inhabitants of soil where growth conditions vary greatly during the course of a day and the course of a year. In Part B, you will examine the effectiveness of common disinfectants and antiseptics for killing *Escherichia coli* and *Staphylococcus epidermidis*. *E. coli* is a Gram-negative, rod-shaped bacterium that does not form endospores. It is an intestinal bacterium. *S. epidermidis* is a Gram-positive coccus that is a normal inhabitant of our skin. In Part B, you will be using a new type of medium called Mueller-Hinton agar.[1] Small disks impregnated with a disinfectant or antiseptic will be placed on inoculated Mueller-Hinton agar medium. As the antimicrobial agent diffuses out of the disk into the medium, a concentration gradient is established such that lower concentrations of the antimicrobial agent are farther away from the disk. At a certain distance from the disk, the microbes will be unaffected by the antimicrobial agent. But closer to the disk, the concentration will be high enough to either kill or inhibit the growth of the microbe. This area of no growth is called a **zone of inhibition** (**Figure 4.2**).

---

[1]Mueller-Hinton agar was developed specifically to test antibiotic and drug susceptibility. It is used here to test other types of antimicrobial agents, although there is no evidence it is necessary to use it exclusively.

PURPOSE

- To examine different methods of disinfection and sterilization
- To determine effectiveness of different disinfectants and antiseptics
- To develop skills in manipulation of bacterial cultures, including aseptic transfers and other aseptic techniques

THE EXERCISE

Part A

MATERIALS:

Two tubes of *B. cereus* broth cultures
Nutrient agar plate
Boiling water bath
Inoculating loop
Autoclave

PROCEDURE: Work in pairs

Day 1

1. Label one tube of *B. cereus* "boil"; label the other "autoclave."

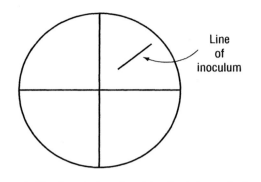

Line
of
inoculum

Figure 4.3   A nutrient agar plate with one section inoculated.

2. Using a wax pencil or marker, divide the bottom of the Petri dish containing nutrient agar into four sections. Label one section "before boiling," one section "after boiling," one section "before autoclaving," and the last section "after autoclaving."
3. Using the aseptic techniques learned in Exercise 3, gently inoculate the nutrient agar with *B. cereus* from the "boil" tube. Use an inoculating loop and make a single line in the center of the "before boiling" quadrant (**Figure 4.3**). Replace the lid on the Petri dish immediately.
4. Heat the "boil" tube in a boiling water bath for 2 minutes.
5. Repeat step 3, this time inoculating the "after boiling" section.
6. Repeat step 3 using the "autoclave" broth culture of *B. cereus* and inoculating the "before autoclaving" section of the medium.
7. Place the "autoclave" tube in a rack in an autoclave. Your instructor will describe how the autoclave is operated and will autoclave the tubes for 15 minutes at 121°C and 15 pounds pressure.
8. After removing the tube from the autoclave, let it cool until it can be easily handled. Then repeat step 3 using the autoclaved culture and inoculating the "after autoclaving" section.
9. Invert the plate and incubate at 37°C.

Day 2
1. Examine your plate to see which sections, if any, exhibit growth.
2. Record your observations in the RESULTS section.

Part B
MATERIALS:
Broth cultures of *E. coli* and *S. epidermidis*
Two Mueller-Hinton agar plates

Sterile swabs
Sterile blank disk
Antiseptics (e.g., mouth wash, antiseptic sprays)
Disinfectants (e.g., bleach, household cleansers)
Forceps soaking in alcohol

PROCEDURE: Work in pairs
1. Using a wax pencil or marker, divide the bottom of one Petri dish into quadrants. Label the plate *E. coli*. Repeat with the second plate, labeling it *S. epidermidis*.
2. Using the aseptic technique demonstrated by your instructor, remove a sterile swab and insert it into the *E. coli* culture.
3. Use the inoculum on the swab to evenly spread bacteria over the entire surface of the medium in the plate labeled *E. coli* (**Figure 4.4**).
4. Repeat steps 2 and 3 using the *S. epidermidis* culture and the corresponding plate.
5. Choose four household disinfectants or antiseptics you would like to test. Label each plate with the names of the antimicrobial agents you have chosen. You will test one antimicrobial agent per quadrant.
6. Remove the forceps from the alcohol and air dry.
7. Use the forceps to pick up a sterile blank disk and moisten it in one of the chosen antimicrobial agents.
8. Place the saturated disk in the appropriate section of the *E. coli* plate.
9. Repeat steps 6 through 8 for the remaining three antimicrobial agents.
10. Repeat steps 6 through 9 this time with the *S. epidermidis* plate. Your plate should look like **Figure 4.5.**
11. Invert the plates and incubate at 37°C.

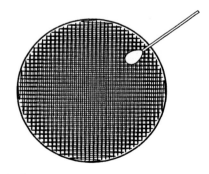

Figure 4.4   Plate divided into quadrants and inoculated by spreading bacteria over the entire plate with a swab.

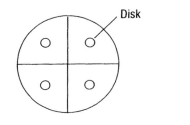

Figure 4.5 Disks saturated with antimicrobial agents and placed on inoculated medium.

Day 2

1. Examine your plates for a zone of inhibition around each disk.
2. Record your observations in the RESULTS section.

REFERENCES

Brock, T.D., et al. *Biology of Microorganisms*, 7th ed. Englewood Cliffs, NJ: Prentice-Hall, 1994.

Prescott, L.M., et al. *Microbiology*, 3rd ed. Dubuque, IA: William C. Brown, Publishers, 1996.

RESULTS

Part A

BB = Before boiling

AB = After boiling

BA = Before autoclaving

AA = After autoclaving

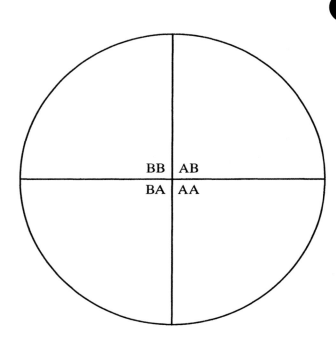

Part B

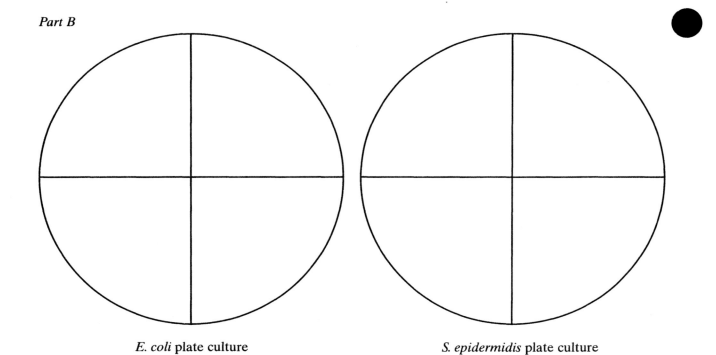

E. coli plate culture   S. epidermidis plate culture

REFLECTIONS

1. Did you predict *B. cereus* would survive boiling? If you repeated Part A with *E. coli* or *S. epidermidis*, would you predict they would survive boiling? Explain.

2. Why would the ability to produce endospores allow bacteria to survive boiling? When were the endospores produced in this experiment: before boiling, or as a result of boiling?

3. Application of heat and chemical agents are not the only procedures used to disinfect, sanitize, or sterilize. List at least three other methods.

4. Choose one of the methods listed in Question 3 and describe how it is used in either the food industry, or in sewage and water treatment facilities.

5. In the description of the preparation of an OR for surgery, bleach rather that alcohol was used to disinfect after delivery of a baby from an HIV-infected mother. What is the mode of killing for both bleach and alcohol? Why was bleach used instead of alcohol?

6. What properties of the disinfectant or antiseptic influence the size of the zone of inhibition?

7. What properties of the bacterium or the medium influence the size of the zone of inhibition?

EXERCISE 5

"SEEING MORE" WITH PHASE MICROSCOPY

You have learned some of the most basic techniques for observing and manipulating microorganisms. In this exercise, you learn about a more sensitive type of microscopy—phase microscopy. To prepare for this exercise, reread Appendix A, which describes some of the physics underlying microscopy.

George could still remember the day his general microbiology instructor lectured about the Rhizobium-*legume mutualistic symbiosis. That lecture led to an undergraduate research project in a laboratory working on* Rhizobium trifolii *and its symbiotic relationship with clover. George's project included videotaping the bacterium as it invaded the clover roots. It was an amazing sequence of events. First, the bacterium attached itself to the root hair (**Figure 5.1**). Second, the root hair curled, in a sense embracing the bacterium and stabilizing the attachment. Third, an infection thread formed through which the bacterium penetrated the plant cells. Finally, the bacterium differentiated into bacteroids and then symbiosomes. Nitrogen fixation occurred in the latter. Although all steps of the invasion process had been documented before, George's videotapes were capturing the process live. Only in this way could such a dynamic process be observed.*

BACKGROUND INFORMATION

Microorganisms carry out many dynamic processes that are best observed with living specimens. However, in many cases, bright-field light microscopy does not resolve the images sufficiently to make clear detailed observations. Fortunately for George, Professor F. Zernike of the University of Copenhagen published a paper in 1934 applying the principles of phase contrast to microscopy. This ultimately led to the development of the first phase microscope, a microscope that creates clear, detailed images of living specimens.

To understand phase microscopy, we must first understand light waves, the ways objects can change light waves, and the effects of combining light waves. We'll begin with light waves and their interactions with objects.

Figure 5.2 shows a light wave and its **wavelength** and **amplitude**. Wavelength determines the color of light, and amplitude determines its intensity or brightness. When light encounters an object, many things can happen to the light depending on the nature of the object. If the object absorbs some of the light, or reflects the light, then the light that passes through the object is decreased in amplitude. Such objects are called amplitude objects, and they appear as dark objects against a light background when examined by bright-field microscopy (**Figure 5.3**). Most biological specimens, however, do not significantly absorb or reflect light. Such specimens are transparent and allow light to pass through without significantly changing amplitude. However, transparent specimens do alter light. The speed of light is slowed or retarded; this retardation is called a **phase shift** (**Figure 5.4**) because the sine curve of the wave is shifted by about 1/4 wavelength (λ). This phase-shifted light can also exhibit another characteristic. If the light ray strikes the edge of an object (e.g., cell or organelle) as it passes through the specimen, its path is changed, producing a **diffracted ray**.

28

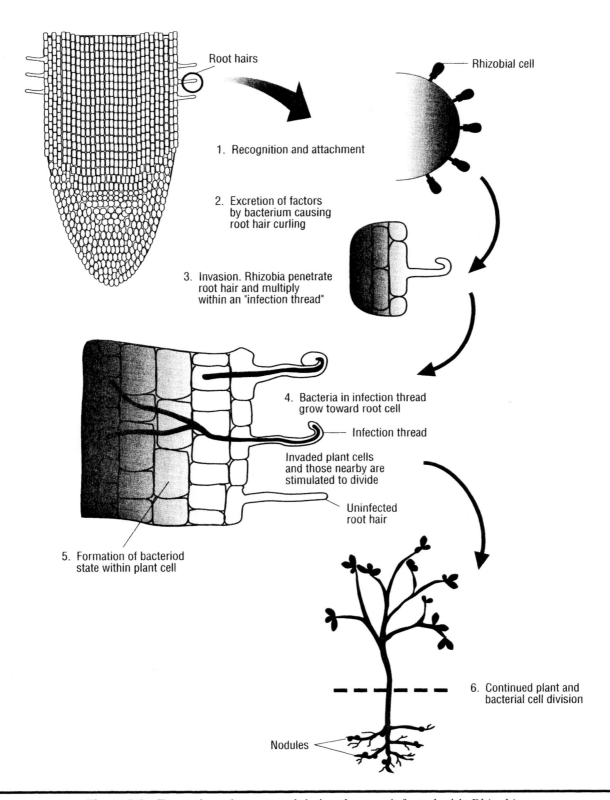

Figure 5.1 Formation of a root nodule in a legume infected with *Rhizobium.*

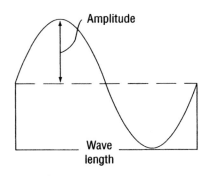

Figure 5.2   A light wave.

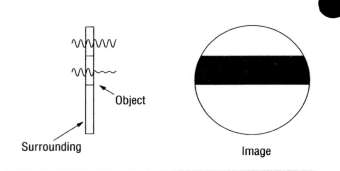

Figure 5.3   Amplitude object. Note that the amplitude of the wave is diminished as it passes through the object.

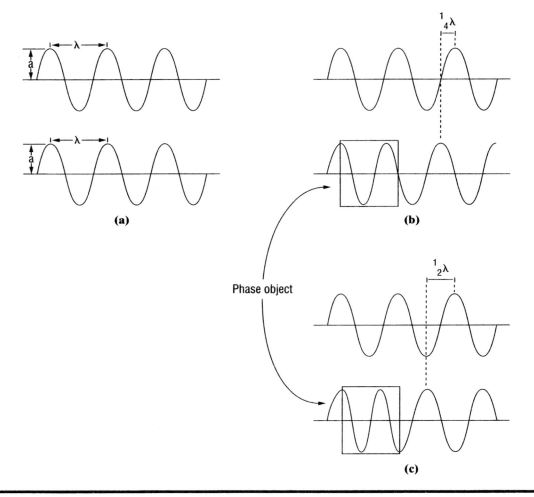

Figure 5.4   Light waves in and out of phase: (a) light waves in phase, (b) light waves out of phase by 1/4 λ, and (c) light waves out of phase by 1/2 λ (reverse phase).

The generation of diffracted rays, rays that deviate from their original path, is very important to the workings of a phase microscope. But there is another light phenomenon of importance—the effect of combining light waves. When two light waves are combined, the resultant wave has an amplitude determined by summing the amplitude of each separate wave. What this means is that when two light waves are in phase, the resultant wave has an amplitude that is greater, and appears brighter than either alone (**Figure 5.5a**). It also means that when two waves are out of phase, the amplitude of the resultant wave is decreased, and is not as bright. This decrease in brightness is not always discernable by the human eye. For instance, phase shifts of 1/4 λ are difficult to detect. However, waves in reverse phase, that is 1/2 λ out of phase, cancel each other out, producing a dark image that is clearly perceived (**Figure 5.5b**).

It should be remembered that microbes are not uniform throughout. Some areas in a cell will cause phase shift and diffraction and some areas will not. Thus, two important types of light rays pass through a biological specimen—diffracted, phase-shifted light rays and direct rays. Most phase microscopes use a special condenser and optics to create a phase shift of 1/2 λ between the diffracted and direct rays. These rays are then superimposed, creating significant contrast which is visible to the eye.

Figure 5.6 shows the optics of a typical phase microscope. There are several features unique to this microscope. The first is the **annular stop,** or annulus, that lies between the light source and the condenser lenses. The annular stop blocks all light except a narrow ring of light. The two condenser lenses focus the light such that the specimen is illuminated by a cone of light that strikes the object obliquely. Notice the diffracted and direct rays that emerge from the specimen. These are focused on the second unique feature of the phase microscope, the **phase plate.** The phase plate is a disk that contains a narrow ring that shifts the phase of any light passing through it. As you can see, the objective lens of the microscope focuses the direct rays on the phase ring, while the diffracted rays miss the phase ring. When the direct and diffracted rays leave the phase plate, their waves are in reverse phase. Above the phase plate is another lens that focuses the direct

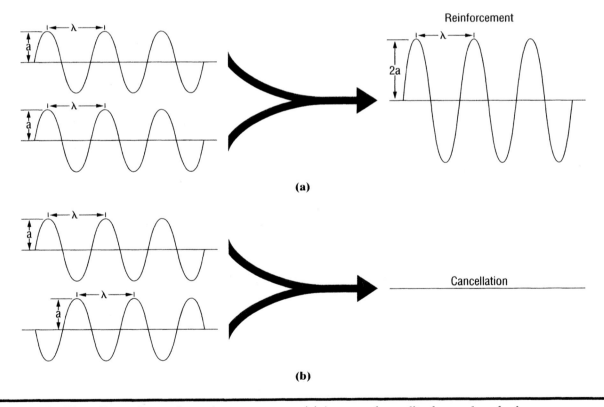

Figure 5.5 The effect of superimposing two waves: (a) increased amplitude produced when waves are in phase, and (b) cancellation produced when waves are 1/2 λ out of phase (reverse phase).

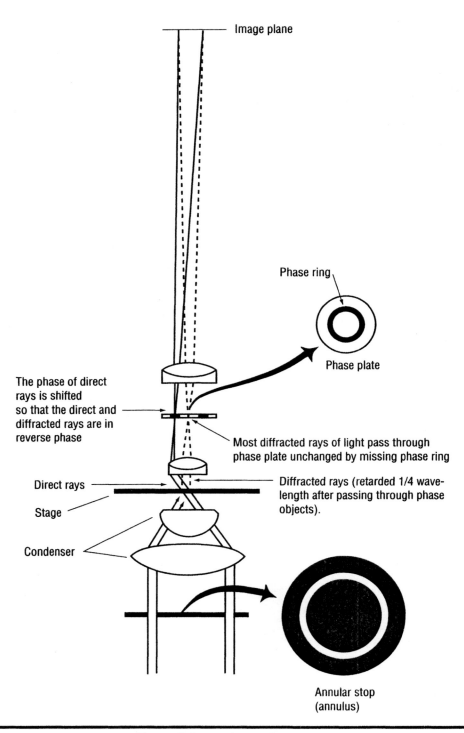

Image plane

Phase ring

Phase plate

The phase of direct rays is shifted so that the direct and diffracted rays are in reverse phase

Most diffracted rays of light pass through phase plate unchanged by missing phase ring

Direct rays

Diffracted rays (retarded 1/4 wavelength after passing through phase objects).

Stage

Condenser

Annular stop (annulus)

Figure 5.6   A phase microscope.

and diffracted rays so they converge at the image plane. Since they are in reverse phase, a dark image appears against a light background.

With these basics in hand, you can now proceed to the exercise. It is divided into two parts. Part A is concerned with adjustment of the phase microscope to properly align the annular stop and phase disk. Correct alignment is critical so that direct rays and diffracted rays are in reverse phase and the specimen is clearly seen. Part B lets you see the difference in an image when the same cell is observed by phase and by bright-field microscopy.

PURPOSE

- To learn how to correctly set up and adjust a phase microscope
- To observe the differences in images produced by bright-field microscopy and phase microscopy

THE EXERCISE

MATERIALS:

Phase microscope
Pond water or hay infusion
Microscope slides
Pasteur pipets or droppers
Phase-focusing telescope
Flat end toothpicks
Coverslips

PROCEDURE:

Part A: Adjusting the Phase Microscope

Note: In most cases, once a phase microscope is properly set up, it remains in alignment for extended periods of time and need only be realigned periodically. However, after heavy use or abuse by individuals having little experience with a phase microscope, realignment may be needed. Thus, it is important to learn this skill.

1. Examine the condenser of the microscope. Notice that it has a rotating disk with labeled positions. Most phase microscopes have three positions, two for phase work and one for regular bright-field work (the blank position). The two phase positions on the condenser disk correspond to specific lenses on the objective nosepiece. The labeling of the lenses and the condenser disk positions varies from microscope to microscope. Your instructor will describe the specifics of your condenser and phase objectives.
2. Examine the light source. Most microscopes have a diaphragm on the light source that can be adjusted. This diaphragm is called the radiant-field diaphragm (**Figure 5.7**). You may or may not have used this light adjustment in previous exercises.
3. Prepare a wet mount of pond water or hay infusion.
4. Focus the microscope as usual using the 10× objective and the condenser disk in its bright-field position.

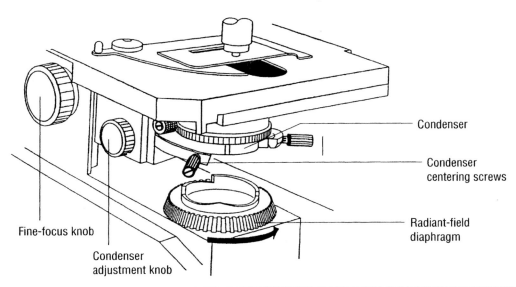

Fine-focus knob
Condenser
adjustment knob

Condenser
Condenser centering screws
Radiant-field diaphragm

Figure 5.7 Substage condenser and radiant-field diaphragm. (Redrawn from Chan, E.C.S., Pelczar, M.J., Jr., and Kreg, N.R.: *Laboratory Exercises in Microbiology,* 6th ed., New York, NY, McGraw-Hill, Inc., 1993. With permission.)

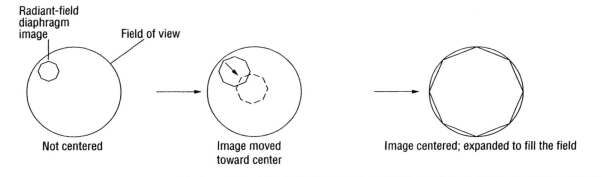

Radiant-field diaphragm image

Field of view

Not centered

Image moved toward center

Image centered; expanded to fill the field

Figure 5.8   Centering a radiant-field diaphragm.

5. Open the condenser diaphragm iris to its widest opening, and close the radiant-field diaphragm to its smallest opening.
6. Look through the eyepiece. You will see a bright shape in the field. Bring it into sharp focus by moving the condenser. Usually this requires lowering the condenser a short distance by rotating the condenser adjustment knob (**Figure 5.7**).
7. Determine if the light is centered in the field. If it is not, turn the condenser centering screws until it is (**Figure 5.8**).
8. Rotate the 40× phase objective into position, and rotate the condenser disk to the appropriate position for that objective.
9. Remove the eyepiece and replace it with the phase-focusing telescope. **Note:** Some microscopes use an aperture viewing prism instead of

a telescope. If your scope is of this type, put it into position instead of the telescope.
10. Look through the telescope. Focus the telescope until you see one of the two images shown in **Figure 5.9.** If the annular stop and phase ring are out of alignment, you will see an image similar to **Figure 5.9a.** If the annular stop and phase ring are in alignment, you will see an image similar to **Figure 5.9b.**
11. If the annular stop and phase ring are out of alignment, you must align them. This is accomplished using either special phase centering screws located on the condenser, or special wrenches. Your instructor will describe the tools you will use. Your goal is to superimpose the ring of light on the phase ring of the phase disk so that an image like that of **Figure 5.9b** is obtained.

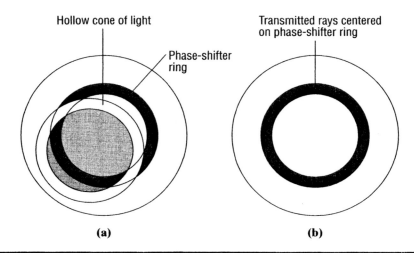

Hollow cone of light

Phase-shifter ring

Transmitted rays centered on phase-shifter ring

(a)

(b)

Figure 5.9   Alignment of the annulus and phase ring: (a) incorrect alignment, and (b) correct alignment.

12. Replace the eyepiece and proceed to the examination of the specimens.

Part B: Examination of the Specimens

1. Rotate the condenser disk to the blank position while the specimen is still focused under the 40× phase objective. Now the microscope is working as a bright-field microscope. **Note:** Phase objectives work well as bright-field objectives when the condenser disk is not in a phase position.

2. Locate an alga or protozoan in the specimen. Try to identify as many details of its cellular structure as possible.

3. Make detailed drawings of your observations in the RESULTS section.

4. While remaining focused on the same microbe, rotate the condenser disk to the position that corresponds to the 40× phase objective. You are now observing a phase image of the microbe.

5. Make detailed drawings of your observations in the RESULTS section.

6. Now examine the specimen for bacteria and compare the image with the phase and bright-field results.

7. Make detailed drawings of your observations in the RESULTS section.

8. Discard the slide of the hay infusion or pond water.

9. Obtain a new microscope slide and coverslip.

10. Place a small drop of water on the microscope slide.

11. Using the flat end of a toothpick, gently scrape the inside of your cheek.

12. Disperse the cheek cells in the drop of water on the microscope slide and overlay with a coverslip.

13. Examine the cheek cells under phase and bright-field.

14. Make detailed drawings of your observations in the RESULTS section.

REFERENCES

Bennett, A.H., et al. *Phase Microscopy.* New York: John Wiley and Sons, Inc., 1951.

Dazzo, F.B., et al. Specific Phases of Root Hair Attachment in the *Rhizobium trifolii*—Clover Symbiosis. *Applied and Environmental Microbiology* 48(1984):1140-1150.

Gerhardt, P. *Methods for General and Molecular Bacteriology.* Washington, DC: American Society for Microbiology Press, 1994.

RESULTS

Draw your observations.

Protozoan or alga

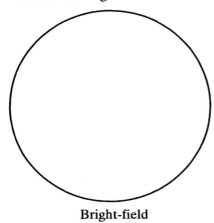

Bright-field

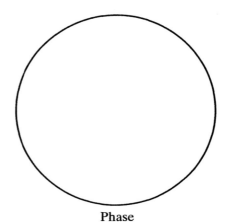

Phase

Bacteria

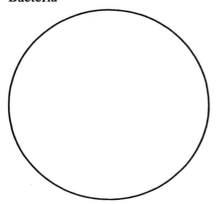

Bright-field

Phase

Cheek cells

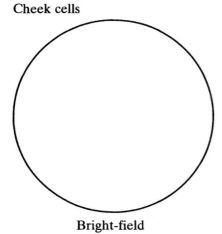

Bright-field

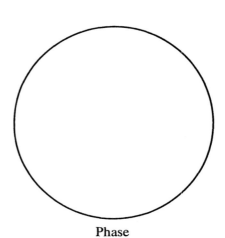

Phase

REFLECTIONS

1. Did you observe any striking differences between the phase and bright-field images of the various cells you observed? What were they?

2. Suppose you did not observe a distinctly different image with the phase objective. What might this mean?

3. Give three examples of organisms or phenomena for which observation by phase microscopy might be preferable to bright-field.

4. Would phase microscopy be of any particular value when examining a stained specimen? Explain.

EXERCISE 6

IMPORTANT MICROBIOLOGICAL STAINS

The previous microscopic examinations allowed you to view microorganisms in a living environment. However, you may have also observed that it is sometimes difficult to see differences in these microbes. This exercise introduces staining procedures that allow you to observe different characteristics of microorganisms and, therefore, start to differentiate between them.

Jenny, a 16-year-old high school student, had complained of a stomach ache and abdominal pain for several days. After 4 days, her pain, which started on her right side, had now spread across her entire abdomen. She also had nausea and some diarrhea. Her mother called Jenny's physician, who advised her to bring Jenny in for an examination. When they arrived, Jenny could hardly stand up because the pain was so intense. A physical examination revealed a temperature of 100.6°F and a blood test showed an increased white blood cell count. These signs indicated appendicitis. Jenny was quickly admitted to the hospital and taken to the operating room where it was discovered that she had a ruptured appendix. A cloudy fluid was taken from the peritoneal cavity near the appendix and was sent to the laboratory. At the same time blood cultures were obtained. Jenny was immediately started on a broad spectrum antibiotic, cephalothin. However, it was important that the laboratory give a preliminary indication of the microorganism(s) causing her infection, since her doctor noticed a lot of inflammation. The peritoneal fluid
*reached the laboratory with a STAT, (immediate) request for a Gram stain and culture. The microbiologist quickly prepared and stained a slide of the fluid for microscopic examination. **Figure 6.1** is a picture similar to the one the microbiologist observed. It shows a small rod-shaped organism that stains Gram-negative (red). It also shows a large number of white blood cells that were found in the peritoneal fluid. The clinical microbiologist called the physician and reported that bacteria resembling a family of bacteria—the Enterobacteriaceae—were observed in large numbers. These bacteria are normal inhabitants of the intestines. Jenny's physician immediately started a different antibiotic—a third generation cephalosporin—which is more active against this group of microorganisms. Within 8 hours, her blood cultures grew a similar Gram-negative rod. The next day her peritoneal culture plates had abundant growth of an organism later identified as Escherichia coli. It was tested for its susceptibility to several different antibiotics including the cephalosporins and was found to be susceptible to all. Jenny gradually improved and was released from the hospital after several days.*

BACKGROUND INFORMATION

The case study illustrates the importance of one of the most widely used and important **differential stains**, the **Gram stain**. It was developed in 1884 by Hans Christian Gram, a Danish pathologist, who introduced the technique of counterstaining after decolorization. He developed the technique to visualize bacteria in tissues, especially purple-staining bacteria. He published the method, and within a few years it became clear that it was of even greater value in classifying bacteria into two major groups.

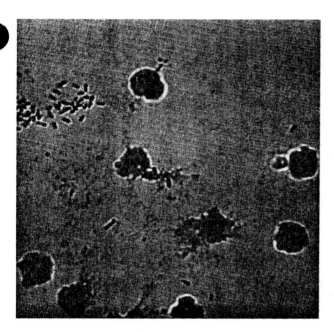

Figure 6.1 Gram stain of *E. coli* from a blood culture. *E. coli* is the small rod-shaped organism that stains Gram-negative (red) and the large cells are polymorphonuclear white blood cells.

Those that retain the dye after decolorizing with alcohol are referred to as **Gram-positive**, and those that lose the dye and stain red with the counterstain, safranin, are referred to as **Gram-negative**.

For many years an understanding of how the Gram stain differentiated species of microbes was not clear. However, it was noticed that the Gram reaction correlated with various important physiological characteristics of bacteria. Now it is known that there are chemical and physical differences in the cell walls of Bacteria that make them unique. Nearly all Bacteria have cell walls with peptidoglycan which is composed of two sugars and several different amino acids (**Figure 6.2**).[1] The Gram-positive Bacteria have thick cell walls consisting of many layers of peptidoglycan. When the basic dye, crystal violet, is added to these cells, it is attracted to the negatively charged surface of the bacterium and it penetrates the peptidoglycan. Iodine, which is added next, also penetrates the cell wall and forms a crystal violet-iodine complex. The

dye-iodine complex is too big to exit through the many layers of peptidoglycan in the cell when alcohol is added in the next step of the procedure. It is also believed that the alcohol dehydrates the pores in the walls, causing them to close. Therefore, in Gram-positive Bacteria the cell wall remains purple, even after counterstaining with the red dye, safranin. However, Gram-negative Bacteria have few layers of peptidoglycan and the dye-iodine complex easily penetrates the outer membrane and underlying peptidoglycan. Since there are so few layers of peptidoglycan, the dye-iodine complex is easily extracted by alcohol. Therefore, Gram-negative Bacteria are counterstained with safranin and appear red. In theory, all Bacteria should be divided into two groups with this method. However, there are instances when a given bacterium is Gram-variable. This is particularly true with older cultures of Gram-positive organisms such as *Bacillus*, which lose their cell wall integrity as they age and become Gram-negative.

The Gram stain is referred to as a complex stain because it uses two dyes to differentiate Bacteria. A simple stain is one in which a single basic dye is used to stain cells. Examples of this stain include crystal violet stain, the first step in the Gram stain procedure, and the methylene blue stain, another basic dye.

Another stain that has been used for years is the indirect or **negative stain.** The advantage of this stain is that it is the simplest and often quickest means of discovering cell shape and possibly refractile inclusions and endospores. It also does not distort bacteria which may happen with the Gram stain, since cells sometimes shrink as a result of heat fixation and alcohol wash. Preparations can easily be made with natural specimens or cultures by mixing them with a

---

[1]There are a few exceptions. Members of the genus *Mycoplasma* lack cell walls.

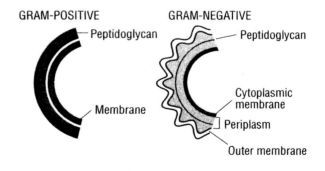

GRAM-POSITIVE — Peptidoglycan — Membrane

GRAM-NEGATIVE — Peptidoglycan — Cytoplasmic membrane — Periplasm — Outer membrane

Figure 6.2 A comparison of the cell walls: (a) Gram-positive Bacteria and (b) Gram-negative Bacteria.

drop of 7% nigrosin solution and making a thin film. The preparation reveals bacteria unstained, standing out brightly against a darker background. Negative stains should not be used to measure cell length or width because some microbes may have capsules or slime layers which do not stain. In addition, some cells may be partially collapsed. Furthermore, at pH 7, nigrosin is negatively charged, just like the bacterial cell surface. Therefore, when the stain dries, the bacteria appear larger than life, even if no capsule exists.

The final stain you will use in this laboratory exercise, **lactophenol cotton blue** (LPCB), is an important eucaryotic stain, especially of fungi. LPCB will stain the thread-like filaments (**hyphae**) of filamentous fungi (**moulds**).[2] In many, it will also stain reproductive structures (**spores**). The hyphae of moulds grow throughout a medium and into the air where they differentiate into spores. Spores are easily dispersed to other locations by air currents, and if the spores land in a location with adequate nutrients (e.g., on bread) they germinate and form hyphae again. **Figure 6.3** shows the hyphae and reproductive structures of two common moulds, *Penicillium* and *Aspergillus*. *Penicillium* is often found on food and most *Penicillium* species produce green colonies. *Aspergillus* can produce many different colored colonies, including green, black and yellow, and is also a common bread mould. Another mould that produces an abundance of "fuzzy growth" is *Rhizopus* (**Figure 6.4**). All three

---

[2]Medical mycologists used the word mould instead of mold to differentiate fungi from preformed molds (e.g., plastic).

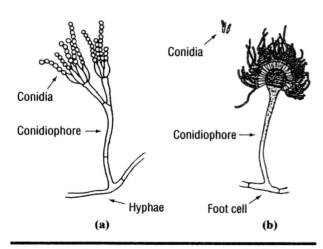

Figure 6.3 The distinctive structures of (a) *Penicillium* and (b) *Aspergillus*.

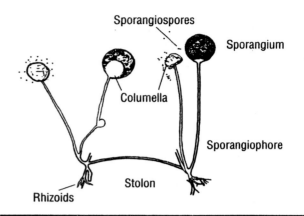

Figure 6.4 *Rhizopus* with a sporangium filled with sporangiospores.

moulds are distinctive and you may be able to find them on some of the food you examine in this laboratory. LPCB is a good stain for fungi because the phenol kills the moulds while the lactic acid preserves the fungal structures. The cotton blue stains chitin in the fungal cell walls a light blue so that they are seen more easily against a light background.

You will use a **transparent tape technique** to prepare your samples for viewing. It is so named because the adhesive side of a clear tape is pressed against a fungal colony. The aerial hyphae cling to the sticky surface and can be gently pulled from the fungal mat. The tape is then placed in a small drop of LPCB on a microscope slide. This technique has an advantage over wet mounts because the original position of the spores and hyphal segments is retained. However, it is of limited value in the study of colonies with a smooth or yeast-like surface, or colonies where sporulation is not present.

PURPOSE

- To examine the characteristics of eucaryotic and procaryotic organisms using staining methods
- To perform three stains: the Gram stain and negative stain on bacteria, and the LPCB stain on fungi

THE EXERCISE

MATERIALS:

Gram stain reagents:
   Crystal violet
   Iodine
   Alcohol
   Safranin

Wash bottles
Inoculating loop
Unknown cultures on nutrient agar plates
Bunsen burner
Mouldy food from your kitchen
7% Nigrosin
LPCB in dropper bottles
Microscope slides
Coverslips
Staining racks
Toothpicks
Nutrient broth cultures of *S. epidermidis* and *E. coli*
Penicillium, Aspergillus, and/or *Rhizopus* growing on
potato dextrose agar

PROCEDURE:

You will perform three important stains and examine the characteristics of organisms with each of these stains:

Part A: Gram Stain

1. Obtain broth cultures of *S. epidermidis* and *E. coli* and a nutrient agar plate with isolated colonies of an unknown organism.
2. Obtain two clean glass slides.
3. Divide one slide in half with a wax pencil or marker.
4. Put a drop or loopful of *E. coli* on one half of the slide and *S. epidermidis* on the other half of the slide. Be sure to identify the organism in each area. Set the slide aside to dry.
5. Divide another slide into thirds.
6. Place a drop of the *E. coli* on one end and *S. epidermidis* on the other end.
7. In the middle space, dispense one drop of distilled water and with a sterile loop, remove a small portion of one colony from your unknown plate and disperse it in the water. **Note:** It is important that a thin smear be made; avoid clumps so that uniform staining can be obtained.
8. Let all smears air dry and heat fix them by quickly passing them through a flame. **Note:** Heating firmly attaches the bacteria to the slide so that they do not wash off when stained.
9. Place the slide on a staining rack and flood the smear with crystal violet. Let it sit on the smear for 1 minute.
10. Gently wash the stain off with water. **Note:** Hold the slide at an angle while washing with water after each step (**Figure 6.5**).
11. Flood the smear with iodine solution and let it sit for 1 minute.

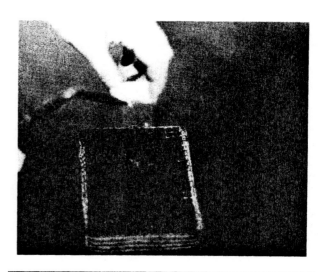

Figure 6.5 Rinsing the slide with water.

12. Gently rinse the slide again with water.
13. Decolorize the smear by tilting the slide and rinsing it with alcohol. The excess crystal violet will wash off and the blue dye will disappear in about 10 seconds. **Note:** This is an important step; do not add too much or too little alcohol to decolorize.
14. Rinse the slide with water to stop the decolorization.
15. Lay the slide flat again and flood the smear with safranin. Let it sit for 30 seconds.
16. Rinse with water and clean the back of the slide with a paper towel. Tilt it to dry or blot dry with absorbent paper.
17. Repeat steps 9 through 16 with the second slide.
18. Observe the slides, first using low power to focus, and then rotating the objectives to high dry and oil immersion. **Note:** Most bacteria are small and need to be viewed in oil immersion to adequately see their Gram reaction and morphology. The *E. coli* are Gram-negative (red) rods while the *S. epidermidis* cells are Gram-positive (purple) cocci. You should observe this Gram reaction for *E. coli* and *S. epidermidis* on both slides. If you do not, repeat the procedure with a new smear. Your unknown can be a Gram-positive or Gram-negative coccus or rod.
19. Record your results in the RESULTS section.

Part B: Negative Stain

1. Place one small drop of 7% nigrosin stain in the center of a coverslip.

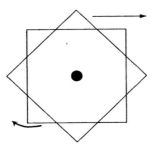

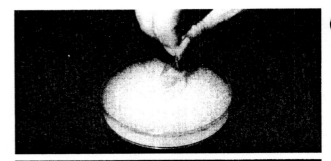

Figure 6.6 Coverslips with suspension of nigrosin between them.

Figure 6.7 Transparent tape with adhesive side out and pressed against fungus.

2. With a toothpick, gently scrape your teeth and gums and mix the material with the nigrosin. You may also remove a small amount of a colony from one of your plates and mix it with the nigrosin.
3. Place another coverslip, rotated at 45°, over the nigrosin (**Figure 6.6**) and slide the two coverslips apart to form a thin film on each.
4. Turn the top coverslip over and let both films dry completely.
5. With another toothpick, add a small amount of vaseline to all four corners of each coverslip to fix the coverslip to the slide.
6. Invert each coverslip on a slide. If you have used small coverslips, you can place both of them on the same slide.
7. Find a very thin area of the film and observe the bacteria under oil immersion. **Note:** Most of the slide will show large cracks from the dried stain, so find an area that has no cracks and observe the clear bacteria against a faint grey background.
8. Record your findings in the RESULTS section.

Part C: LPCB Stain

Your were told you may bring in moulds you wish to examine. Bread or food from your refrigerator are good sources. You will also have the opportunity to examine plate cultures of an *Aspergillus*, *Penicillium*, or *Rhizopus*.

1. Place a small drop of LPCB stain in the middle of a glass slide.
2. Obtain a 4-cm strip of transparent adhesive tape. Loop the tape and hold it between your thumb and index finger with the adhesive side out.
3. Firmly press the adhesive side to the surface of the fungus to be studied (**Figure 6.7**).
4. Gently pull the tape from the surface and place it on the slide with LPCB (**Figure 6.8**). The tape acts

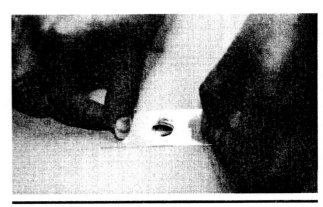

Figure 6.8 Inoculated adhesive tape placed over a drop of LPCB.

as a coverslip so press it as flat as possible, avoiding air bubbles. However, do not press too firmly or the hyphal structures will be disturbed. One technique is to start at one end of the tape and gently lay it across the slide.

5. Observe the preparations under low power and high power and draw any structures you see in the RESULTS section. Try to find hyphae and spores and, if you can, find intact structures such as hyphae with conidiophores and conidia, or sporangiophores, sporangia and rhizoids.
6. Prepare several slides of your moulds or the moulds from the culture plates. Do not be concerned if you cannot attach a name to your fungi, but see if they have any similarities to the known moulds you have been supplied with. Take some time observing the various structures of the different species. Further investigation of moulds will be done in Exercise 13.
7. Record your observations in the RESULTS section.

REFERENCES

Brock, T.D., et al. *Biology of Microorganisms,* 7th ed. Englewood Cliffs, NJ: Prentice Hall 1994.

Collard, P. *The Development of Microbiology.* Cambridge: Cambridge University Press, 1976.

Gerhardt, P., et al. *Methods for General and Molecular Bacteriology.* Washington, DC: American Society for Microbiology Press, 1994.

Koneman, E. and Roberts, G. *Practical Laboratory Mycology*, 3rd ed. Baltimore: Williams & Wilkins, 1985.

RESULTS

Part A: Gram Stain

Record the morphology and Gram reactions below:

E. coli_____

S. epidermidis_____

Unknown #_____   _____

Part B: Negative Stain

Draw the microorganisms and background you observed. Also record the objective used to observe these specimens.

Teeth scrapings:_____   Culture: _____

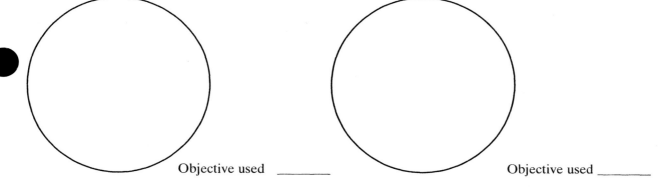

Objective used _____   Objective used _____

Part C: LPCB Stain

Draw any fungal structures you saw in the mould. Also, show their variation in size and shape.

Food type: _____   Culture: _____

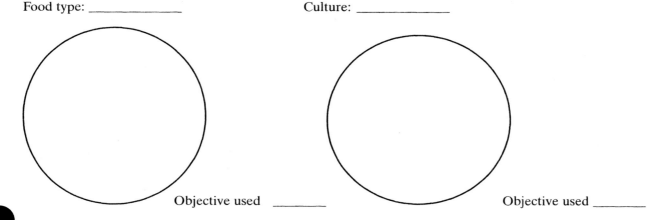

Objective used _____   Objective used _____

REFLECTIONS

1. You were instructed to redo the unknown if the known bacteria did not stain properly. Explain why you were instructed to do so.

2. Briefly explain during each of the four steps of the Gram stain what the Gram-positive and Gram-negative bacteria will look like.

3. What microorganism that you observed has species that produce an antibiotic? What is the antibiotic?

4. Which dye will not kill microorganisms if a wet preparation is made? Why?

5. Preparing stains of microorganisms takes time. Why do we do it?

6. What is dental plaque? What is the role of bacteria in the production of dental caries?

7. You were instructed to use only young cultures for Gram staining. Why?

MODERN STAINING PROCEDURES

As you have learned in previous exercises, stains are routinely used in the microscopic examination of microbes to aid in visualizing the microbes and to differentiate one microbe from another. Over the years, staining procedures have improved tremendously. One major breakthrough has been the development of fluorescent dyes to visualize specific cell structures. You will gain experience in the use of two of these dyes, DAPI and Calcofluor, in this exercise.

Rhonda[1] had a problem. She was doing an undergraduate research project on the fungal pathogen of barley, Ustilago hordei. *When Rhonda began her work, the prevailing belief was that* U. hordei *was only pathogenic after it had mated and formed a dikaryon, a cell with two haploid nuclei. The question Rhonda was trying to answer was, "Can a monokaryon having one diploid nucleus initiate infection as well?" Rhonda's task was to create diploid monokaryons in the lab. However, she was not certain if the procedure she planned to use would give the desired results. The only way Rhonda would know for sure was to look at the cells after completing the procedure and determine if they contained one or two nuclei. The nuclei of* U. hordei *are not easily seen in a wet mount, so Rhonda needed to stain them. She began by trying DAPI, a fluorescent dye that binds DNA. After staining cells with*

---

[1]This story is based on the experience of a real student. No names have been changed. Rhonda is now a clinical laboratory scientist in a hospital in eastern Montana.

DAPI, she could see nuclei clearly but she had forgotten that the rest of the cell would not fluoresce. Therefore, it was difficult to determine if two fluorescing bodies (i.e., nuclei) close to each other were the two nuclei of a dikaryon, or the two nuclei of overlapping or adjacent monokaryotic cells. To solve her problem, Rhonda used another dye, Calcofluor, to specifically stain the cell walls. The two dyes together solved her problem. She could easily distinguish dikaryons from monokaryons. Rhonda's experiments subsequently showed that diploids are also pathogenic.

BACKGROUND INFORMATION

There are many applications for **specific stains**—stains of specific cells or cell structures—besides those illustrated by Rhonda's research. Many of the most commonly used specific stains use **fluorescent dyes** or fluorochromes. Fluorescent dyes are complex organic molecules that absorb light at one wavelength, the excitatory wavelength, and emit light at another, longer wavelength, the emission wavelength. The intensity of the fluorescence is always much less than the excitatory light intensity, so specially designed microscopes are required to illuminate and view the stained specimen. Different methods of illumination have been developed, but the most useful is incident illumination, where light is reflected onto an object, rather than transmitted through an object. This is more commonly called **epi-illumination.** Fluorescent microscopy using epi-illumination is called **epi-fluorescence.** In epi-fluorescence microscopy, specialized objective lenses act as both objective lenses and condensers. The excitatory beam of light is directed down through the objective lens onto the specimen, but only the fluorescent emissions are directed back to the eye.

This is accomplished by the use of filter sets that produce the correct excitatory wavelength and only allow transmission to the eye of the emission wavelength.

In this exercise, you will examine a yeast, *Saccharomyces cerevisiae*, stained by two different fluorochromes. The first, DAPI (4',6'-Diamidino-2-phenylindole · 2HCl) binds DNA by an unknown binding mechanism (**Figure 7.1a**). DAPI is excited at wavelength 350 nanometers (nm) and emits at 450 nm. Although *S. cerevisiae* is not dikaryotic, its DNA is easily stained by DAPI, and under the right growth conditions, the nuclear divisions of mitosis and meiosis can be observed. The second fluorochrome, Calcofluor (also known as Calcofluor White M2R, Fluorescent Brightener 28, and Cellufluor) is excited and emits light at about the same wavelengths as DAPI (**Figure 7.1b**). Calcofluor is known to stain chitin, a polysaccharide common to the cell walls of many fungi, but it is also useful for staining cellulose in plant and algal cell walls.

PURPOSE

• To learn to use a fluorescent microscope
• To examine cell structures stained by fluorescent dyes

THE EXERCISE

MATERIALS:
Epi-fluorescence microscope
1 mg/ml stock solution of DAPI
1 mg/ml stock solution of Calcofluor
1.5 ml microcentrifuge tube
1 ml pipets
Microscope slides
Disposable gloves
Actively growing (log phase) culture of *S. cerevisiae*
Disposable test tube (12 × 75 mm) and lid
Micropipetter and pipet tips
Microcentrifuge
Coverslips
Microcentrifuge tube

PROCEDURE: Work in groups designated by your instructor

Part A: DAPI

1. Pipet 0.5 ml of the *S. cerevisiae* culture into a disposable test tube.
2. Add 1 ml of 95% ethanol. Vortex and let the cells fix for 10 minutes. **Note:** The addition of alcohol to the cells prevents the cells from progressing any further through cell division. It also makes the cells more permeable to the dye.
   CAUTION: Before starting the next step, put on a pair of gloves. The toxicity and carcinogenicity of DAPI has not been carefully studied. However, it is safe to assume that any DNA-binding molecule such as DAPI has the potential to be hazardous.
3. Add 10 µl of the DAPI stock solution to the alcohol fixed cells. Vortex to mix.
4. Prepare a wet mount of the stained cells (see Exercise 2).

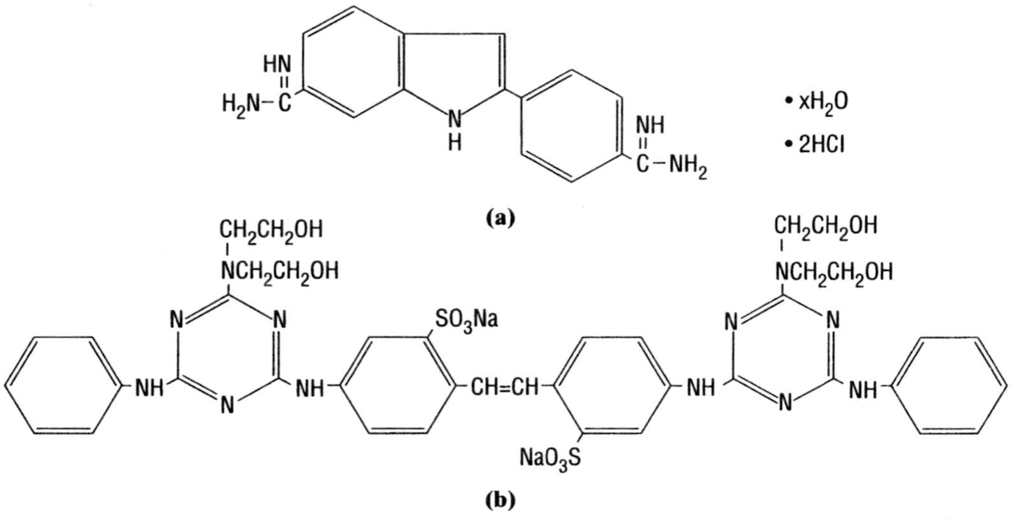

Figure 7.1 Molecular structure of fluorochromes: (a) DAPI and (b) Calcofluor.

5. Examine the cells using bright-field microscopy. Note the small buds (**Figure 7.2**) emerging on many of the larger cells.
6. Focus clearly on one budding cell and draw what you see in the RESULTS section.
7. Switch to epi-fluorescence illumination. Your instructor will tell you which filter set to use if there is more than one set on the microscope. You should now be able to see the nucleus of the budding cell. You should also look for the nucleus of the bud. **Note:** Since each microscope is a little different, your instructor will demonstrate how to switch from transmitted light to epi-illumination.
8. Draw the cells in the RESULTS section.

Part B: Calcofluor

1. Pipet 1 ml of the yeast culture into a micro centrifuge tube.
2. Spin the cells at top speed for 5 minutes. Discard the supernatant.
3. Resuspend the cell pellet in 1 ml of the Calcofluor solution.
4. Incubate at room temperature for 5 minutes.
5. Observe the stained cells as you did for the DAPI-stained cells.
6. Record your observations in the RESULTS section.

Part C: Optional

1. Try designing a procedure to repeat Rhonda's experiment with *S. cerevisiae,* staining cells with

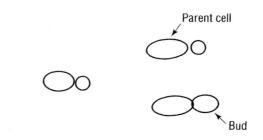

Figure 7.2 Budding yeast cells.

both DAPI and Calcofluor. If supplies are available, test your protocol.
2. Record your observations in the RESULTS section.

REFERENCES

Gerhardt, P. *Methods for General and Molecular Bacteriology.* Washington, DC: American Society for Microbiology Press, 1994.

Guthrie, C. and Fink, G.R. *Guide to Yeast Genetics and Molecular Biology.* San Diego: Harcourt, Brace Jovanovich, 1991.

Pringle, J.R. Staining of Bud Scars and Other Cell Wall Chitin With Calcofluor. *Methods in Enzymology* 194(1991):732-735.

Pringle, J.R., et al. Immunofluorescence Methods for Yeast. *Methods in Enzymology* 194(1991):565-601.

RESULTS

Draw the images you observed.

DAPI:

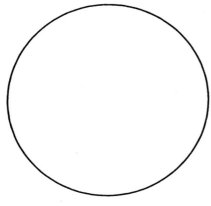

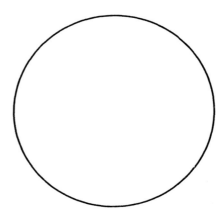

Bright-field   Epi-fluorescence

Calcofluor:

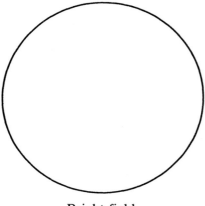

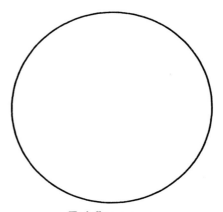

Bright-field   Epi-fluorescence

Results of optional experiment:

REFLECTIONS

1. Did you observe any DAPI-stained cells that look like this? Suggest what you may have been observing.

   Bright-field ∞

   Epi-fluorescence   ●∷●

2. In Exercise 6, you used a nonfluorescent dye that specifically stains chitin in fungal cell walls. What was that dye? Would double-staining cells with that dye and DAPI have solved Rhonda's problem? Explain.

3. List three other fluorescent stains. What is the usefulness of each?

4. Describe how simple staining and fluorescence staining are similar and how they are different. What are the advantages of each?

5. If you did the optional part of the exercise, did your staining protocol work? If it didn't, what changes would you need to make to enable you to see both the cell outline and the nucleus?

EXERCISE 8

SOME LIKE IT HOT!

As you begin to investigate microbes more closely, one of the things you will discover is their incredible diversity. They live everywhere, including in extreme environments. During this exercise, you will explore some of the diverse environmental conditions in which microorganisms live. It may also give you some idea of how scientists can exploit this diversity for many uses.

Yellowstone National Park—Newsflash!

"Researchers who develop commercial microbes from bubbling hot springs in Yellowstone National Park will have to share their profits with the taxpayers," said John Varley, Director of the Yellowstone Center for Resources, as he spoke to a conference of about 125 scientists. No longer will pharmaceutical and bioengineering companies be allowed to take Yellowstone microbes and claim exclusive use without paying royalties. The microbes in question are called thermophiles and live at extreme temperatures in boiling hot springs in the park. They can be used in industrial applications requiring heat.

The idea of a royalty system drew some complaints by scientists. "'Bioprospectors' disturb nothing and take nothing irreplaceable—often just a few vials of water from hot springs," some said. "Any microbes removed are quickly replaced as their survivors multiply." Others said microbes are so ubiquitous that "tourists can carry them away on their shoes."[1]

Little did Thomas D. Brock and Hudson Freeze know that in the 1960s when they isolated a microbe they

---

[1]Article from September 24, 1995, *Great Falls Tribune*, Great Falls, Montana.

named Thermus aquaticus *from several hot springs in Yellowstone that they would be creating such a fuss. This microbe has an optimum growth temperature of 70°C and produces a heat-resistant enzyme called DNA polymerase which was characterized in 1976. This enzyme is important in a process developed in 1983 called polymerase chain reaction (PCR). Its inventor, Kary Mullis, won a Nobel Prize for PCR in 1993. PCR is a surprisingly simple method for making unlimited copies of DNA fragments. The applications for PCR have spread throughout the biological sciences, and include DNA fingerprinting, an important forensic technique. The DNA polymerase of* T. aquaticus *(Taq) is stable at high temperatures. The use of Taq polymerase allowed PCR to be automated. Taq polymerase has also generated millions of dollars for Hoffman-LaRoche, a pharmaceutical giant that owns the patent for the process.*

Currently, many other thermophiles are being investigated for use as road de-icers, degraders of oil spills, and for improvement of gold mine processes. Interestingly E. coli *has now been engineered to produce abundant quantities of Taq polymerase. In fact, many scientists believe that it may no longer be necessary to collect microorganisms because standard laboratory strains such as* E. coli *can be redesigned in laboratories by genetic engineering. Another interesting point is that at the same time Brock and his colleagues isolated* T. aquaticus *from the geothermal springs, they also isolated it from man-made thermal habitats, including the hot water taps at Indiana University.*

BACKGROUND INFORMATION

The story above illustrates only one of the extreme environments in which microorganisms can live. The microorganisms that thrive at body temperatures and ambient air temperatures are abundant and often studied. These organisms are called

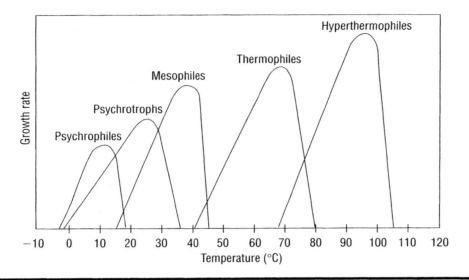

Figure 8.1 The range of temperatures for microbial growth.

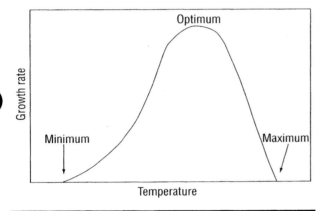

Figure 8.2 The relationship of temperature to growth rate.

mesophiles and grow at temperatures from 13°C to 45°C. The **thermophiles** discussed above grow in temperatures ranging from 42°C to 100°C or more. At temperatures above 80°C, the Archaea predominate (see Exercise 16). Another group of microorganisms, called **psychrophiles**, grow at temperatures ranging from −3°C to 20°C (**Figure 8.1**). All organisms have ranges of temperature at which there is a minimum amount of growth called minimum temperature; a temperature above which, growth is not possible, called maximum temperature; and an optimum growth temperature, the temperature at which growth is most rapid (**Figure 8.2**). Also, microorganisms can grow across a range of temperatures. For example, they can be tolerant of low temperatures but prefer a mesophilic temperature (psychrotolerant).

In addition to temperature differences, microorganisms have also adapted to different levels of acidity and alkalinity. A few microorganisms, such as *Sulfolobus* and *Thiobacillus,* grow in extreme acid niches (pH 1 to 2) and oxidize sulfide minerals producing sulfuric acid. These microorganisms are called **acidophiles**. Other microorganisms live in naturally occurring alkaline environments such as soda lakes and deserts where pH values above 10 are common. These **alkalophiles** are well known and include *Rhizobium, Bacillus,* several enteric bacteria and cyanobacteria. Each microorganism also has a pH range and an optimum pH for growth. In general, fungi tend to be more acid tolerant than bacteria.

Another parameter that affects microbial growth is the presence or absence of oxygen. Some microorganisms require oxygen as a terminal electron acceptor and are called **aerobes**. Others lack a respiratory system (electron transport chain) and cannot use oxygen. These organisms are called **anaerobes**. Here too, we have organisms existing over a spectrum of oxygen requirements. See **Table 8.1** for the terms used to describe the oxygen relationships of microorganisms. One of the ways to study anaerobes in the laboratory is to add a reducing agent to a medium which reacts with oxygen, excluding it from the medium. Sodium thioglycollate is such an agent. When added to a tubed medium, it will react with oxygen throughout the tube and as a result, oxygen is

TABLE 8.1 Terms Used to Describe Oxygen Relationships of Microorganisms

Group	O_2 Effect
Aerobes	
Obligate	Required
Facultative	Not required, but growth better with O_2
Microaerophilic	Required, but at levels lower than atmospheric
Anaerobes	
Aerotolerant	Not required, and growth no better when O_2 present
Obligate (strict) anaerobes	Harmful or lethal

only found at the top where the medium contacts air. Oxygen presence turns the redox dye resazurin pink.

The last parameter we will investigate in this exercise is the availability of water, the solvent of life for all organisms. When salts or sugars are dissolved in water they have an affinity for and interact with water. The water interacting with such solutes is unavailable to microbes. That is why most organisms do not grow well in high-solute concentrations. However, some organisms known as **halophiles** require high sodium concentrations to survive. Many of these microorganisms belong to the Archaea. There are many places on Earth that contain an increased concentration of sodium such as in seawater, salty soils and on our skin, and these microorganisms live in such environments. There are also some microorganisms capable of living in high sugar environments, called **osmophiles**, and dry environments, known as **xerophiles**.

Even though the effects of each environmental factor listed above are easy to understand when considered alone, in natural environments the combined influence of these factors is not always as straightforward. For example, a change in one parameter, like a cold temperature, can influence a change in another factor, such as oxygen availability. Therefore, studying microorganisms living in natural environments continues to be a challenge to microbiologists.

PURPOSE

- To determine the effects of temperature, pH, oxygen and salt concentrations (water availability) on the growth of bacteria

THE EXERCISE

Part A

MATERIALS:

Nutrient agar plates

Thioglycollate broth tubes

Nutrient agar plates with 5% NaCl, 10% NaCl, and 15% NaCl

Yeast extract glucose broth tubes at pH 3.0, 5.0, 7.0 and 9.0

Organisms: Temperature effects—*E. coli, Pseudomonas fluorescens,* and *Bacillus stearothermophilus*

pH effects—*E. coli, Saccharomyces cerevisiae,* and *Alcaligenes faecalis*

Oxygen effects—*E. coli, P. fluorescens,* and *Clostridium butryicum*

Salt effects—*E. coli, S. epidermidis, S. cerevisiae,* and *Bacillus subtilis*

PROCEDURE: Work in groups as designated by your instructor.

1. Design a set of experiments which will test four environmental influences on bacterial growth: temperature, pH, oxygen and salt concentration. Listed above are the media available to you and the microorganisms we recommend for testing each parameter. Design a protocol for testing each parameter. Each experimental protocol should include the media you will use and incubation conditions.

2. Submit your experimental protocols to your instructor for approval before proceeding.

3. Record your results in the RESULTS section in the form of tables. Also record the results obtained by others, if you tested only one of the environmental factors.

4. Write a laboratory report explaining the testing procedures and results. Follow the format used in scientific journals including an introduction, experimental methods, results, and conclusions, to write your paper (see Appendix B). Be sure to include the results for all four environmental factors in your report.

REFERENCES

Brock, T.D. and Freeze, H. *Thermus aquaticus* gen.n. and sp.n., a Non-sporulating Extreme Thermophile. *Journal of Bacteriology* 98(1969):289-297.

Chien, A., et al. Deoxyribonucleic Acid Polymerase From the Extreme Thermophile *Thermus aquaticus.* *Journal of Bacteriology* 127(1976):1550-1557.

Mullis, K. The Unusual Origin of the Polymerase Chain Reaction. *Scientific American* (April, 1990): 56-65.

Innis, M., et al. DNA Sequencing With *Thermus aquaticus* DNA Polymerase and Direct Sequencing of PCR-amplified DNA. *Proceedings of the National Academy of Sciences* 85(1988):9436-9440.

Lawyer, F., et al. Isolation, Characterization, and Expression in *Escherichia coli* of the DNA Polymerase Gene From *Thermus aquaticus.* *Journal of Biological Chemistry* 264(1989):6427-6436.

RESULTS

Temperature effects:

pH effects:

Oxygen effects:

Salt differences:

REFLECTIONS

1. What is your opinion about the ruling of Yellowstone National Park officials who say that profits from biotechnology firms that obtain materials from thermal springs should be shared with taxpayers?

2. *E. coli* is tested in all four experiments. Write a profile of this organism describing its growth characteristics under all four of these conditions.

3. What do you think will happen to the thioglycollate broth if the tube is left standing at room temperature, uninoculated, for several days? What if the tube was refrigerated?

4. List an environmental variable involved in food preservation and give an example of the food.

EXERCISE 9

MICROBE SAFARI

In previous exercises, you have learned a variety of techniques routinely used to study and characterize microorganisms. You have also observed many different microbes. In this exercise, you will put your newly acquired knowledge and skills to work to isolate and study microbes from a small section of the microbial universe—the habitats in and near your science building.

BACKGROUND INFORMATION

In previous exercises, you have observed and manipulated a variety of different microbes. Have you wondered where they came from? All microbes used in laboratories were originally isolated from their natural habitat and then cultivated in artificial environments. It is believed that only a small fraction of microbial species has been isolated and identified. Most species are yet to be discovered! In recent years, scientists have increasingly argued the importance of cataloguing all species of life on Earth to get a clearer picture of biodiversity and to learn more about how organisms evolve and persist or become extinct. Numerous research projects have been proposed to assess microbial diversity. In this exercise, you will in your own way contribute to this assessment by isolating and characterizing microbes in or near your science building. To complete the exercise, you need to develop a research plan with other members of a group. In developing your plan you should remember that both animate objects (e.g., humans and plants) and inanimate objects (e.g., toilets, door handles, and bench tops) are potential habitats. So grab an inoculating loop and enjoy this microbe safari!

PURPOSE

- To put to use some of the techniques learned in previous exercises
- To explore possible habitats for microbes
- To discover the diversity of microbes in the environment
- To gain experience in working with groups to develop and implement a research plan

THE EXERCISE

MATERIALS:

Sterile swabs
Tube of sterile distilled water
Sterile Pasteur pipets
Sterile applicator sticks
Inoculating loop
Nutrient agar plates
Other materials you may request

PROCEDURE:

Part A: Beginning the Exercise: Work in groups of 5

1. As a group develop a plan to sample 5 different sites in or near your laboratory building. In the plan, determine what materials will be needed for sampling each site and how the sampling will be done. **Note:** It may be helpful for you to read steps 3 and 6 in the next section as you develop your sampling plan.
2. Discuss your group's sampling plan with other groups in the class. Your instructor will lead this discussion. Your group may want to modify its sampling plan following the discussion.

Part B: Completing the Exercise

1. Sample the sites chosen in your research plan.
2. Incubate the samples in an appropriate location.

3. During the incubation period, all members of the group should review the techniques learned in previous exercises. The group should then meet to develop a research plan to characterize the microbes isolated from each sampling site. **Note:** This need not involve time outside your normal laboratory time. For instance, if time allows in the first laboratory period devoted to "Microbe Safari," you can meet during that period. The research plan should address the following issues:
   - How to assess the number of microbes from each sampling site
   - How to assess the diversity of microbes at each sampling site
   - How to characterize the microbes at each sampling site
   - What materials will be needed to complete the project
   - A time line for completion of the project
4. Give a copy of your group's research plan to your instructor to critique. You may want to modify the plan after getting feedback.
5. Implement the plan, collect, organize, and analyze the data. **Note:** An excellent description for recording experiments in a research notebook is found in *A Short Guide to Writing About Science* by David Porush (see REFERENCES).
6. Write a formal laboratory report (see Appendix B) on the results of your project. Be sure to address the following issues in your report:
   - Why were the 5 sampled sites chosen? Did the group have any preconceived notions regarding the relative numbers and diversity of microbes which might be found at each sampling site?
   - What were the characteristics of each sampling site at the time of sampling? Are these characteristic known to change over time?
   - What were the relative numbers of microbes at each site? Estimate the number of different microbes at each site. What were their major characteristics? If you had any preconceived notions about a site, were the results consistent with them?
   - Does the group think the microbes identified at each site were transients or normal inhabitants of the site? Why?
   - Based on what the group learned about each microbe characterized, what statements could be made regarding its energy source?
   - How quantitative are your results? Can legitimate comparisons regarding numbers of microbes at different sites be made? Why or why not?
   - Can any general statements be made about the types of environments that best support microbial life?
   - Were any sampling sites devoid of life? What were those sites like? Could microbes have been present at those sites and not detected? Why or why not?

REFERENCES

Porush, D. Writing From the Moment of Observation. In *A Short Guide to Writing About Science*. New York: HarperCollins College Publishers, 1995.

SECTION II

THE MICROBES

In the "Getting Started" section, you learned some of the ways microbes are manipulated in a laboratory setting so they can be studied. In each of these exercises you have observed microorganisms, and have begun to discover the diversity of microbes on Earth. In this section, we turn our attention to a more formal consideration of the microbes.

EXERCISE 10

THE CLASSIFICATION GAME

Before considering individual groups of microbes, it is worthwhile to examine how microorganisms have been sorted into taxons. In this exercise, you will devise a classification scheme to identify and establish relatedness among microbes from a complex microbial ecosystem. From this experience, you will hopefully gain a better appreciation not only of microbial diversity, but of the difficult task taxonomists face when classifying microorganisms.

As chief science officer of the Federation Star Ship Beagle *you have led the science team to the surface of Orcim, a newly discovered planet in the Delta quadrant. The assessment of biodiversity on the planet is almost done, but the hard part remains—determining the number of microscopic organisms on the planet. The team has brought back numerous environmental samples from likely habitats for the many microorganisms thought to inhabit Orcim. As a specialist in microscopic life forms, you are especially eager to start examining the samples collected.*

BACKGROUND INFORMATION

One of the important milestones in childhood development is learning to sort objects into groups based on their similarities. This skill never wanes and manifests itself perhaps most clearly in our sorting of life forms, a process scientists refer to as **taxonomy**. Taxonomic schemes do more than sort, however. They also attempt to show the evolutionary relationships of organisms. Thus, organisms thought to be closely related share many characteristics; they are placed in the same taxonomic group and are considered to have diverged from a common ancestor.

Your challenge in this exercise is to examine a complex community of microorganisms and to sort them into taxonomic groups. This is important because people often view taxonomy and classification schemes as being written in stone. The truth is that taxonomy is a constantly changing and frequently controversial area of science.

PURPOSE

- To develop a scheme for classifying and identifying microorganisms
- To assess microbial biodiversity in an environmental sample

THE EXERCISE

MATERIALS:

Sample of a complex microbial ecosystem
Microscope slides
Carboxymethyl cellulose
Coverslips

PROCEDURE: Work in groups of three to four

1. As a group, prepare one wet mount from the sample and take turns examining the life forms in it. Your observations of microbial diversity will prepare you for the next step. **Note:** If the microbes are moving too quickly to examine carefully, add a drop of carboxymethylcellulose to the wet mount. Carboxymethylcellulose is a viscous solution that impedes the movement of motile microorganisms.

2. After examining the sample for a minute or two, discuss the most striking characteristics of the microorganisms you observed.

3. Develop a plan for classifying the microorganisms in the sample. **Note:** The time allotted for executing your plan will be 30 minutes, unless your instructor tells you otherwise. Therefore, try to approach your task in a way that is efficient and avoids duplication of effort (i.e., divide the labor in some way). One thing to remember as you develop your plan is that the microorganisms in the sample could range in size from 2 to 250 micrometers (μm). Think about the magnification that would be best for observing microbes in the 2 to 4 μm size range. Take about 10 minutes to develop your plan.

4. In the next 30 minutes, use your plan to classify the microbes and assess the biodiversity in your sample. Describe as many different "species" of microbes as possible in your sample in the 30 minute time limit.

5. Report your group's findings to the class in a discussion led by your instructor. Share this information on the sample you examined: a list of characteristics used to differentiate "species," the number of different "species" observed, and a description of one "species."

6. The box shows a dichotomous key used to identify conifers in Yellowstone National Park and the surrounding area. As a group, formalize your classification scheme as a dichotomous key.

A Dichotomous Scheme to Identify Conifers of the Yellowstone Area

I. Needles at least 2 to 3 inches long; needles in bundles of two or more
   A. Needles in bundles of two; small woody cones, open or tightly closed ..... *Lodgepole pine*
   B. Needles in bundles of two, three or five; cones open, quite large and woody or falling apart
      1. Needles in bundles of two to three; needles 4 to 6 inches long; cones with barbs on scales .... *Ponderosa pine*
      2. Needles in bundles of five
         a. Cones large, woody; usually with sticky sap; tree grows at low elevations .... *Limber pine*
         b. Cones broken apart when mature, purplish when immature; tree grows at high elevations .... *Whitebark pine*

II. Needles shorter than 2 inches or tiny scales; needles or scales single on the stem, not in bundles
   A. Leaves very tiny scales or short wedge-shaped needles; small purple berries; tree grows at lower elevations
      1. Tree-like growth habit with scales as leaves .... *Rocky Mountain juniper*
      2. Low shrub with wedge-shaped leaves .... *Common juniper*
   B. Leaves are single needles, either flat or pointed; trees usually with cones
      1. Needles sharp and pointed, square in cross-section; cones with flexible scales; cones usually grow at top of tree .... *Spruce*
      2. Needles flat, not square in cross-section
         a. Needles soft and flat; cones form at top of tree but disintegrate at maturity; tree grows at higher elevations; winter buds rounded .... *Subalpine fir*
         b. Needles flat; cones with three-pointed papery bracts between scales; winter buds pointed; cones form from top to bottom of tree .... *Douglas fir*

RESULTS

Specimen examined:_____

Species   *Description*

The dichotomous key developed by your group:

REFLECTIONS

1. Describe the plan your group used to assess biodiversity in the specimen you examined.

2. How did you ensure that the same "species" was not counted more than once?

3. What characteristics were better at distinguishing "species"? What characteristics were common to all or most of the "species"?

4. Do you think you have underestimated or overestimated the number of "species" in your sample? Explain your answer.

5. Currently, there are several issues in taxonomy that are being hotly debated. Identify one of these issues. What are the arguments on each side?

EXERCISE 11

PROTOZOA—
FRIEND AND FOE

Previous exercises have allowed you to study procaryotes (bacteria) and some eucaryotes. This exercise begins a more in-depth study of one group of the eucaryotic microorganisms, the protozoa. These eucaryotes are usually larger and easier to observe microscopically. Even though they are unicellular, they have some interesting characteristics that make observing them fun.

In the early 1990s, a scourge of rainbow trout finally reached a pristine river of Montana—the Madison River. The disease is called whirling disease (WD) and is caused by the protozoan parasite Myxobolus cerebralis. Montana is the last of the lower 48 states to get this worldwide trout disease because Montana, for the most part, still manages wild reproduction of trout without using hatchery supplementation, especially in the Madison. M. cerebralis was isolated in young fish after a 90% reduction of rainbow trout was noted over a 3-year period (1992-1994). The term "whirling" comes from the characteristic whirling behavior the young fish exhibit before dying. Necrosis of cartilage, especially that of the brain case and spine, leads to inflammation and pinched nerves, which causes the small trout to whirl uncontrollably.

M. cerebralis has an interesting life cycle that was not completely understood until 1983. The spores of the parasite are shed from diseased or dead fish (**Figure 11.1a**). The spores can lay dormant in the bottom sediment for up to 30 years until they are ingested by a small tubeworm, Tubifex tubifex, which resides in the mud (**Figure 11.1b**). The spores mature in the gut of the worm into another form of the protozoan, the Triactinomyxon (TAM) stage (**Figure 11.1c**). The TAM have a spore head and three hook appendages. When TAM are excreted by the worm, they invade the fish through their skin, gills, or digestive tract (**Figure 11.1d**). TAM live for only 3 to 4 days if they cannot find a host. Each TAM contains 30 to 60 sporozoites, which are released inside the fish and migrate to areas rich in cartilage. There they multiply, produce spores, and deform or kill the fish. (**Figure 11.1e**). The disease process takes 50 to 150 days before the fish die or are eaten by predators. Young trout (less than 6 months old) are most susceptible to the disease because they have immature cartilage. When exposed to high doses of TAM, adult fish can be infected but are asymptomatic and the severity of infection decreases with increasing age of the fish.

The discovery of WD has led to heated controversy. The controversy stems from the belief held by many scientists that the parasite was introduced into the river by transplanted infected fish. How this happened is unknown. What can be done to stop WD outbreaks is being investigated. Stricter laws concerning transport of live trout across state lines are being proposed. A national and international search for rainbow populations which are naturally resistant to the parasite is in progress. Such an approach was useful for salmon infected with the parasite Ceratomyxa shasta. Experimental studies of brown trout, which are resistant to WD, may shed some light on how rainbow trout can be bred for resistance. A vaccine is also being researched which would confer immunity upon healthy rainbow trout. Finally, because little is known about the tubeworms, attention is being focused on this intermediate host of the parasite's life cycle. Perhaps breaking the parasitic cycle without major ecological consequences to the river is another possibility. Nevertheless, whatever the steps taken to stop WD, this small protozoan is another example of a microorganism that not only changes a trout's ecosystem, but also causes economic hardship on an area dependent upon fishing and tourism.

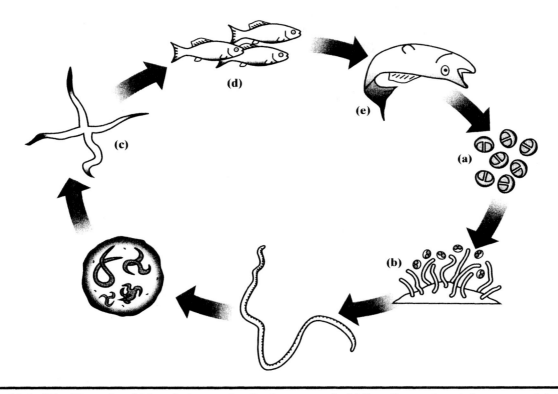

Figure 11.1 The life cycle of *Myxobolus cerebralis,* the cause of whirling disease in rainbow trout: (a) spores, (b) spores ingested by tubificid worm, (c) spores mature in gut to TAM, (d) fish infected with TAM, and (e) fish with whirling disease.

BACKGROUND INFORMATION

Many protozoa are **symbiotic** and spend a portion or all of their lives associated with another species. The protozoan *Myxobolus* described above is a **parasite** and harms the host it lives in. Other examples of parasites that cause disease in humans include *Giardia, Toxoplasma, Cryptospordium,* and *Plasmodium,* a malarial parasite. Many protozoa live as **commensals** and benefit from living with another organism but do not harm it. A third type of symbiosis exhibited by protozoa is **mutualism,** which is a relationship where both organisms benefit from living with each other. Protozoa live in freshwater, marine, soil and aerial habitats, on the surfaces of trees. They are also important members of the community of microorganisms in wastewater treatment facilities.

Protozoa are unicellular, eucaryotic organisms. They have several defining characteristics that differentiate them from other eucaryotic organisms: they lack chlorophyll, have no cell walls, and are usually motile. In fact, motility has traditionally been used to distinguish the various subgroups of protozoa (e.g., ciliates, flagellates, and amoeba). However, recent comparisons at the genetic level (such as 18s rRNA sequences) indicate there are several more distinct lines of decent of protozoa than was previously known (**Figure 11.2**).

A good example of "friendly" symbiotic protozoa are those that live in ruminant animals, such as cows, sheep, goats, and deer. Mammals and most animals lack enzymes necessary to digest cellulose. Therefore, ruminant animals that subsist on grasses and leafy plants use microorganisms to metabolize the insoluble polysaccharides. The microbes in the rumen of these animals are anaerobes and include bacteria, fungi, and protozoa. The rumen protozoa, which are ciliates for the most part, play an important role in the digestion of cellulose to disaccharides and glucose. They are also a source of nitrogen for the host, more than bacteria. For this reason, ruminants are not as dependent on outside protein sources as non-ruminant animals. Ciliated protozoa move by means of numerous hair-like appendages called cilia. The best known ciliate is from the genus *Paramecium* (**Figure 11.3**). Paramecia ingest food through a distinct oral region or mouth. The

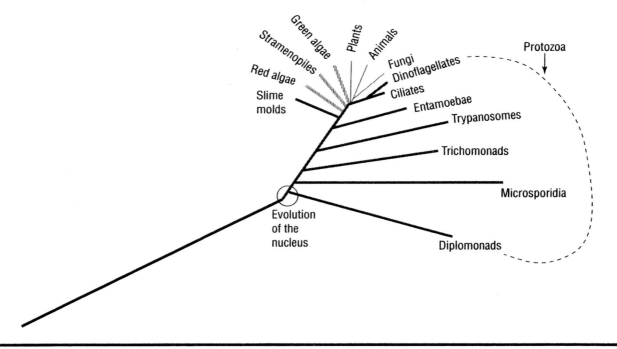

Figure 11.2 The phylogenetic tree of the Eucarya as determined by 18s rRNA sequencing, showing many branches which contain protozoa. Compare this tree to the universal rooted tree in Exercise 16. (Courtesy of David Ward.)

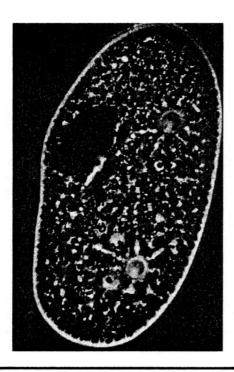

Figure 11.3 A scanning electron micrograph of *Paramecium.*

food moves through a gullet and into the cytoplasm where food vacuoles containing enzymes help digest the particles.

Another example of symbiosis is the mutualistic relationship of flagellated protozoa and termites. These flagellates live in the gut of the termite and amazingly subsist entirely on the wood particles ingested by the termite. The flagellates digest and metabolize cellulose in the wood particles to acetate and other products that the termite utilizes. Because the termite does not produce cellulases—enzymes that hydrolyze cellulose, it depends on the flagellates for its existence.

In this exercise you will observe protozoa from a number of different sources. In Part A you will observe them as they ingest and perhaps digest yeast cells. The yeast are dyed with Congo red, an indicator dye which is red at pH 7, orange at pH 5, and blue at pH 3. Adding a light suspension of the yeast to a sample will allow you to observe how protozoa move about and ingest other organisms. If you observe the protozoa long enough (for at least 20 minutes), you may see some of the ingested yeast start to be digested and turn a different color. If your sample is from a natural source, like pond water, hay infusion or rumen fluid, observe the many other microorganisms and particulate matter that the protozoa may be feeding on. In Part B you will examine the hindgut contents of termite's. The hindgut is a swollen segment of the single, long chord that can be pulled out of the termites body. The swollen sac can be pierced with a dissecting needle and the fluid spread over a slide for observation. In Part C you will observe prepared slides of protozoa, if available.

PURPOSE

• To observe the characteristics of some protozoa, including motility and ingestion of particulate matter

THE EXERCISE

MATERIALS:

Protozoa from hay infusion, pond water, or rumen fluid
Culture of *Paramecium* or other ciliates
Tweezers
Microscope slides
Toothpicks
Prepared slides of different protozoa
Termites
Suspension of bakers' yeast dyed with Congo red water
Dissecting needles
Coverslips
Disposable pipets
Saline solution

PROCEDURE:

Part A

1. With a pipet, place a drop of the sample (pond water, hay infusion, rumen fluid or culture of paramecia) on a glass slide.
2. With another pipet, transfer a small drop of red yeast to the suspension and mix with a toothpick.
3. Place a coverslip on the mixture. **Note:** The volume of the mixture should be just enough to fill the entire coverslip and no more.
4. Begin microscopic examination of the wet mount at low power and then proceed to high dry magnification. The protozoa are 10 to 20 times larger than bacteria and should be easily observed feeding on the yeast at these magnifications.
5. Optional: Prepare a hanging drop slide (see Exercise 2) and observe the slide periodically as the protozoa are feeding. You may be able to see some digestion of the yeast cells.

6. Describe your observations in the RESULTS section by drawing as many different protozoa feeding on yeast as possible.

Part B

1. Obtain a termite and place it on a microscope slide.
2. Use two tweezers to grasp both ends of the termite and pull. The termite's head should separate from the rest of the body. Attached to the head will be the digestive tract, a single long chord. About halfway along its length should be a swollen segment. This is the hindgut.
3. Pierce the hindgut with a dissecting needle and smear the fluid on a slide.
4. Add one drop of saline solution to the fluid and mix with a toothpick. **Note:** Adding saline preserves the anaerobic parasites for a longer period of time.
5. Immediately place a coverslip on the fluid and observe, first on low power magnification and then on high dry.
6. Observe their motility and describe as many different gut protozoa as possible in the RESULTS section. **Note:** You may also be able to observe spirochete bacteria, common in termites.

Part C

1. Observe prepared slides of protozoa. You should be able to observe organelles using these slides but, of course, not their motility.

REFERENCES

Markiw, M. and Wolf, K. *Myxosoma cerebralis* (Myxozoa:Myxosporea) Etiologic Agent of Salmonid Whirling Disease Requires Tubificid Worm (Annelida:Oligochaeta) in Its Life Cycle. *Journal of Protozology* 30 (1983):561-564.

Markiw, M. Experimentally Induced Whirling Disease I. Dose Response of Fry and Adults of Rainbow Trout Exposed to the Triactinomyson Stage of *Myxobolus cerebralis. Journal of Aquatic Health* 4(1992):40-43.

Knapp, S., et al. *Bibliography of Whirling Disease in Salmonid Fishes.* Bozeman, MT: Montana State University Montana Department of Fish, Wildlife and Parks, 1995.

Ogimoto, K. and Imai, S. *Atlas of Rumen Microbiology.* Tokyo: Japan Scientific Societies Press, 1981.

RESULTS

Draw your observations of ciliates feeding on yeast cells and the flagellates from the termite hindgut. If possible, note any organelles you see in the protozoa. Try to differentiate between the types of protozoa you observe.

Part A: Sample from natural source

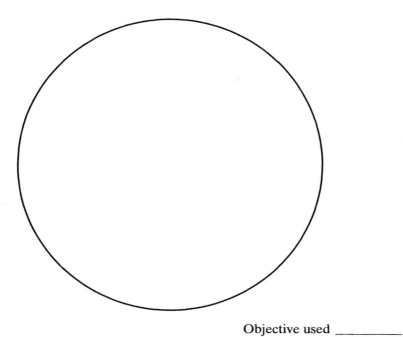

Objective used _____

Part B: Termite hindgut

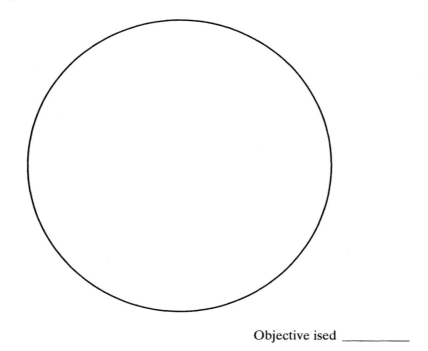

Objective ised _____

REFECTIONS

1. If you observed the protozoa feeding for 20 minutes or longer, did you detect digestion of yeast?

2. How do ciliates ingest their food?

3. If you observed other protozoa besides ciliates, how do the nonciliates move?

4. In the cytoplasm and nucleus of many protozoa are bacteria that live symbiotically. Speculate on the role these endosymbiont bacteria may play. Why are they there?

EXERCISE 12

ALGAE

In the previous exercise, you examined animal-like eucaryotic microbes—the protozoa. In this exercise we turn our attention to photosynthetic, plant-like microbes—the algae. Algae can be either unicellular or multicellular. The unicellular, microalgae are of most interest to microbiologists. However, their importance as phytoplankton in bodies of water brings them to the attention of biologists as well.

This was heaven to Sarah—a cottage on a secluded ocean beach, and two weeks of nothing to do except relax. Sarah sighed with pleasure as she drank her morning coffee and looked out at the sea. Her mind wandered from one thought to another until she was drawn from her ruminations by a large shape floating quite a distance from shore. She could not determine what the object was and continued to watch it as it came closer and closer. Finally, Sarah left the cottage and walked out to the beach to get a better look. It was a whale—a dead whale. Sarah ran to the cottage and called local authorities. This marked the end of her tranquil vacation. Over the next two weeks, seven more dead whales washed ashore. Her secluded beach was overrun with local authorities, scientists, and others trying to figure out what was killing these beautiful animals. The verdict: death due to ingestion of a neurotoxin produced by the alga Alexandrium tamarense *(**Figure 12.1**).*

BACKGROUND INFORMATION

Although stories of toxic algal blooms make great headlines, the beneficial attributes of algae far outweigh the bad. Algae are oxygenic, photosynthetic, eucaryotic microbes that are found in almost any environment where water and light are in good supply. Light is absorbed by chlorophyll and other pigments in the chloroplasts of algae and used as an energy source for driving carbon dioxide fixation. The end products of photosynthesis, organic molecules such as glucose and sucrose, are chemical sources of energy that fuel the activities of **chemotrophs** in the ecosystem. By converting light energy into chemical energy, algae serve the same function in aquatic environments that plants do in terrestrial environments. That is, they are the **primary producers** and form the base of the food chain. Algae also provide food for humans, especially in oriental countries. Edible alge are called nori in Japan, dulse in Canada and the United States, and sloke in Ireland. Furthermore, compounds derived from algae are used in the food industry as stabilizers and thickeners. A classic example is carrageenan, which is used in ice cream and other products. An entirely different use is made of the remains of **diatoms,** which are algae

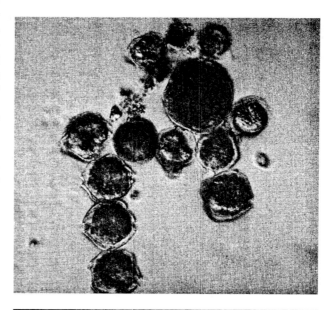

Figure 12.1 The alga of *Alexandrium tamarense.* (Courtesy of D.M. Anderson.)

having cell walls made of silica. When these organisms die, they fall to the sediments underlying a body of water. Because their cell walls are recalcitrant to decay, they remain essentially intact for centuries. At certain sites, the sediments formed from dead diatoms are so extensive that they can be mined as diatomaceous earth. Diatomaceous earth is used in toothpaste, swimming pool filters, and a variety of polishing agents. There is another algal product of utmost importance to microbiologists. That product is agar, an agent routinely used to solidify media.

Algae are a diverse group of organisms that vary greatly in size, shape, and other features. Some are unicellular, some colonial and others multicellular (**Figure 12.2**). Many of the multicellular forms are large and have complicated bodies that closely resemble true plants. However, these multicellular forms lack the vascular systems (phloem and xylem) that are characteristic of plants. Many algae are motile, at least during some stage of their life cycle. Although cellulose is the most common cell wall material observed in algae,

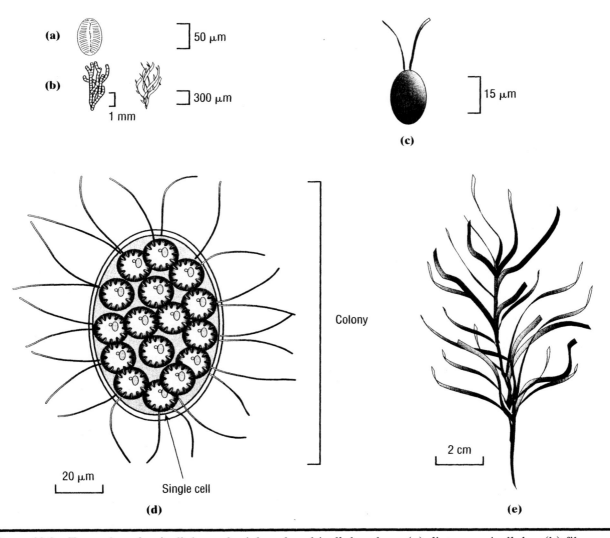

Figure 12.2 Examples of unicellular, colonial, and multicellular algae: (a) diatom, unicellular, (b) filamentous green algae, multicellular, (c) *Chloromonas* sp., green algae, unicellular, (d) *Pandorina unicocca*, green algae, colonial, and (e) *Dumontia incrassata*, red algae, multicellular.

some algal cell walls are composed of silica and other molecules.

The diversity of form exhibited by algae reflects their phylogenetic diversity. Although much more research is needed, current data indicate that there are three major lines of descent for algae: the green algae, the red algae, and a conglomerate of algae that includes the diatoms, golden-brown algae, and brown algae (**Figure 12.3**). There have also been some surprises from these studies on the phylogeny of algae. The dinoflagellates, long considered to be algae (and the reason Sarah's bucolic vacation was disrupted), appear to be more closely related to ciliated protozoa than to any of the algae.

In this exercise you will isolate microalgae, especially diatoms. These microbes readily attach to surfaces and move across them with a gliding motion. Because diatoms are **phototrophs**, which use light as a source of energy, they migrate upwards when illuminated from above. You will take advantage of this characteristic by placing coverslips on top of sediments from an aquatic environment and illuminating the sediments from above. The diatoms will move through the sediments and attach themselves to the underside of the coverslip. In this exercise, you will also isolate microalgae in pure culture using the same streak plate method employed in Exercise 3.

PURPOSE

- To observe microalgae
- To cultivate microalgae

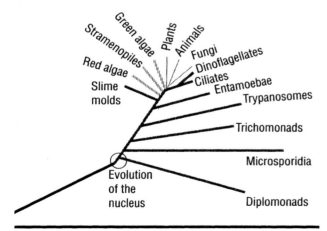

Figure 12.3 The placement of algae on the universal phylogenetic tree. (Courtesy of David Ward.)

THE EXERCISE

Part A: Isolation of Microalgae from Aquatic Ecosystems

MATERIALS:

Water
Sediments
Microbial mat material from either a freshwater or marine ecosystem, including fish tanks
Petri dishes
Coverslips
Forceps
Illuminated growth chamber
Microscope slides
Microscopes

PROCEDURE:

Day 1

1. Place a layer of sediments from an aquatic ecosystem in the bottom of a Petri dish. Add water (from the same source) just to cover.
2. Using forceps, place a coverslip on the sediments.
3. Incubate at room temperature (RT) in a growth chamber with illumination from above. The Petri dishes should be placed about 12 inches from the light source.
4. Incubate for 2 to 10 days. Check the Petri dishes regularly and add water (from the original source) as needed to keep the sediments moist.

Day 2

1. Using forceps, remove the coverslip from the Petri dish and place it, sediment-side down, on a microscope slide.
2. Use low power to scan the specimen and determine the diversity of microbes attached to the coverslip. In addition to algae, you may also observe a variety of protozoa, especially those that adhere to surfaces. Examine individual microbes of interest under high power.
3. Record your observations in the RESULTS section.

Part B: Isolation of Microalgae in Pure Culture

MATERIALS:

Coverslip from Day 2 of Part A
Plastic tube containing 1 ml of either freshwater algal broth or marine algal broth
Freshwater algal plates or marine algal plates
Bunsen burner
Illuminated growth chamber
Inoculating loop

Dissecting microscope
Inoculating needle
Vortex mixer
Microscope slides
Coverslips

PROCEDURE:

Day 1

1. Hold one coverslip from Part A: Day 2 with two forceps and bend the coverslip until it breaks.
2. Place the pieces of the coverslip in the tube of algal broth.
3. Vortex the coverslip in the algal broth for about 10 seconds to detach the cells from the coverslip and create a suspension of cells.
4. Using the streak plate method described in Exercise 3, streak a loopful of inoculum from the suspension on the freshwater or marine algal plates.
5. Place the plates in a clear plastic box and incubate them 4 to 10 days under illumination as you did in Part A. **Note:** By incubating the plates in a plastic box, less moisture is lost from the medium during the long incubation period.

Day 2

1. Examine the plates for growth.
2. Observe the colonies under a dissecting microscope at about 20× magnification.
3. Using an inoculating needle, prepare a wet mount from a colony you believe to be an algal colony. **Note:** The fucoxanthin and β-carotene pigments of diatoms mask the chlorophyll. Therefore, diatom colonies have a golden-brown to dark brown appearance (**Figure 12.4**). In green algal cells, chlorophyll predominates and the colonies appear green. White or translucent colonies are probably bacterial colonies.

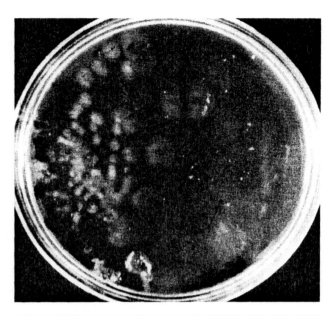

Figure 12.4   Two diatom colonies, indicated by arrows.

3. Examine the wet mount first under low power and then with the high-power objective lens.
4. Record your observations in the RESULTS section.

REFERENCES

Anderson, D.M. "Red Tides." *Scientific American* 271(1994):62-67.

Bold, H.C. and Wynne, M.J. *Introduction to the Algae.* Englewood Cliffs, NJ: Prentice-Hall, 1985.

Fogg, G.E. *Algal Cultures and Phytoplankton Ecology.* Madison, Wisc.: University of Wisconsin Press, 1975.

Stein, J.R. *Handbook of Phycological Methods. Culture Methods and Growth Measurements.* Cambridge: Cambridge University Press, 1973.

RESULTS

Record your observations of:

Algae and other organisms (Part A)

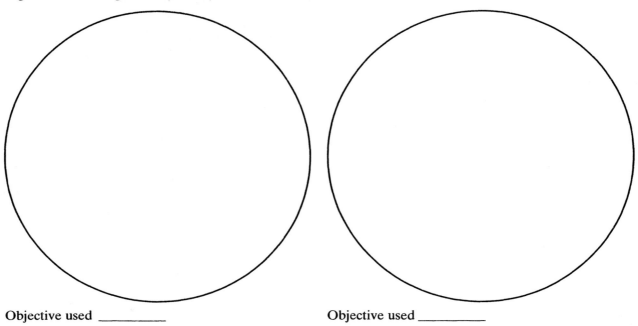

Objective used _____   Objective used _____

Algae isolated in pure culture (Part B)

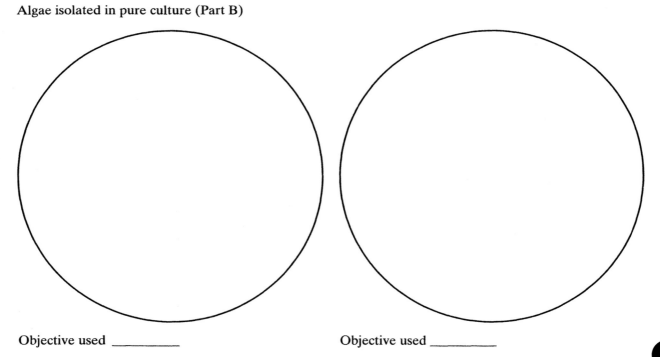

Objective used _____   Objective used _____

REFLECTIONS

1. In Part A, you were instructed to incubate the Petri dishes with illumination from above. Why was this stipulated?

2. On the coverslips from Part A, you probably observed protozoa as well as algae. What characteristics did you use to decide if you were observing protozoa or algae?

3. Some phycologists (scientists who study algae) include cyanobacteria in their field of study. What are cyanobacteria, and why are they often grouped with algae? Why is it incorrect to do so? (Hint: See **Figure 16.3** in Exercise 16.)

EXERCISE 13

A FUNGUS AMONG US

The last of the eucaryotic microbes you will examine are the fungi. In Exercise 6 you used the transparent tape technique and LPCB to look at hyphal characteristics of these organisms. Now you will examine more closely several representative fungi using other techniques. This closer look should give you a better appreciation of these unique and interesting microorganisms.

Joe rushed into the locker room and panted out of breath, "I forgot my tennis shoes!" It was just an hour before the basketball game and he was the star guard for his high school team. His friend John said, "Here, wear these! I have an extra pair." Joe played most of the game wearing his friend's shoes and thanked him later because he scored fifteen points in a winning cause. It must have been the shoes.

About a week later, Joe's feet began to bother him. They itched and were inflamed, especially in the web between the fourth and fifth toes. He tolerated the itching for another week until he noticed the itching and inflammation had spread to other toes. The skin on his toes started to scale and continued to be red and itchy, but Joe continued to play basketball and shower in the locker room. About 3 weeks later, his feet became unbearable and he showed them to his mother. She gasped and immediately made an appointment with their doctor. Their physician diagnosed Joe as probably having "athlete's foot" or tinea pedis. The doctor recommended a topical cream to treat the fungal disease and recommended Joe call him back if the treatment didn't work. The fungus that usually causes this condition is called Trichophyton mentagrophytes. Joe and his doctor discussed how he may have acquired the fungus. The most obvious means of transmission was the borrowed tennis shoes, but Joe also may have contracted the fungus from scales of skin shed by other athletes in the shower or on the locker room floor.

Joe diligently applied the recommended topical anti-fungal agent, miconazole, for 2 to 3 weeks and recovered from the fungal infection. He also found out that his friend John had athlete's foot as well and was using a similar cream. Both talked to their coach who warned the rest of the team about the disease. Whether Joe got the dermatophyte (fungus of the skin) from the borrowed shoes or from the locker room floor is not known, but you can be sure he won't borrow someone's shoes again.

BACKGROUND INFORMATION

The fungi are eucaryotic organisms which are non-motile, have cell walls, have no chlorophyll (so are not photosynthetic), and reproduce by means of spores. The spores are produced either sexually or asexually and germinate on or in appropriate substrates. Fungi grow primarily as filamentous structures (**moulds**), as unicellular budding forms (**yeast**), or as a combination of both yeast forms and moulds (**dimorphic fungi**). **Mushrooms** are filamentous fungi that form large fruiting bodies, which are the edible part of the mushroom. Most fungi are saprophytes, that is, they live on decaying organic matter and play a crucial role in the degradation of organic carbon. Without these microorganisms, we would literally drown in our own wastes. A few fungi, however, can cause significant plant and animal diseases. Of the more than 250,000 fungal species, only about 150 are known to cause human infections. These infections seem to be an accident for the fungus and are a dead end for them, because most fungal infections, with a few exceptions, are not transmitted from human to human.

Fungi are highly diverse and exhibit a variety of shapes, sizes, pigments, and other characteristics. This variety, both macroscopically and microscopically, helps to differentiate one fungus from another. Historically, fungi have been classified and named based on reproductive characteristics—asexual or sexual. In many cases, the sexual form of the fungus was not known until after the asexual form was named and well documented. This resulted in two names for the same organism—one for its sexual form and one for its asexual form. The development of DNA technologies has allowed us to determine evolutionary relationships based on genetic comparisons. (For more information on this, see Exercise 16.) **Table 13.1** is a brief classification scheme used by some mycologists. The strength of this scheme resides in the fact that the subdivisions have been determined by 18S rRNA gene sequences and the two division names are more informative. As molecular analyses continue, this scheme will change and mycologists may finally be able to combine sexual and asexual fungi into one classification scheme, making the study of fungi less confusing.

You will study and identify structural characteristics of four different fungi, including the dermatophyte that most often causes athletes foot, *T. mentagrophytes.* The purpose of this exercise is not to make you experts at identifying fungi, but to give you some appreciation of the diverse structures these microorganisms exhibit. A description, drawing, and picture of each of the four fungi follows **Table 13.1.**

Fungi like natural substrates and are easily grown on media such as potato dextrose agar. With the exception of some yeast, they do not grow as fast as bacteria (2 to 14 or more days). They produce a variety of colonial types, from fuzzy, cottony, and wrinkled (moulds), to mucoid and round (yeast). You will learn several new techniques to study these microorganisms. They include a tease preparation, which is a rapid procedure, and a slide culture, which is slower but provides better preservation of structures. Each is described in the exercise. With practice, these procedures will allow you to study the microscopic and sporulating characteristics of the fungi. The yeast *Candida albicans* will be easy to observe by making a wet prep. You will also grow this yeast in the presence of animal serum, which stimulates germ tube hyphal and pseudohyphal formation (**Figure 13.4**).

TABLE 13.1 Classification and Characteristics of Some Fungi[a]

Taxonomic Group	Characteristics	Examples
Division: *Coenomycota*	Hyphae with no septa	
Subdivision: *Chytridiomycotina*	Mostly aquatic, sometimes form hyphae, flagellated	*Blastocladiales*—water moulds
Subdivision: *Zygomycotina*	Sexual reproduction with zygospores; asexual reproduction with sporangia	*Rhizopus* *Mucor* *Absidia*
Division: *Dikaryomycota*	Hyphae have septa which separates binucleated segments	
Subdivision: *Ascomycotina*	Sexual reproduction within asci (ascospores formed); ~75% of all described fungi	*Sordaria* *Ajellomyces* (sexual form of *Histoplasma* and *Blastomyces*) *Saccharomyces*
Subdivision: *Basidiomycotina*	Sexual reproduction within basidium (basidiospores formed)	*Amanita* and *Agaricus* (mushrooms) *Filobasidiella* (sexual form of *Cryptococcus*), *Ustilago*
Form-Subdivision:[b] *Deuteromycotina*	Asexual reproduction within conidiophores (conidiospores), yeast (budding) or fruiting bodies; structures pigmented and unpigmented	*Aspergillus* *Penicillium* *Candida* *Trichophyton* *Alternaria* *Fusarium*

[a]Mitchell, T.G., Cutler, J.E., Deepe, G.S., and Hazen, K.C. Principles of Medical Mycology. Washington, D.C.: American Society for Microbiology, forthcoming.

[b]This subdivision not a true taxon.

Rhizopus

This fungus grows to mature within 4 days producing a dense cottony type of growth. At first the colony is white and then turns grey or yellow-brown. When the reverse side is examined, the mycelial mat is white. During microscopic examination, *Rhizopus* has aseptate hyphae with numerous sporangiophores which are connected by stolons, analogous to a strawberry plant. At the base of the sporangiophores are root-like hyphae called rhizoids. The sporangiophores are long and brown, and each terminates in a dark round sporangium where asexual reproduction occurs. The sporangium contains a columella and many oval spores, called sporangiospores. Occasionally sexual reproduction occurs when hyphae of different mating types (+ and − strains) make contact and form a thick-walled zygosporangium (zygospore) and a diploid zygote (**Figure 13.1**). *Rhizopus* is a common contaminate in the laboratory and home, but may cause serious disease (sinusitis, pneumonia, wound infections, and brain lesions) in patients with underlying conditions such as severe diabetes, malignant blood disorders such as leukemia, and in intravenous drug users. As with other fungi, they are among the many emerging opportunistic pathogens attacking immunocompromised patients.

Alternaria

This fungus is an example of a melanin-producing, dark-pigmented, or dematiaceous fungus. It matures within 5 days and its surface is woolly with a greenish black or brown color and grey aerial hyphae. The reverse is black, a distinctive characteristic of dematiaceous fungi. When examined microscopically, *Alternaria* have hyphae that are septate and dark (**Figure 13.2**). The conidiophores are also septate and sometimes have a zigzag appearance. They produce distinctively different conidia which are large, brown, and have longitudinal and transverse septations. The conidia can be found alone or in chains and are club shaped. *Alternaria* are normally part of our environment and are commonly considered contaminants. On occasion, however, they have been implicated in diseases called phaeohyphomycoses. This term is applied to disease caused by dematiaceous fungi that produce cutaneous (skin), subcutaneous (beneath the skin), or systemic (throughout the body) infection in humans.

Trichophyton mentagrophytes

Trichophyton and the other dermatophytes are usually slower growing fungi. They sometimes require 2 to 3 weeks to grow. *T. mentagrophytes* is a moderate grower and matures within 7 to 10 days. The colony morphology of this fungus varies greatly. It can be pink or yellow, and have tan and powdery or white and downy surfaces. The powdery forms can be wrinkled. The reverse is usually tan but may be colorless, yellow, or red. This fungus can rapidly become sterile (no conidiation) and produce a cottony appearance if grown too long. Under

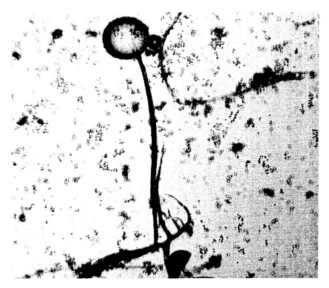

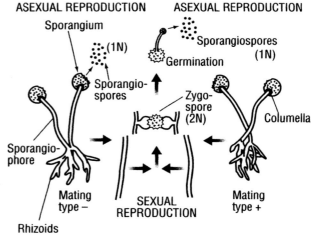

Figure 13.1 *Rhizopus oryzae.*

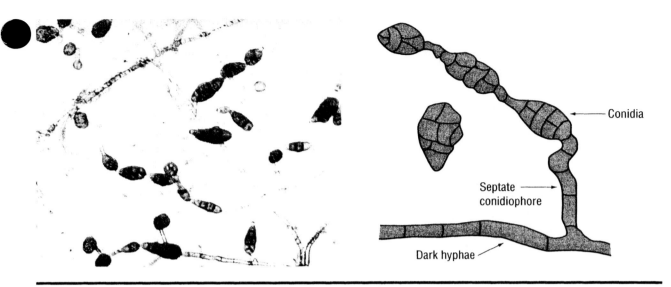

Figure 13.2   *Alternaria* sp.

microscopic examination, *T. mentagrophytes* has hyphae that are septate and nonpigmented (**Figure 13.3**). The hyphae tend to coil more than other dermatophytes. Sometimes it will produce cigar-shaped, thin-walled macroconidia that attach directly to the hyphae. These macroconidia contain one to six cells and are found in young cultures 5 to 10 days old. They also produce microconidia that are small and round and may cluster on branched conidiophores. *T. mentagrophytes* will live on any part of the outermost layer of skin, including hair and nails. It is one of several dermatophytes that digest and obtain nutrients from keratin in skin and do not usually invade living tissue. It is unusual because it can be transmitted from human to human and depends on human or animal infection for survival. As Joe found out, it is one of the most common causes of athlete's foot. The dermatophytes as a group are the most common infectious agents of humans. The diseases are called tinea or ringworm. Fortunately, ringworm is treatable and not life threatening.

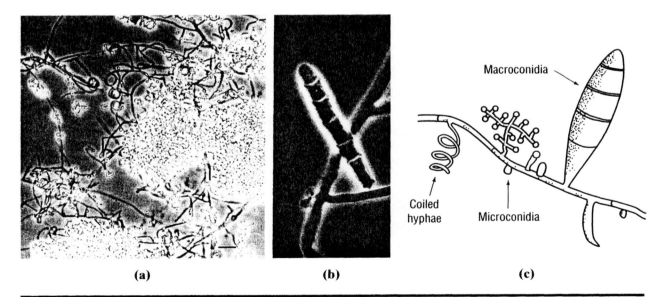

(a)   (b)   (c)

Figure 13.3   *Trichophyton mentagrophytes* (a and b courtesy of St-Germain, G. and Summerbell, R. *Identifying Filamentous Fungi: A Clinical Laboratory Handbook,* Belmont, CA: Star Publishing Co., 1996. With permission.).

Candida albicans

C. *albicans* is a rapidly growing yeast and produces cream-colored, smooth colonies in 2 to 3
days. It reproduces by budding and forms true
hyphae and pseudohyphae when the buds, called
blastoconidia, elongate and remain attached to the
parent cell forming chains of cells (**Figure 13.4**).
Under certain laboratory conditions it produces
true hyphae as well. When incubated in serum, it
produces germ tubes that become true hyphae. *C.*
albicans is one of the few fungi found as normal
microbiota of the mucous membranes (e.g., the gastrointestinal tract and vagina). Therefore, it is difficult to determine its significance when isolated in
the clinical laboratory. *C. albicans* can cause a localized infection or disseminated disease and is considered an opportunistic pathogen in patients with
impaired immune systems. These patients include
AIDS patients, people on prolonged treatment
with antibiotics and other cytotoxic drugs, people
with underlying diseases such as diabetes, intravenous drug users, and people with catheters. Candidiasis (infection with any *Candida* sp.*)* is
increasing in this country and is now the fourth-
leading cause of nosocomial or hospital-acquired
blood infections. *C. albicans* is the cause of approximately 60% of all cases of candidiasis.

PURPOSE

- To examine a variety of characteristics of fungi,
  including their hyphae and spores
- To learn techniques used for growth and microscopic examination of fungi
- To learn how several common fungi are classified
  and identified

**CAUTION: Certain precautions should be taken when
working with fungi. Care should be taken not to expose
people at risk to inhalation of spores of moulds, particularly those people having impaired immune systems
or allergies. Keep the lids of all cultures closed and dis-
pose of the slides and plates properly.**

THE EXERCISE

MATERIALS:

Cultures of *Rhizopus oryzae, Alternaria* sp., *T. menta-
    grophytes,* and *C. albicans* growing on PDA plates
LPCB
Slide culture chamber (sterile Petri dish with bent
    glass rod, filter paper, slide, and coverslip)
PDA plates
0.5 to 1.0 ml of sterile rabbit plasma or bovine serum
Inoculating needle or sterile wooden applicator sticks
Dissecting microscope

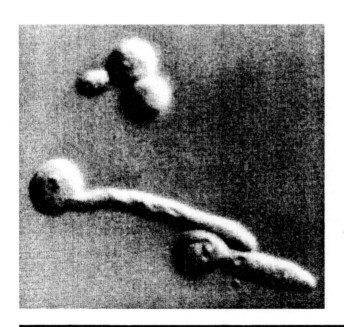

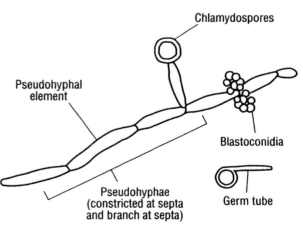

Figure 13.4 *Candida albicans.*

Microscope slides
Coverslips
Two dissecting needles (one with bent tip)
Metal spatula or scalpel
Forceps
Pasteur pipets

PROCEDURE: Work in groups of two or three

Part A: Examination of Mould Cultures Using the Tease Prep Method

1. Observe the colony morphology of each mould, including the color of the upper surface and the reverse of the plate. Record this information in the RESULTS section.
2. If available, observe the moulds on the plates with a dissecting microscope.
3. Prepare a **tease prep** of each of the three moulds following the procedure below:
   a. Place a drop of LPCB on a clean glass slide.
   b. With a sterile bent dissecting needle, gently remove 1 to 2 mm of the colony where sporulation is taking place. It is often the area that is pigmented and located about 1 cm inside the edge of the colony.
   c. Gently transfer the colony fragment to the drop of LPCB.
   d. Using both sterile dissecting needles, *gently* separate the hyphae. The fungal spores are extremely fragile, but too little teasing will not separate the filaments enough to observe characteristic structures such as conidia.
   e. After you have teased the hyphae apart, add a coverslip to the prep, and sterilize the dissecting needles by inserting them in a flame.
4. Examine your preps under low power and then high power to see the structures in detail. Mould structures are usually large enough to view without the use of oil immersion. **Note:** Making tease preps requires patience and practice, so make another prep if your first is unsuccessful. Unfortunately, this method does not always preserve the original position and structures of the hyphae and conidia, but it is a very rapid method. If your instructor agrees, you may also make preps using the transparent tape method described in Exercise 6.
5. Draw your observations in the RESULTS section.

Part B: Examination of Moulds Using the Slide Culture Method

1. Select one of the mould cultures to prepare a **slide culture.**

2. Obtain a sterile slide culture chamber that has a sterile glass slide, coverslip, bent rod, and filter paper (**Figure 13.5**).
3. Moisten the filter paper with 3 to 4 ml of sterile water.
4. Obtain an uninoculated plate of PDA and cut a 1 × 1 cm block with a flame sterilized spatula or scalpel. Transfer the block to the center of the glass slide.
5. With a sterile dissecting needle or applicator stick, inoculate the fungus on the four sides of the agar block (**Figure 13.5**).
6. Using flame sterilized forceps, place the coverslip over the inoculated agar block. Apply slight pressure to ensure adherence.
7. Replace the lid of the Petri dish and incubate at room temperature or 28°C for 3 to 10 days.
8. Examine the slide culture periodically for growth and add water if the filter paper begins to dry.
9. After sufficient growth is noted (the mould will grow on the surface of the slide and on the undersurface of the coverslip), carefully remove the coverslip with forceps and place it on another slide that has a drop of LPCB.
10. With an applicator stick or needle, gently lift the block of agar off the original slide and discard the agar in a container of antifungal disinfectant. Add a drop of LPCB to the slide and place a new coverslip on it.
11. Examine the preps under low- and high-power magnification. These preps, if done properly, should give you a better look at undisturbed structures. **Note:** Both slide preps can be sealed around the edges with nail polish or mounting fluid if you desire to keep the preparations for further study.
12. Record your observations in the RESULTS section.

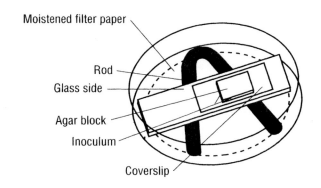

Moistened filter paper

Rod

Glass side

Agar block

Inoculum

Coverslip

Figure 13.5   A slide culture chamber and inoculum.

Part C: Examination of the Yeast C. albicans

1. Examine the plate with *C. albicans* and record the colony morphology in the RESULTS section.
2. Prepare a **wet mount** of *C. albicans* by suspending a portion of a colony of the yeast in a drop of water on a slide. Place a coverslip on the suspension and examine the slide for budding yeast.
3. Conduct a **germ tube test** by making a *very light* suspension (one colony) of the yeast in the sterile serum. Too many cells ($>10^6$ per ml) will cause a significant decrease in the percentage of cells forming germ tubes.
4. Incubate the tube at 35°C for 2 hours.
5. With a pipet, place a drop of the suspension on a slide and overlay with a coverslip.
6. Immediately examine under high dry power for the presence of germ tubes (**Figure 13.4**). **Note:** With very few exceptions, no other yeast will form germ tubes under these conditions. They appear as tubes or filaments that are not constricted at their point of origin on the parent cell.
7. Record your microscopic observations of *C. albicans* in the RESULTS section.

REFERENCES

Kwong-Chun, K.J. and Bennett, J.E. *Medical Mycology*. Philadelphia: Lea & Febiger, 1992.

Larone, D.H. *Medically Important Fungi, A Guide to Identification*, 3rd ed. Washington, DC: American Society for Microbiology Press, 1995.

Mitchel, T.G., et al. *Principles of Medical Mycology*. Washington, DC: American Society for Microbiology Press, forthcoming.

St-Germain, G., and Summerbell, R. *Identifying Filamentous Fungi, A Clinical Laboratory Handbook*. Belmont, CA: Star Publishing Co., 1996.

RESULTS

Record your observations below.

Rhizopus oryzae
Colony morphology:

Alternaria
Colony morphology:

Microscopic observations:

Microscopic observations:

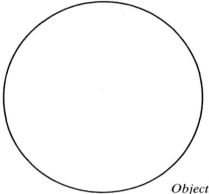

Objective used _____

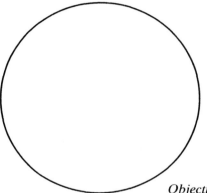

Objective used _____

T. mentagrophytes
Colony morphology:

C. albicans
Colony morphology:

Microscopic observations:

Microscopic observations:

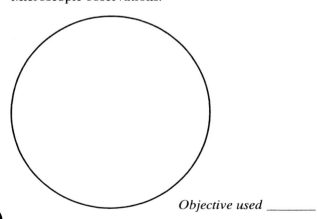

Objective used _____

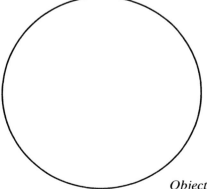

Objective used _____

REFLECTIONS

1. Fungi secrete many chemicals that are beneficial to humans. Name two of these chemicals and the fungi that produce them.

2. What is meant by an opportunistic pathogen?

3. Aflatoxins are a problem in the food industry and agriculture. Name a fungus that produces them. Why are aflatoxins such a concern?

4. Why are vaginal yeast infections common in some women after they have been treated with antibiotics?

IDENTIFYING STRUCTURAL FEATURES OF BACTERIA USING SPECIAL STAINS

This is the first exercise in which procaryotes are studied exclusively. During this exercise the structural differences that differentiate and identify bacteria will be examined. This can be done using special stains other than the Gram stain. These stains, although sometimes not diagnostic, are useful tools in the initial identification and characterization of a microorganism.

Kathy had just started her first microbiology course when her instructor announced a special project to be completed by the end of the term. Each student was required to isolate a bacterium from the environment. The environment could be anything: a diseased plant, dirty water, soil, food, or the surface of a sink. Whatever the source, the task was to isolate and identify a bacterium—not a fungus—and write a report on it.

The only tools that Kathy had been exposed to so far were the microscope, some staining procedures, and media for growing bacteria. She decided to ask for a nutrient agar plate, a sterile swab, and sterile water. Her thought was to swab the surface of something and she wanted sterile materials to make sure that what grew came from that source. She also knew that many different bacteria will grow on nutrient agar and her chance of isolating at least one was good.

On the way home with her materials, Kathy tried to decide what to culture. Once home, she went to the

refrigerator to get something to eat and reached for a carrot in a vegetable container. She noticed one of the carrots looked like it was rotting, because it had dark mushy spots. Wouldn't it be interesting to find out what was causing the carrot to go soft? She carefully sliced off a piece of soft carrot and using the moistened sterile swab, swabbed its surface. Kathy then swept the swab across the nutrient plate and inverted it. She kept the plate in a warm place and the next day took it to the laboratory. Several colonies grew after 2 days. She chose one and streaked it for isolation on another nutrient agar plate.

During the next laboratory period, Kathy's instructor introduced several new staining procedures in addition to the Gram stain that they had already learned. Kathy decided to use some of these stains to characterize her bacterium. The stains would tell her if the bacterium had a capsule, endospores, inclusion bodies, and the composition of its cell wall (increased lipids or polysaccharides). The Gram stain was the first stain she did and it revealed Gram-negative rods. Unfortunately, as Kathy started to look up references about Gram-negative rods, she realized it could be one of many different species. She proceeded with the other stains but they were all negative, so were of little help. What would she do now? At least she knew it was a Gram-negative, non–endospore-forming rod. Maybe in future laboratories, her instructor would give additional methods for identifying organisms.[1]

-----

[1]Kathy's story will be continued in the next exercise.

BACKGROUND INFORMATION

Bacteria are procaryotes that can be characterized by the presence or absence of certain structural features. Some of these structures help them survive in unfriendly environments. A good example of this is the **capsule** produced by the bacterium *Streptococcus pneumoniae*, a Gram-positive diplococcus which causes pneumonia. The capsule is composed of a relatively unstructured network of polysaccharides that covers the surface of the bacterium. The capsule protects the bacterium from being opsonized by complement (see Exercise 39) and therefore, the bacterium is not engulfed, or **phagocytized**, as efficiently by the body's phagocytes. Another bacterium that produces a capsule is *Klebsiella pneumoniae,* a Gram-negative, rod-shaped microorganism.

During this exercise you will perform and examine a number of stains that help visualize several structural features of bacteria. You will begin by doing a capsule stain on *K. pneumoniae* and observing its capsule. Capsule formation by this bacterium is enhanced by growing it in milk. Milk also contains particles that allow the background of the smear to be stained and observed. The staining process consists of adding crystal violet to a prepared smear of *K. pneumoniae* grown in milk. The capsule stains a lighter blue than the background material or the cell. When copper sulfate is added, the dye is removed faster from the capsule than it is from the particles in the background or the cell. As a result, the capsule becomes colorless and the cells and background are stained (**Figure 14.1**).

Another characteristic you will observe is the ability to form an **endospore**, a spore that forms within the cell. Endospores are dormant forms of bacteria that are extremely resistant to harsh environmental conditions such as drying, heat, or chemicals. They are formed by certain bacteria as they reach the end of their growth phase. These round, thick-walled, durable bodies are eventually the only thing left as the rest of cell, the **vegetative** part, dies. Endospores can survive for years until, given the right environmental conditions, they germinate to produce a vegetative cell (**Figure 14.2a**). Endospores can be positioned terminally, subterminally, or centrally within the cell. (**Figure 14.2b**).

An example of an endospore-forming bacterium and the one we will use in this exercise is *Bacillus cereus*. It is a Gram-positive bacillus commonly found in soil. If *B. cereus* cells are heated while being stained with malachite green, the stain penetrates the endospore, dyeing it green. When the cells are counterstained with safranin, the vegetative part of the cell stains pink or red.

Movement, another characteristic of some bacteria, is most often accomplished by means of **flagella.** Flagella are rigid, coiled tubes composed of the protein flagellin. Flagella are attached to the cell wall and membrane of a bacterium. By rotating like a propeller, these appendages cause the cell to move. **Figure 14.3** shows the different distribution of one or

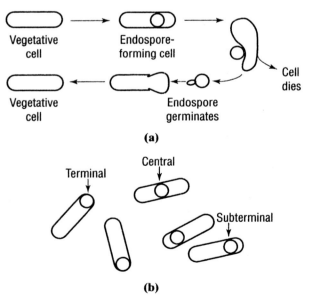

(a)

(b)

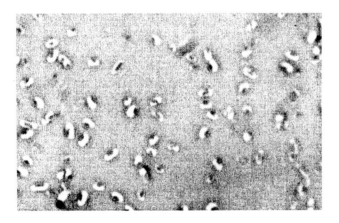

Figure 14.1 A capsule stain of *K. pneumoniae* grown in milk. Note the clearing around the cell; this is the capsule.

Figure 14.2 (a) Life cycle of an endo spore-forming bacterium; (b) location of endospores within a vegetative cell.

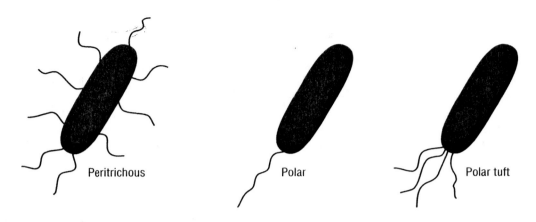

Peritrichous

Polar

Polar tuft

Figure 14.3 The various locations of flagella on bacteria.

more flagella on cells. Flagella are not easy to stain because they are easily sheared off during cell preparation. They also have a very small diameter and must be heavily stained to make them visible by light microscopy. Because there is still no easy or reliable method for staining flagella, you will view prepared slides of bacteria with flagella.

Under certain culture conditions, many bacteria will produce deposits within their cytoplasm called **inclusions**. Inclusions serve as storage molecules for energy and structural building blocks of the cell. They are deposits of fats, polysaccharides, sulfur and phosphate granules, and **poly-β-hydroxybutyrate (PHB)**. PHB is a lipid-like compound consisting of monomers of **β-hydroxybutyrate** joined by ester linkages. PHB granules are storage depots for carbon and energy and are used by the cell when it is in a low-nutrient environment. They appear as blue-black droplets within a cell when stained with Sudan black B. The rest of the cytoplasm appears pink when counterstained with safranin. You will stain and observe PHB inclusion bodies in the bacterium *B. cereus*.

The last characteristic to be examined is the difference in cell wall composition of some bacteria. You have already learned the importance of the Gram stain, which distinguishes cells with a Gram-negative cell wall from cells with a Gram-positive cell wall. But not all bacteria stain with Gram stain reagents like crystal violet or safranin. These bacteria have large amounts of lipid (in particular mycolic acid) in their cell walls. These lipids form stable complexes with certain dyes such as fuchsin. It is thought that when exposed to heat and phenol in the primary stain, the carbolfuchsin penetrates the cell wall. The mycolic acids in the cell wall retain the stain even when exposed to acid-alcohol, a

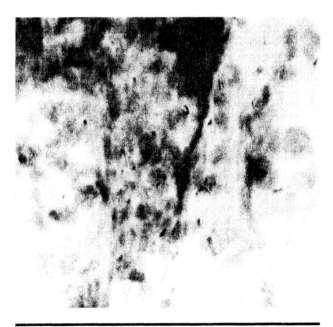

Figure 14.4 Acid-fast mycobacteria in a stained smear of sputum from a patient with *M. tuberculosis.*

strong decolorizing agent. Because of this, these bacteria are named **acid-fast bacteria (AFB)** and the stain is an acid–fast stain. A counterstain of methylene blue is used to stain the non–acid-fast bacteria for easier microscopic recognition (**Figure 14.4**). The most common AFB are the mycobacteria, notably *Mycobacterium tuberculosis* and *M. leprae,* the causative agents of tuberculosis and leprosy, respectively. The acid-fast stain is a rapid test for identifying these organisms in clinical samples from diseased patients. You will stain a mycobacterium, *M. gordonae*, which is a nonpathogenic species widely distributed in soil and water.

PURPOSE

- To learn about structures of bacteria: endospores, capsules, flagella, and inclusion bodies
- To examine bacteria with an increased lipid content in their cell walls using the acid-fast stain
- To learn new staining procedures for examining different structures of bacteria

THE EXERCISE

MATERIALS:

Culture of *K. pneumoniae* in milk
Two nutrient agar plates of *B. cereus*—one more than 24 hours old and one less than 48 hours old
Slant culture of *M. gordonae*
20% copper sulfate
Safranin solution (same as in Gram stain)
95% acid-alcohol
Sudan black B stain
Boiling water bath with staining rack
Inoculating loops
Culture of *E. coli* in milk
Slant or plate culture of *E. coli*
Microscope slides
Forceps
Aqueous crystal violet
5% malachite green
Carbolfuschin stain
1% methylene blue
Xylene
Prepared slides of bacteria with flagella
Microscopes

PROCEDURE:

You will be performing four special stains—capsule, endospore, PHB, and acid-fast—and observing the stained smears microscopically. You will also observe prepared slides of microorganisms that have flagella. Follow the procedure below for each stain.

Part A: Capsule Stain

1. Obtain a culture of *K. pneumoniae* grown in milk and aseptically remove a loopful of the culture.
2. Spread the inoculum on a slide, making a thin smear over one half of the slide (**Figure 14.5**).
3. Obtain a loopful of *E. coli* grown in milk and make a thin smear on the other half of the slide.
4. Let the slide air dry.
5. Flood the smear with aqueous crystal violet and let stand 2 minutes.
6. Wash the slide with copious quantities of 20% copper sulfate solution and blot dry.
7. Examine the smear under oil immersion, searching for an area that is thinly stained.
8. Draw and label the cells and their surrounding capsules (if present) in the RESULTS section. Also indicate the color of the organisms.

Part B: Endospore Stain

1. Obtain an old culture (more than 48 hours old) of *B. cereus* and make a smear on one half of a glass slide.
2. On the other half of the slide, make a smear with *E. coli*.
3. Let the slide air dry and heat fix the smear.
4. Place the slide on a staining rack over a boiling water bath.
5. Flood the smear with malachite green solution for 5 minutes. **Note:** Replace any evaporated stain with fresh dye so that it doesn't become dry.
   CAUTION: Handle the hot slide with forceps and not your fingers.
6. Remove the slide from the rack and allow the slide to cool to room temperature.
7. Rinse with water, drain the slide, and then flood the smear with safranin for 1 to 2 minutes.
8. Rinse the slide with water and blot dry.

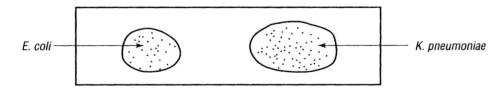

Figure 14.5   Smear with *E. coli* and *K. pneumoniae*.

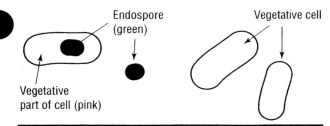

Figure 14.6 Endospores after staining with malachite green.

9. Observe the cells under oil immersion. The endospores are green and the vegetative cells are pink or red (**Figure 14.6**). **Note:** Not all cells produce endospores at the same time. Therefore, some bacteria may have endospores while others do not.
10. Record your observations by making drawings of both bacteria in the RESULTS section.

Part C: AFB Stain (Ziehl-Neelsen)

1. Obtain a prepared and heat fixed smear of *M. gordonae* and *B. cereus* on a numbered slide. The slide is divided in half by a line and one side is marked A and the other B. Record your slide number.
   CAUTION: Use gloves when performing this staining procedure. Avoid contact with your eyes, skin, and clothing because all three reagents are irritants. The staining procedure should also be done in rooms with adequate ventilation.
2. Put the slide on a boiling water bath and flood the slide with carbolfuchsin stain for 1 minute. Do not permit the stain to boil or evaporate completely.
   CAUTION: Handle the hot slide with forceps and not your fingers.
3. Remove the slide from the heat and allow the stain to remain on the slide for an additional 4 to 5 minutes. Place it on another staining rack.
4. Rinse the slide well with distilled water and tilt to drain.
5. Decolorize the slide with acid-alcohol for 3 minutes.
6. Rinse the slide well with distilled water and tilt to drain.
7. Flood the slide with methylene blue for 1 minute.
8. Rinse the slide well with distilled water and allow to air dry.
9. Examine the slide under oil immersion for acid-fast rods. They will appear as small, red, slightly curved, possibly beaded cells with tapered ends against a blue background. The non–acid-fast rods are blue against a blue background.

10. Determine which bacterium (A or B) is AFB positive and record your results in the RESULTS section.

Part D: Inclusion Body Staining (Sudan Black B for PHB)

1. Prepare a smear with two bacteria, *B. cereus* and *E. coli*. Each bacterium should be on one-half of the smear as in the endospore stain.
2. Heat fix the smear.
3. Immerse the slide in Sudan black B for 15 minutes.
4. Remove the slide, let it drain and air dry by leaning it against a rack on an absorbent paper towel.
5. Immerse the slide several times in a staining jar containing xylene.
   CAUTION: Use a covered jar of xylene and immediately cover the jar after using. Xylene fumes are noxious or harmful to your health.
6. Blot the slide dry with bibulous paper or let air dry.
7. Counterstain the slide by placing it on a staining rack and flooding the smear with safranin for 10 seconds.
8. Rinse the slide thoroughly with tap water several times and blot dry with bibulous paper.
9. Examine the slide using oil immersion. The inclusion bodies are small, black, and refractile, and form chains inside the rods. You may have to focus up and down to see the small bodies which may not appear in every cell.
10. Record your observations of both bacteria in the RESULTS section.

Part E: Flagella Stain

1. Obtain the prepared slides provided by your instructor and observe the flagella.
2. Record your observations of these hair-like projections and how they occur on different types of bacteria (if available) in the RESULTS section.

REFERENCES

Baron, E.J. et al., *Bailey and Scott's Diagnostic Microbiology*, 9th ed. St. Louis: Mosby–Year Book, Inc., 1994.

Gerhardt, P., et al. *Methods for General and Molecular Bacteriology*. Washington, DC: American Society for Microbiology Press, 1994.

Salyers, A.A. and Whitt, D.D. *Bacterial Pathogenesis, A Molecular Approach*. Washington, DC: American Society for Microbiology Press, 1994.

RESULTS

Record your observations after each staining procedure below:

Capsule stain:

E. coli

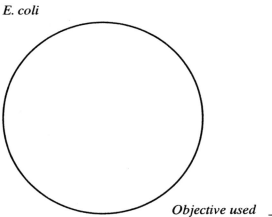

Objective used _____

K. pneumoniae

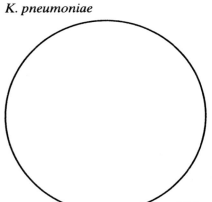

Objective used _____

Endospore stain:

E. coli

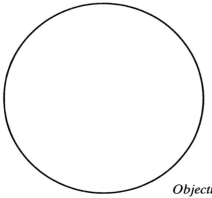

Objective used _____

B. cereus

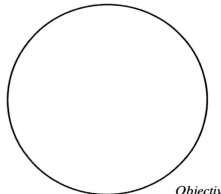

Objective used _____

Inclusion body stain:

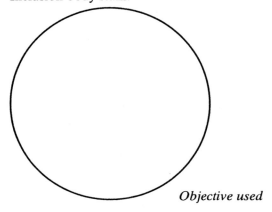

Objective used _____

Flagella stain:

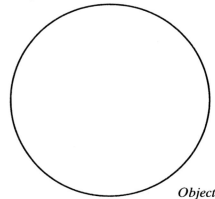

Objective used _____

AFB staining results:

Unknown smear # _____

A. _____ (AFB positive or negative)   B. _____ (AFB positive or negative)

REFLECTIONS

1. Certain endospore-forming bacteria are a particular concern of the canned food industry. Name one of these bacteria and explain why it is of such concern.

2. PHBs and related compounds such as PHAs (poly-hydroxy-alkanates) are plastic-like molecules that are of great interest to industrial microbiologists. Why is there so much interest in microbially produced plastics?

3. Is the production of an endospore by a bacterium considered a method of reproduction?

4. Why do capsules make bacteria so resistant to phagocytosis?

5. Why is the AFB stain so important when diagnosing leprosy?

EXERCISE 15

IDENTIFYING BACTERIA USING METABOLIC CHARACTERISTICS

This exercise continues the study of bacteria and how they are identified. The tests performed in this exercise illustrate some of the classic biochemical characteristics that are used to identify bacteria. These patterns of metabolism have been used for years to differentiate many bacteria and have given us phenotypic profiles of bacteria. It is only recently that molecular methods have allowed us to compare the genetic makeup of bacteria at the level of nucleotide sequences and give us an even more precise genotypic relationship of bacteria and other organisms. We will explore these methods in the next exercise.

Kathy was anxious to begin this laboratory exercise. From her previous work (Exercise 14), she knew the bacterium she had isolated from the rotting carrot was a Gram-negative rod. But sadly, she discovered there are hundreds of Gram-negative rods. This exercise would introduce the use of metabolic characteristics in identification of bacteria. So today, Kathy would learn about tests that may enable her to identify her bacterium.

Kathy's instructor carefully explained the metabolic characteristics the class would use. The instructor demonstrated how to inoculate the differential media contained in tubes. Kathy inoculated several tubed media with known bacteria her instructor provided and with her unidentified carrot pathogen. After incubating the media, she examined the tubes and recorded their reactions. Kathy was glad to have the known iso-

lates because, even though her instructor describ(what a positive and negative reaction looked like, was nice to see them first-hand. After recording ea(reaction, Kathy proceeded to investigate several bi chemical tables that gave results for Gram-negati· rods. Kathy's investigation led her to the fami Enterobacteriaceae, although her bacterium did n give many positive reactions to the biochemical tes she performed, including indole production, carboh drate fermentations, and urease production. The carr(rot bacterium did resemble one of the known bacteri a Pseudomonas. Kathy decided to investigate the lite ature focusing on the most common causes of ve(etable spoilage, known as soft rot. Several books me(tioned two Gram-negative rods belonging to th genera Pseudomonas and Erwinia. She discovered th oxidase test was particularly helpful in distinguishin between these two organisms. She reviewed her not(and fortunately it was one of the tests she had don(Her microbe was negative and so is Erwinia. Pse(domonas spp. are primarily oxidase positive, especiall those species that cause soft rot in vegetables. To pos(tively identify her bacterium, Kathy would have to d further biochemical testing. However, after talking t her instructor, she felt reasonably sure that the microb that caused her carrots to rot was Erwinia carotovor(Her final task was to report her results and hand in he lab report. Needless to say, because of Kathy thoughtful thinking, testing, and reporting, she receive(high marks.[1]

------

[1]Kathy's story does not end here, but continues in the nex exercise.

BACKGROUND INFORMATION

Bacteria have relatively few morphological features useful for identification. Therefore, metabolic characteristics are very important. As noted in Exercise 14, evolutionary relationships (phylogeny) of organisms are best established by making genetic comparisons. However, there are many instances where an organism needs to be identified and this is generally accomplished by observing phenotypic characteristics. For instance, in a clinical setting, the position of a pathogen in a phylogenetic tree is of little importance. What is important is the identity of the pathogen so that a patient can be treated.

Metabolism is the sum total of all chemical reactions carried out by cells. These reactions or processes include those by which cells convert nutrients into cellular components using energy, known as biosynthetic processes or **anabolism,** and the processes by which cells degrade nutrients producing waste products and energy known as degradative processes or **catabolism.** In many cases the intermediates of catabolic pathways serve as carbon skeletons for the anabolic biosynthesis of new cellular components. By studying if and how bacteria degrade a range of compounds, we can generate a phenotypic profile of its metabolic characteristics. These metabolic characteristics are the classical means of identifying bacteria.

Numerous biochemical characteristics are used to distinguish bacteria. You will observe only a few of those used to differentiate several Gram-negative rods. These characteristics include a bacterium's ability to ferment carbohydrates, produce specific enzymes, catabolize amino acids, and use compounds to respire. Each of these characteristics can be determined by a specific **differential** medium. These media contain compounds that enable us to detect a particular metabolic process. The mechanism of the reaction of each tubed media is explained in the procedure section, as is the method of inoculation and interpretation.

Carbohydrate Fermentation (Glucose, Lactose, and Sucrose)

Many organisms ferment carbohydrates such as glucose, lactose, and sucrose. Carbohydrates are used by most microorganisms as a source of carbon and energy. The end products of carbohydrate fermentation are often acids such as pyruvic acid and lactic acid. These acids can be detected by using a brom cresol purple dye that changes from purple to yellow when the medium becomes acidic. Glucose, a monosaccharide, is fermented by many bacteria and, depending on the pathway, end products such as pyruvic acid, lactic acid, hydrogen, carbon dioxide, and ethanol are produced. Lactose is a disaccharide composed of glucose and galactose. It is only fermented if the organism produces an enzyme called β-galactosidase. This enzyme cleaves the bond between glucose and galactose, and then normal glucose fermentation and galactose fermentation take place. Similarly, sucrose is a disaccharide of glucose and fructose. Microorganisms that have the enzyme sucrase cleave the bond between glucose and fructose and the same fermentation pathways are followed (fructose is an isomer of glucose and can be changed into glucose easily).

Mixed Acid Fermentation (Methyl Red Test) and Acetoin Production (Voges-Proskauer Test)

Under anaerobic conditions, some bacteria, such as *E. coli*, produce large amounts of organic acids (acetic, lactic, formic, and succinic) when glucose is the sole source of carbon. This catabolic pathway is known as the **mixed acid fermentation pathway.** These bacteria make so much of these strong acids (with only a small amount reutilized) that the acids drop the pH of the medium to 4 or 5, even overcoming the buffering system of the medium. By adding an indicator such as methyl red to a culture as in the ***Methyl Red (MR) test***, these strong acid producers can be detected. By contrast, other Gram-negative rods (e.g., *Klebsiella)* when grown in the same medium (MR-VP broth) produce small amounts of acids. However, they produce large amounts of neutral products in the form of butanediol and ethanol via a pathway known as the **butanediol fermentation pathway (Figure 15.1).** An intermediate in the production of butanediol is acetoin (acetylmethylcarbinol). The **Voges-Proskauer (VP) test** is used to detect the presence of this intermediate. MR-VP broth contains glucose, protein, and phosphate buffer.

Catabolism of the Amino Acids Tryptophan (Indole Production) and Lysine

In addition to using glucose as an energy source, some microorganisms also utilize certain amino acids for energy. One of these amino acids is tryptophan. Microorganisms (e.g., *E. coli*) with the enzyme tryptophanase, degrade tryptophan to indole, pyruvic acid, and ammonia.

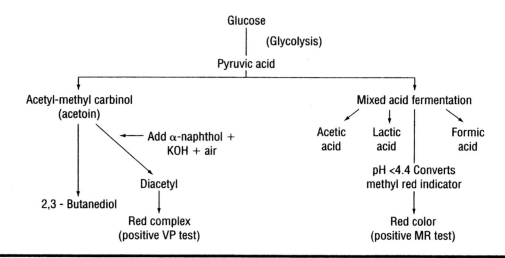

Figure 15.1   The two glucose fermentation pathways detected by the MR-VP test.

Indole is a waste product of the microorganism, pyruvic acid is used by the cell as a carbon and energy source, and ammonia dissipates or is used to make other amino acids. To determine whether an organism has catabolized tryptophan, we can test for the production of indole with the **indole test.**

Another amino acid which microorganisms may utilize is lysine. Some microorganisms (*E. coli* again) decarboxylate lysine because they produce the enzyme **lysine decarboxylase.** The result is the production of the amine, cadaverine, and carbon dioxide.

During initial studies of decarboxylation reactions, it was determined that the medium used to detect any of the decarboxylation reactions (e.g., lysine, ornithine, arginine, and glutamic acid) must be acidic. Therefore, a small amount of glucose is added to the medium so that after the bacterium ferments glucose, a suitable acid environment is produced. To this basal medium is then added the specific amino acid and brom cresol purple, a pH indicator.

Detection of Specific Enzymes (Urease and Oxidase)

The above metabolic reactions all have specific enzymes which are involved in catabolism. Two other important enzymes which facilitate catabolism of substrates are **urease** and **oxidase**. If a microorganism has the enzyme urease (e.g., *Proteus*), it hydrolyzes urea to ammonia, CO_2 and water. The reaction is as follows:

The ammonia formed makes the medium alkaline and increases the pH.

The **oxidase test** determines if an organism has cytochrome *c* oxidase as a respiratory enzyme. Cytochrome *c* oxidase is a heme-containing protein, which is one of the enzymes responsible for reactions taking place during oxidative phosphorylation. Cytochrome *c* is one of several different cytochromes organisms can have. Bacteria capable of either aerobic or anaerobic respiration have one or more cytochromes in their electron transport system. Cytochrome *c* oxidase catalyzes the oxidation of cytochrome *c* as follows:

$$2 \text{ reduced cytochrome } c \; + \; 2 \, H^+ \; + \; \tfrac{1}{2} O_2$$

$$\downarrow \text{Cytochrome } c \text{ oxidase}$$

$$2 \text{ oxidized cytochrome } c \; + \; H_2O$$

Nitrate Reduction (for Synthesis of Amino Acids or for Energy Metabolism)

Certain bacteria such as those from the family *Enterobacteriaceae* reduce nitrate to nitrite and ultimately to ammonia or nitrogen gas. This is done through the action of enzymes called nitrate reductases. Some bacteria utilize the ammonia to produce amino acids or other nitrogenous compounds. This is known as assimilatory nitrate reduction. Other bacteria (e.g., *Pseudomonas*) utilize nitrate or nitrite as the terminal electron acceptor for a respiratory chain when O_2 is not available (anaerobic respiration). Therefore, these normally aerobic organisms are capable of nitrate respiration and will grow anaerobically. This is known as dissimilatory nitrate reduction. The reactions involved in nitrate reduction are as follows:

$$NO_3^- \xrightarrow[\text{Reductase}]{\text{Nitrate}} NO_2^- \xrightarrow[\text{Reductase}]{\text{Nitrate}} NH_3 \quad \text{or} \quad N_2$$

Nitrate   Nitrite   Ammonia or Nitrogen gas

PURPOSE

* To explore the importance of metabolic characteristics in identifying bacteria
* To use differential media to test a bacterium's ability to produce certain enzymes, catabolize amino acids, and to ferment and respire carbohydrates, both anaerobically and aerobically

THE EXERCISE

MATERIALS:

Glucose, lactose, and sucrose fermentation tubes
Christensen's urease agar slants
Moeller decarboxylase broth base with 1% lysine
Filter paper strips
Pasteur pipets
Plate cultures of *E. coli, Klebsiella pneumoniae, Proteus vulgaris* and *Pseudomonas aeruginosa*
One unknown culture plate
Kovac's reagent (p-dimethyl-aminobenzaldehyde)
Oxidase reagent (tetramethyl-p-phenylenediamine dihydrochloride)
Tryptone broth
MR-VP tubes
Moeller decarboxylase broth base
Nitrate broth
Sterile mineral oil in tubes
Inoculating needles
Small, empty sterile tubes

Methyl red reagent
40% KOH
5% α-naphthol
Nitrate reagents (sulfanilic acid and α-naphthylamine)
Zinc dust

CAUTION: The reagents listed above are for the most part either potential irritants and/or toxic. Alpha-napthol is highly toxic and possibly carcinogenic. Handle all of them with care. Avoid contact with your skin and eyes.

PROCEDURE:

You will be given the four Gram-negative rods listed above and your task is to inoculate the nine tubed media and perform the oxidase test on each of these bacteria. You will also receive an unknown bacterium that you will be expected to identify; it is one of the four listed above. Follow the directions below on how to perform and interpret each test result.

Part A: Carbohydrate Fermentation Tubes:
1% glucose, 1% lactose, and 1% sucrose

1. Obtain one tube of each of the carbohydrate fermentation tubes for each of the four bacteria and label them appropriately. **Note:** Each medium contains brom cresol purple indicator for pH changes.
2. With a sterile inoculating needle, obtain an isolated colony from one bacterium and inoculate the broth tube.
3. Repeat step 2 for each of the remaining three bacteria and your unknown.
4. Incubate the tubes at 35°C for 18 to 24 hours. **Note:** A negative test can be reincubated for up to 4 days. If acids are produced due to fermentation of the carbohydrate, the brom cresol indicator will turn from purple to yellow.
   Interpretation:
   Positive: Acidification of the broth with a change in color from purple to yellow
   Negative: No acidification; the broth remains a purple color
5. Record your results in the RESULTS section.

Part B: Indole Test

1. Obtain one tube of tryptone broth for each of the four bacteria and your unknown. Label them appropriately.
2. With a sterile inoculating needle, obtain an isolated colony from one of your plates and inoculate the broth tube.
3. Repeat step 2 for all of the organisms.

4. Incubate the tubes at 35°C for 18 to 24 hours.
5. Add 1 to 2 drops of Kovac's reagent and determine indole production. **Note:** Do not shake the tube. Kovac's reagent is an acidic alcoholic solution of p-dimethyl-aminobenzaldehyde that combines with indole to form a red-colored complex at the interface of the medium and reagent.
   Interpretation:
   Positive: Red color in upper aqueous layer (at the interface)
   Negative: Light yellow color in the upper aqueous layer
6. Record your results in the RESULTS section.

Part C: Methyl Red–Voges–Proskauer (MR-VP) Test

1. Obtain one tube of MR-VP broth (2 ml) for each of the four bacteria and your unknown culture and label them appropriately. **Note:** Only one tube is necessary for both tests.
2. Heavily inoculate each broth with an isolated colony.
3. Incubate the broth at 35°C for 24 to 48 hours.
4. Obtain another sterile empty tube and carefully transfer 1 ml of the broth to it. **Note:** Use a pipet to transfer the broth to prevent unnecessary spills.
5. To perform the methyl red test, add 2 drops of methyl red indicator to one of the tubes and observe the color at the surface of the medium. **Note:** The production of strong acids will drop the pH to 4 or 5 and this acidity can be detected by the methyl red indicator.
   Interpretation:
   Positive: A stable red color develops immediately
   Negative: The color of the reagent turns yellow
6. To perform the Voges-Proskauer test, add 6 drops of α-naphthol to the second tube.
7. Then add 3 drops of 40% KOH to the tube.
8. Shake the tube to expose the broth culture to atmospheric oxygen and let it stand undisturbed for 10 to 15 minutes. **Note:** The two reagents in the presence of oxygen react with acetoin producing diacetyl. Diacetyl reacts with peptones in the broth to form a red-colored complex (**Figure 15.1**). The α-naphthol serves as a catalyst and color intensifier.
   Interpretation:
   Positive: A red color develops after 15 minutes indicating the presence of diacetyl. **Note:** This test should *not* be read after 1 hour because of the potential for false positive interpretations (a copper-red color)
   Negative: No color development
9. Record your results in the RESULTS section.

Part D: Urease Test

1. Obtain one Christensen's urea agar slant for each of the four bacteria and your unknown culture and label them appropriately.
2. Streak the surface of each agar slant with a portion of an isolated colony. Replace the caps of the tubes loosely.
3. Incubate the tubes for 18 to 24 hours at 35°C. A negative test can be reincubated and observed for up to 4 days. **Note:** The hydrolysis of urea produces ammonia which increases the pH of the medium. The pH shift is detected by the indicator phenol red, which is light orange at pH 6.8 and turns magenta at pH 8.1. The medium is buffered and contains certain nutrients that increase the sensitivity of the test for species that produce only a small amount of urease.
   Interpretation:
   Positive: The medium turns from light orange to magenta; the degree of color depends on the amount of ammonia that diffuses throughout the medium. *Proteus* sp. may give a positive result within 1 to 6 hours
   Negative: The medium remains light orange throughout
4. Record your results in the RESULTS section.

Part E: Lysine Decarboxylase Test

1. Obtain two tubes for each of the four bacteria and your unknown (a decarboxylase broth base tube and decarboxylase broth base with 1% lysine) and label them appropriately.
2. Inoculate both the control tubes (broth base) and test broth tubes (base with lysine) with an isolated colony of each bacterium. **Note:** A control tube without lysine is used for each bacterium tested. It should remain yellow. This is done to verify that the organism is an acid-producing, glucose fermenter (it produces acids so that the decarboxylation reaction can take place). If it is not a glucose fermenter, the test is not useful for identification.
3. Overlay all tubes with sterile mineral oil to approximately 1 cm above the surface. **Note:** To prevent oxidation of glucose at the surface of the tube (surface reverting to purple color), the metabolic process must be anaerobic. This can be accomplished by overlaying the medium with sterile mineral oil.
4. Incubate all tubes for 24 to 48 hours at 35°C. **Note:** Because this reaction is a two-step process, 48 hours may be needed to complete the reaction. If

the bacterium ferments glucose, it will first turn the indicator yellow (acids are produced). Then if the bacterium decarboxylates lysine, the cadaverine that is produced neutralizes the acids from fermentation and turns the indicator back to its original purple color.

Interpretation:

Control tube: The broth has converted from a purple to yellow color; **Note:** Conversion of this tube indicates the organism is viable, is a fermenter, and that the pH of the medium has been lowered sufficiently to activate the decarboxylase enzyme

Positive: Reversion of the medium back to a purple color

Negative: The medium turns yellow except for a possible small rim of purple at the top of the broth

Record your results in the RESULTS section.

rt F: Nitrate Reduction Test

Obtain one nitrate broth tube for each bacterium and your unknown culture and label them appropriately. Nitrate broth contains 0.1% potassium nitrate, which serves as a nitrogen source for assimilatory nitrate reduction and as a terminal electron acceptor for dissimilatory nitrate reduction.

Inoculate each broth with a portion of an isolated colony from each plate.

Incubate the tubes at 35°C for 24 to 48 hours.

Add 3 drops of sulfanilic acid and 3 drops of α-naphthylamine to each tube.

CAUTION: α-naphthylamine is a potential carcinogen and sulfonic acid is an irritant. Wear gloves when handling both of these reagents.

Look for a red color which should develop in 1 to 2 minutes. **Note:** These reagents react with nitrite to form a red color indicating the bacterium has reduced nitrate to nitrite.

If no color has developed, add zinc dust to the tube. **Note:** Since these two reagents only detect the presence of nitrite and not nitrogen or ammonia, a small amount of zinc dust is added to tubes that do not develop a red color. Zinc reacts with nitrate and forms a red color complex. Therefore, a red color after zinc is added means nitrate

reduction has *not* occurred. No red color after the zinc is added means there was further reduction of nitrate to nitrogen or ammonia gas.

Interpretation:

Positive (reduction of nitrate to nitrite): red color develops after addition of both reagents

Positive (reduction of nitrate to nitrogen gas or ammonia): no red color change after addition of both reagents and the zinc dust

Negative (no nitrate reduction): no red color after addition of both reagents, but a red color after addition of zinc dust

7. Record your results in the RESULTS section.

Part G. Oxidase Test

1. Obtain a piece of filter paper and saturate it with oxidase reagent. **Note:** You may have commercial oxidase strips or disks already impregnated with the reagent.

2. Obtain an inoculum with a *platinum* loop or wooden applicator stick and rub it into the impregnated filter paper. **Note:** If cytochrome *c* oxidase is present, cytochrome *c* will be in the oxidized form. Oxidized cytochrome *c* then reacts with the substrate tetramethyl-p-phenylenediamine in the oxidase reagent, producing a purple color. A platinum loop instead of a nichrome loop is necessary because nichrome itself can cause oxidation of the reagent.

Interpretation:

Positive: Strip or disk turns purple within 10 seconds

Negative: No purple color develops

3. Record your results in the RESULTS section.

REFERENCES

Baron, E.J., et. al. *Bailey and Scott's Diagnostic Microbiology*, 9th ed., St. Louis: Mosby–Year Book, 1994.

Barry, A.L., et. al. Improved 18-Hour Methyl Red Test. *Applied Microbiology* 20(1970):866.

Blazevic, D.J. and Ederer, G.M. *Principles of Biochemical Tests in Diagnostic Microbiology*. New York: Wiley and Sons, 1975.

McFaddin, J.F. *Biochemical Tests for Identification of Medical Bacteria*, 2nd ed., Baltimore: Williams and Wilkins, 1980.

RESULTS

Record your results and identify your unknown culture.

Test	E. coli	Klebsiella pneumoniae	Proteus vulgaris	Pseudomonas aeruginosa	Unknown #
Acid from glucose					
Acid from lactose					
Acid from sucrose					
Indole production					
Methyl red (MR)					
Voges-Proskauer (VP)					
Urease					
Lysine decarboxylase					
Decarboxylase control					
Nitrate reduction					
Oxidase					

Unknown # _____

Identification _____

REFLECTIONS

1. As an organism hydrolyzes tryptophan, it produces indole, pyruvic acid, and ammonia. Why is it that we measure indole and not the other end products, pyruvic acid or ammonia, to tell us if this reaction took place?

2. Based on your knowledge of biochemical pathways, which of the bacteria are capable of only respiratory types of metabolism and which are fermentative? Are any of the bacteria strict aerobes?

3. Which test suggests that a bacterium respires aerobically? Explain.

EXERCISE 16

NEW DIRECTIONS IN CLASSIFICATION AND IDENTIFICATION

Structural and metabolic characteristics of organisms have been the basis of taxonomic classification. The advent of protein and nucleic acid sequencing technologies has led to a better understanding of the evolutionary relationships of organisms, which in turn is clarifying how evolution occurs. It has also allowed us to identify microorganisms without isolating and culturing them. As a result, taxonomy is in tremendous turmoil. Several new classification schemes have been proposed. Only time and more hard work will settle the arguments.

Kathy was feeling very proud of herself. She had received an "A" for her work to identify the pathogen causing soft rot in a carrot (Exercises 14 and 15). She clearly had the business of bacterial identification under control. The next day Kathy's instructor opened the lecture by saying, "It has been estimated that only a very small fraction of microbes have been identified and classified. For the most part, those that have been are those we are able to culture. Why have we identified and classified so few? How does this fact impact our ability to understand complex ecosystems such as soil?"

Kathy thought over her recent experience in identification of a bacterium. She had begun by doing a few simple stains—but only after she had obtained a pure culture of the bacterium. Then she characterized the bacterium metabolically—but most of the metabolic

tests depended on the ability of the bacterium to grow on a variety of differential media. Kathy was stumped. How could she have identified her microbe if she couldn't grow it in culture? With thousands of different species in soil, water, and other microbial communities, how could one determine the exact number of microbes and their identity without obtaining pure cultures of each? Kathy hoped the answer would be provided in her instructor's lecture.

BACKGROUND INFORMATION

The questions Kathy's instructor posed have plagued microbiologists for decades. Then in the 1970s, procedures were developed for sequencing nucleic acids. These techniques, coupled with procedures for isolating nucleic acids from complex samples such as soil, meant microbiologists no longer had to culture microbes before the makeup of a microbial community could be determined.

The development of sequencing techniques had another, perhaps more far-reaching, impact on microbial taxonomy. Throughout the history of biology, taxonomists have used phenotypic characteristics to sort organisms into taxonomic groups, called **taxons**. Their goal was to establish a scheme that reflected and demonstrated the evolution of each taxon.

Numerous phenotypic classification schemes have been proposed. The first divided all life into two kingdoms, Plantae and Animalia. But as the study of microbes progressed, it became apparent that microbes could not be easily placed in either of these two categories. For one thing, many microbes have both plant-like *and* animal-like characteristics. As you observed in Exercise 12, for instance, all algae are photosynthetic (plant-like), but many are also motile (animal-like). A second problem was the fact that some microbes are procaryotic whereas others are eucaryotic. It was difficult to place such fundamentally different cell types within the same kingdom.

In 1969, Robert Whittaker proposed what is now a widely accepted scheme having five kingdoms (**Figure 16.1**). In this scheme, the procaryotic microorganisms are placed in a kingdom (Procaryotae; Monera). Most of the protozoa and algae are placed in a separate kingdom (Protista) and fungi, plants, and animals each have their own kingdoms. Although this scheme solved some of the problems of the two-

kingdom system, several questions still remained. Do schemes based on phenotypic characteristics accurately represent the evolutionary relationship of organisms? Would the relationships hold if organisms could be examined at the genetic level? In other words, do organisms with similar phenotypes necessarily share a common ancestor? And if they do (or do not), what does this tell us about evolutionary processes?

The examination of gene sequences allows us to make inferences about the evolutionary history of a species, known as **phylogeny**. This, in turn, allows us to more correctly assign organisms to taxons and to order them in a taxonomic hierarchy. Species evolve as the result of changes that occur in genetic material over time. These changes include base pair substitutions, deletions, insertions, duplications, and rearrangements. **Figure 16.2** shows in very simple terms how

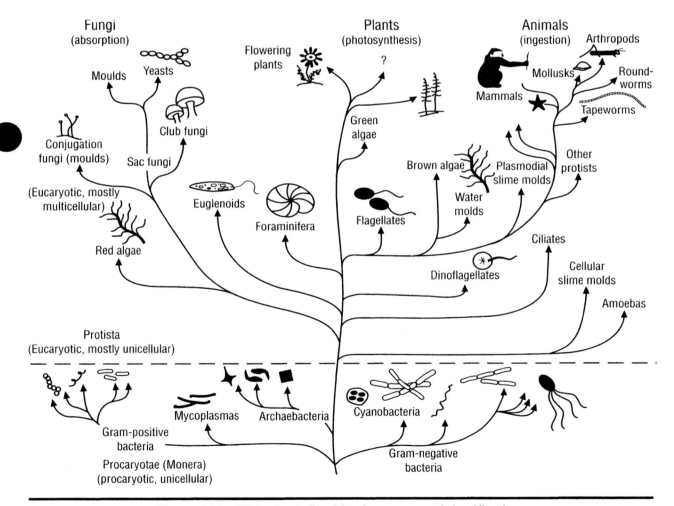

Figure 16.1 Whittaker's five-kingdom system of classification.

several species might evolve from a common ancestor as a result of base pair substitutions. It is important to remember that "one substitution does not a new species make." However, you can see from **Figure 16.2** and **Table 16.1** that the more closely related organisms are, the more recently they diverged from a common ancestor and the more similar their sequences of nucleic acids.

There are relatively few rules for choosing genes to compare. One rule, of course, is that the same genes be compared; that apples be compared with apples, not oranges. Put another way, the tryptophanase gene of one organism would be compared with the tryptophanase gene of another organism, but not to the other organism's β-galactosidase gene. Genes such as the tryptophanase and β-galactosidase are not found in all organisms. Therefore, genes common to all organisms are most often used for genetic comparisons, especially when broad phylogenetic relationships are being established. Such genes include the gene for 16S rRNA, one of the rRNA molecules found in the small subunit of procaryotic ribosomes, and its counterpart in eucaryotic ribosomes, the gene for 18S rRNA.

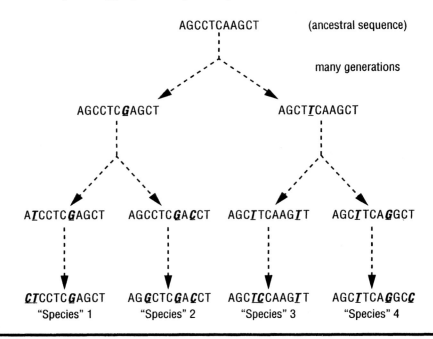

Figure 16.2 A very simple example of how different species might diverge from a common ancestor by base pair substitutions. In reality, more extensive changes than those shown would occur before a new species evolved. The base pair substitutions are shown in bold italics and are underlined. All arrows represent many generations and years. For ease of presentation, we have shown only one of the DNA strands.

TABLE 16.1 Percent Similarity of the Sequences Shown in Figure 16.2

	Ancestral sequence	Species 1	Species 2	Species 3	Species 4
Ancestral sequence	100%	73%	73%	73%	73%
Species 1		100%	64%	45%	45%
Species 2			100%	45%	45%
Species 3				100%	64%
Species 4					100%

Comparisons of 16S and 18S rRNA sequences are now being used to devise phylogenetic trees. Phylogenetic trees are created by a variety of different approaches, but all begin by aligning the sequences being compared and calculating some measure of similarity. As you might imagine, such alignments and calculations were not easily done before the development of high-speed computers. As more and more sequences were compared and catalogued, taxonomists discovered that Whittaker's five-kingdom classification scheme (**Figure 16.1**) does not effectively classify the procaryotic microbes known as the Archaebacteria. In the late 1970s, Carl Woese proposed a three-kingdom system (**Figure 16.3**) that recognized the vast phylogenetic difference between the Archaebacteria and the Eubacteria. Over the last twenty years, this tree has been refined and recently a new universal phylogenetic tree proposed (**Figure 16.4**).

Today, newly determined 16S or 18S rRNA sequences can be compared to previously determined sequences archived in a databank. One such databank is maintained by the Ribosomal Database Project (RDP) located at the University of Illinois. In this exercise, you will be given a rRNA sequence from the small subunit of the ribosomes of an unknown organism. By comparing that sequence to the RDP database, you will identify the unknown.

PURPOSE

- To explore the use of molecular techniques in bacterial taxonomy
- To gain experience in accessing and using electronic databases
- To identify an unknown organism from its small subunit rRNA sequence (16S or 18S rRNA)

THE EXERCISE

MATERIALS:

Computer, printer, modem, and appropriate software to access and navigate the World Wide Web (WWW) rRNA sequence of an unknown organism

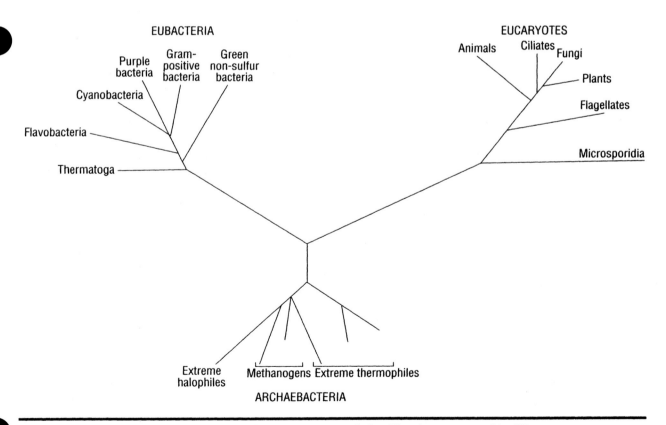

Figure 16.3 The three-kingdom system of classification proposed by Woese.

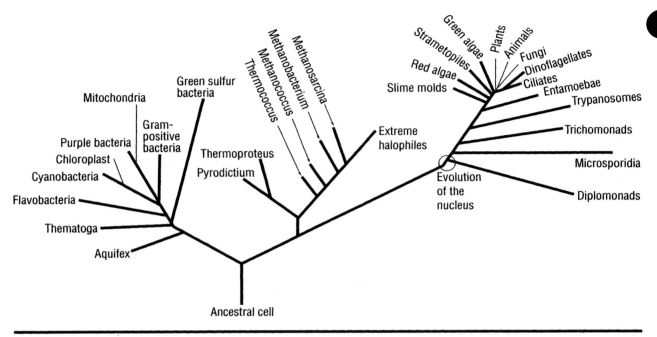

Figure 16.4 The three-domain classification system.

PROCEDURE: Work in pairs

1. Access the World Wide Web (WWW, also known as the Web) and go to the RDP home page (**Figure 16.5**). Its Web address is *http://rdpwww.life.uiuc.edu.* **Note:** Most colleges and universities have a home page that includes information about the WWW. If you have no experience exploring the Web, you may want to begin learning more about it. The RDP home page also has information about the WWW.

2. Once you reach the RDP home page, read it carefully. This home page allows you to connect quickly with other Web pages at the RDP site. Check a few of them out. We especially recommend "Frequently Asked Questions." **Note:** Most Web navigation software allows you to move to new Web sites or pages by pointing to highlighted phrases with a mouse and clicking on them. For others, move the cursor to the phrase, then give a command that takes you to the desired site. Your instructor will explain your software to you.

3. After exploring the RDP Web pages to get oriented, you are now ready to begin your project. If you are not already there, return to the RDP home page (**Figure 16.5**).

4. Go to the RDP Web page for the **Small Ribosomal Subunit (SSU)** database (**Figure 16.6**).

5. When you get to the **SSU** database, scroll down the page to the section titled **Analysis Services** (**Figure 16.6**).

6. In **Analysis Services,** find the service called **Similarity Rank.** Go to that Web page (**Figure 16.7**). This page allows you to enter the rRNA sequence of your unknown culture and have it compared to other sequences in the database. As a result of this comparison, you will be given the names of organisms with sequences most similar to yours.

7. Since you do not know what type of organism you have, begin by searching the SSU_Prok database. Do this by selecting that database (**Figure 16.7**).

8. To check all the organisms in that database, select "All organisms in the database" (**Figure 16.7**).

9. Scroll down the page a little further and enter a name for your sequence (e.g., Garibaldi, Joe, Susan) (**Figure 16.7**).

10. Just below the space for entering the sequence name is space for typing in the actual nucleotide sequence. Type the sequence in that space (**Figure 16.7**).

11. Below the sequence space is the section of the page called **Output Formatting.** Indicate that you want a list of the 20 most similar sequences.

12. Next indicate that you *do not* want to obtain a similarity ranking on the complement of your sequence.

Text continued on p. 106.

Ribosomal Database Project
University of Illinois at Urbana-Champaign
Department of Microbiology

←———————— GO HERE (Step 3)

The Ribosomal Database Project is supported by the National Science Foundation
Division of Biological Instrumentation and Resources (BIR 93-14392)

The Ribosomal Database Project offers curated ribosome related data, analysis services, and software.

Users should cite *Nucleic Acids Res.* 24:82-85 (1996) (which is the same as Medline ID 96174604) in publications that benefit from RDP services.

Welcome to the RDP's redesigned web pages! More changes will continue to be made over the next few months, including a release of new data. See the What's new section for more details.

If you are using Netscape 2.0 or other web browsers that support frames without easy movement between frames, look at Navigating Frames for some additional assistance.

General Information

Help!   Frequently-Asked Questions   Mail Us!   Register and Comment

Data

SSU Home Page   LSU Home Page

←————————————————————————————— GO HERE (Step 4)

Analysis Functions

Subalign   Subtree   Check Probe   Check Chimera

Similarity Rank   Align Sequence   Suggest Tree

Software

Other WWW Sites of Interest

Stay informed about the RDP by registering for the RDP email list.

Last modified October 25, 1996. Click! and BLM

Figure 16.5 The RDP home page.

Small Subunit Ribosomal   http://rdpwww.life.uiuc.edu/RDP/data/ssu.html

Small Subunit ribosomal RNA

The Ribosomal Database Project
Department of Microbiology, University of Illinois at Urbana-Champaign, USA.

Users should cite *Nucleic Acids Res.* 24:82-85 (1996) (which is the same as Medline ID 96174604) in publications that benefit from RDP services.

The SSU rRNA data files were last updated on 17-MAY-1995.

The Small Subunit rRNA data are divided into two functional groups, the Prokaryotic group and the Eukaryotic group. Each group has an associated alignment. New sequences that have not been curated or aligned can still be used for analysis functions; they are placed in the Unaligned group until they can be curated.

Organisms in the RDP Database

More than 3000 organisms occur in the RDP SSU rRNA data files. Most, but not all, of these organisms are available in aligned form and placed on a phylogenetic tree. Lists of the available organisms are provided as follows:

Prokaryotes in taxonomic or alphabetical order ◄─────────── GO HERE (Step 17)
Eukaryotes in taxonomic or alphabetical order
All organisms (including unaligned sequences) in alphabetical order

Data

The SSU alignments are offered in both GenBank and AE2 formats. **Caution:** these alignments are large. Select and download them only if you have enough disk space to do so.

Prokaryotic alignment in GenBank [12 MB] or AE2 [12 MB] format
Eukaryotic alignment in GenBank [2.6 MB] or AE2[2.6 MB] format
Phylogenetic tree of Prokaryotic organisms in
    PostScript(tm) format
    newick format
    text format
Phylogenetic tree of Eukaryotic organisms in
    PostScript(tm) format
    newick format
    text format
Secondary structure diagrams

Analysis Services ◄─────────────────────────── GO HERE (Step 5)

Most of the analysis services offered by the RDP can function on any organism found in the lists above. In many cases, such as probe checking, it will make sense for the user to perform the analysis on the entire database. However, it is often useful to restrict the operations of commands to smaller groups of organisms, i.e. only the Crenarchaeota. An organism selection utility is provided for this purpose, but users should see the organism selection instructions for details on how this utility works.

Extract a portion of an alignment (SUBALIGN)

Extract a portion of a phylogenetic tree (SUBTREE)

Check a probe (CHECK_PROBE)

Check a sequence for chimeras (CHECK_CHIMERA)

Find the most similar sequence (SIMILARITY_RANK) ◄─────────── GO HERE (Step 6)

Align a sequence (ALIGN_SEQUENCE)

Place an organism on a subtree (SUGGEST_TREE)

Help!

Any questions may be mailed to rdp@phylo.life.uiuc.edu.
Last modified October 25, 1996. Click! and BLM

Figure 16.6   Small ribosomal subunit RNA database home page.

Finding Similar Sequences http://rdpwww.life.uiuc.edu/RDP/commands/rank.html

Finding Similar Sequences (Similarity_rank)

The Ribosomal Database Project
Department of Microbiology, University of Illinois at Urbana-Champaign, USA.

This form allows you to find organisms in the RDP alignment that have sequences similar to your test sequence.

Source Selection

Which rRNA database would you like to search?

1. Small Subunit Prokaryotes (SSU_Prok). ← SELECT THIS FIRST (Step 7)
2. Small Subunit Eukaryotes (SSU_Euk).
3. All Small Subunit rRNAs from the unaligned database (SSU_Unal).
4. Large Subunit rRNAs (LSU_rRNA).
5. All Large Subunit rRNAs from the unaligned database (LSU_Unal).

Select the organism sequences you would like to rank your sequence against:

1. All organisms in the database. ← SELECT THIS (Step 8)
2. My custom list.
   Enter the Login name you saved your list under here: .
   If you need to configure a custom IDlist, visit the RDP organism selection page.
3. The RDP shortID: .

To restrict the analysis to a small range of positions that correspond to base positions in a specific organism, e.g. E. coli, enter an RDP organism shortID and position range below.

Organism RDP ShortID:

Start Column:

End Column:

Enter your sequence name: ← MAKE UP AND ENTER A NAME FOR YOUR SEQUENCE HERE (Step 9)

Enter your sequence here:

← TYPE YOUR SEQUENCE IN THIS SPACE (Step 10)

Output Formatting

When you submit this form, the server will compare your sequence to the RDP database and return a list of the most similar sequences. How long would you like this list to be? ← LIMIT THE LIST TO THE 20 MOST SIMILAR SEQUENCES (STEP 11)

Would you like to rank the complement of your sequence also?

No. ← YOU DO NOT WANT TO RANK THE COMPLEMENT (Step 12)
Yes.

To rank your sequence, press this button:. ← GO HERE (Step 13)

To reset this page to its default values, press this button:.

Help!

The SIMILARITY_RANK software PAL was written by Niels Larsen.

Any questions may be mailed to rdp@phylo.life.uiuc.edu.
Last modified October 25, 1996. Click! and BLM

Figure 16.7 Finding similar sequences home page.

13. Press the "Submit" button. Within a few moments, a page will appear with the list of most similar sequences.
14. Examine the list prepared for you by the RDP. The numbers next to each organism in the list are measures of similarity. A similarity value of 1.0 means your sequence is identical to the sequence in the database for that organism. If the number is very low (e.g., below 0.6), your organism is not a procaryote, and you will need to repeat the procedure, this time using the eucaryotic database.
15. Record the top five organisms in the list and the corresponding similarity values in the RESULTS section.
16. Return to the SSU rRNA database page (**Figure 16.6**).
17. Scroll down the page to the section titled **Organisms in the RDP Database**. From this section you can access information about the organisms that are most similar to yours.
18. Find your organism in either the procaryotic or eucaryotic alphabetical list and go to its Web page. Each organism's Web page provides considerable information.

19. Record the required information in the RESULTS section. If possible, look up the journal articles cited at the organism's Web page. The articles often describe the characteristics of the organism, how the sequence was obtained, and the research project that led to the archiving of this sequence.

REFERENCES

Brock, et. al. *Biology of Microorganisms*, 7th ed., Englewood Cliffs, NJ: Prentice-Hall, 1994.

Felsenstein, J. Phylogenies From Molecular Sequences: Inference and Reliability. *Annual Review of Genetics* 22(1988):521-565.

Maidek, B.L., et al. The Ribosomal Database Project. *Nucleic Acids Research* 22(1994):3485-3487.

Woese, C.R. Bacterial Evolution. *Microbiological Reviews* 51(1987):221-271.

Woese, C.R. et al. Towards a Natural System of Organisms: Proposal for the Domains Archaea, Bacteria, and Eucarya. *Proceedings of the National Academy of Sciences* 87(1990):4576-4579.

RESULTS

List the top five most similar organisms and their similarity rankings:

Information about your unknown:

Name: _____

Date sequence entered into database: _____

Articles cited: _____

Domain to which your organism belongs: _____

If Eukarya, was your sequence from cytoplasmic ribosomes, mitochondrial ribosomes, or chloroplast ribosomes?

REFLECTIONS

1. If your unknown is a procaryote, look it up in *Bergey's Manual of Systematic Bacteriology*. What are the major phenotypic characteristics of your organism?

2. If your unknown is a eucaryote, which line of descent would it be located along (e.g., ciliate, green algae, diplomonads) (See **Figure 16.4**) What are the major phenotypic features of this group?

3. In general, biologists prefer Whittaker's classification scheme to Woese's scheme. Why do you think this might be the case?

4. Recently, Woese's three-kingdom system (**Figure 16.3**) has been modified to a three-domain (or empire) system (**Figure 16.4**). Why might this modification be more acceptable to biologists?

5. In a sense, you may have acted as an evolutionary force on the rRNA gene that you worked with in this exercise. How is that so? (Hint: Think about your typing skills.)

EXERCISE 17

GROWING VIRUSES

In the previous exercises, you have learned about those microbes that are cellular and obviously alive. Now you will turn your attention to a group of microbes that are acellular and do not exhibit all the characteristics of life—the viruses.

Samantha plopped her tired, hot, and slightly sunburned body into her favorite chair. She sipped cold lemonade as she checked her "Yard Things to Do" list. It had been a busy month. First, her graduation from college with a degree in chemical engineering. Then, starting her new job at DuPont and preparing for her wedding. Samantha had spent the last week cleaning the backyard for the wedding. With the yard work done, she had 2 days to rest before the big day. Samantha leaned her head back and dozed briefly. Half asleep, she barely noticed a slight tingling sensation on her upper lip. Instinctively, she reached up and rubbed the spot a few times.

The next morning Samantha slept in. "I need my beauty sleep," she had joked with her mother the night before. It had been a long and restful night. As she yawned and stretched awake, she felt a strong itching sensation on her upper lip. She reached up to scratch it. "Ouch!" She sat straight up in bed and carefully probed the spot on her lip. "Oh, no!" she yelled as she jumped out of bed and ran to the mirror. "Not a cold sore!"

BACKGROUND INFORMATION

Samantha's cold sore, caused by herpes simplex virus I (HSV I), clearly demonstrates that viruses can cause diseases in humans. HSV I, like all other viruses, is an obligate intracellular parasite. That is,

viruses can only reproduce inside cells of a host organism. Humans aren't the only organisms infected by viruses. Non-human animals, plants, algae, fungi, and bacteria are also infected. Viruses that infect and reproduce within bacteria are known as **bacteriophages** or **phages** for short. Most bacteriophages, like most human viruses, harm their host cells. Despite their harmful effects, it is important to note that much of our understanding of DNA replication and the control of gene expression has come from studies of viral replication.

Working with an animal virus such as HSV I is not feasible in a general microbiology teaching. Bacteriophages, however, can be manipulated by students quite easily and successfully. In this exercise you will work with the bacteriophage T_4 (**Figure 17.1**). T_4's host is the bacterium *Escherichia coli*. If T_4 viruses are mixed with *E. coli* cells, the

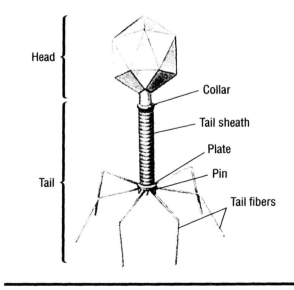

Figure 17.1 Bacteriophage T_4.

viruses attach to cells and inject their DNA. Once inside the cell, the T_4 DNA enables the phage to take over the cell's genetic machinery and use it to generate more T_4 particles. At the end of this reproductive process, each infected cell is literally packed with new virus particles; the cell bursts in a phenomenon called **lysis** and the viruses are released (**Figure 17.2**). The released viruses can then infect other nearby *E. coli* cells.

If T_4 infects bacteria growing on a solid surface, it is possible to see the result of lysing the bacterial cells. Imagine bacterial cells spread so close to each other on a medium that after incubation they produce **confluent growth** covering the entire medium. Microbial geneticists often call this a lawn of bacteria. Now imagine that one cell in the lawn is infected with T_4. That cell will eventually lyse, releasing new viruses. These viruses will infect cells nearby. Those cells will lyse and release more viruses, and so on. When the lawn of cells is examined after an appropriate incubation period, it is confluent everywhere except where the infected cell was located. In that area, a small clear spot is seen; it contains no bacteria because they have been lysed. This clear spot is called a **plaque**. Though a plaque appears empty, it is in fact loaded with virus particles, which can be, if desired, isolated from the plaque.

In this exercise, you will prepare a soft agar overlay containing T_4 and *E. coli*. This creates an even, confluent lawn against which plaques are easily seen. In addition, it spreads the viruses out so that isolated plaques are observed. The T_4 stock you will use contains between 1×10^9 to 1×10^{11} virus particles/ml. Therefore, the sample must be diluted so that between 30 and 300 plaques are observed.[1] You will prepare the phage stock for plating by making a set of dilutions called **serial dilutions** (**Figure 17.3**). To ensure that the proper number of plaques per plate is observed (i.e., 30 to 300), 0.1 ml aliquots from three different dilutions will be plated.

PURPOSE

- To illustrate that viruses can be propagated or grown in culture
- To enable you to see one effect viruses have on their host cells—the lysis of cells and the formation of plaques

---

[1] The range 30 to 300 is one you will encounter not only when counting plaques, but when enumerating bacteria by the plate count method (see Exercise 20). This range is used for three reasons. First, 30 is high enough to be statistically accurate. Second, 300 colonies or plaques are easily counted with relatively little error. Finally, when dealing with colonies, having only 300 or fewer colonies forming on a plate avoids nutrient competition that might result if the colonies are more densely packed on the medium.

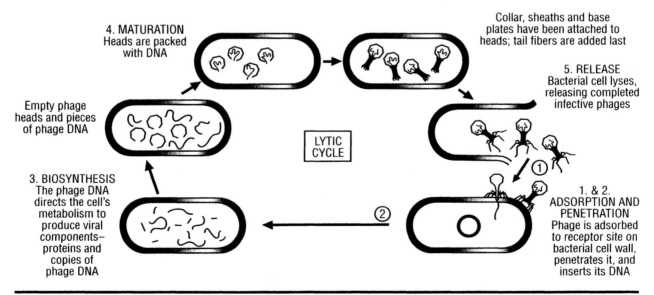

Figure 17.2 The life cycle of T_4 virus.

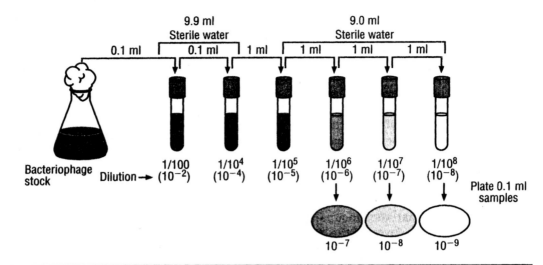

Figure 17.3 Preparing serial dilutions of the T_4 phage stock.

THE EXERCISE

MATERIALS:

Overnight culture of *E. coli* strain B

Two tubes of 9.9 ml dilution blanks

Three *T*ryptone sodium chloride (*N*aCl) *A*gar plates, (TNA plates) warmed to 37°C

Three tubes of molten *T*ryptone *N*aCl soft agar (TN soft agar) held at 50°C

Sample of T_4 stock

Four tubes of 9.0 ml dilution blanks

0.1 ml pipets, 1.0 ml pipets, and pipet aids or micropipetters and pipet tips

50°C water bath

PROCEDURE: Work in groups of two or three

Day 1

1. Arrange the dilution blanks in a rack in the order shown in **Figure 17.3.** Label the tubes as indicated (e.g., 10^{-2}, 10^{-4}, etc.).
2. Label the three TNA plates 10^{-7}, 10^{-8}, 10^{-9}. Also label the plates with your name and date.
3. Use a micropipetter or 0.1 ml pipet to transfer 100 microliters (µl) (0.1 ml) of the phage stock into the tube labeled 10^{-2}. Adding 0.1 ml of the sample to 9.9 ml of the diluent gives a 1/100 (1:100) dilution. Mix gently by rolling the tube between your hands or flicking the bottom of the tube with your fingers. **Note:** Your instructor will demonstrate the use of the micropipetter (or the 0.1 ml pipet and pipet aid). Use a new pipet tip (or pipet) for each step of the dilution series. This

is important because if the same tip or pip used, viruses attached to that tip or pipet wi transferred to the next tube along with viruses that are supposed to be transferre subsequent dilution steps. As a result, the tions are incorrect.

4. Transfer 0.1 ml of the 10^{-2} dilution into the labeled 10^{-4}. Adding 0.1 ml of the 10^{-2} dilt to 9.9 ml of diluent further dilutes the stock factor of 1/100, giving a final dilution of Mix gently.
5. Transfer 1.0 ml of the 10^{-4} dilution into the labeled 10^{-5}. Adding 1.0 ml of the 10^{-4} dilt to 9 ml of diluent further dilutes the stock factor of 1/10 (1:10), giving a final dilutic 10^{-5}. Mix gently.
6. Continue making serial dilutions as show **Figure 17.3.**
7. Add 0.1 ml of *E. coli* strain B to a tube of TN agar. **Note:** The TN soft agar tubes are in a : water bath and should be kept in the water until ready to pour into the TNA plates. The solidifies very quickly once removed from water bath.
8. Add 0.1 ml of the 10^{-6} dilution of T_4 to the soft agar.
9. Quickly mix the agar, cells, and viruse: flicking the bottom of the tube or rolling the between your hands, then pour into the ' plate labeled 10^{-7}.
10. Repeat steps 7 through 9 for the 10^{-7} dilt and 10^{-8} TNA plate.

11. Repeat steps 7 through 9 for the 10^{-8} dilution and 10^{-9} TNA plate.
12. When the agar hardens, invert the plates and incubate at 37°C overnight.

Day 2

1. Examine your group's plates by holding them up to the light and looking through them. Notice that most of the medium is opaque due to the confluent growth of *E. coli*, but that scattered around the medium are small transparent areas. These are plaques.

2. Count the number of plaques on each plate and record your results. If a plate has more than 300 plaques, the plaques are considered to be too numerous to count (TNTC), and the count for that plate should be recorded as such.

REFERENCES

Brock, T.D., et al. *Biology of Microorganisms*, 7th ed., Englewood Cliffs, NJ: Prentice-Hall, 1994.

Mathews, C. *Bacteriophage* T_4. Washington, DC: American Society for Microbiology Press, 1983.

RESULTS

Record the number of plaques observed:

10^{-7} plate _____

10^{-8} plate _____

10^{-9} plate _____

REFLECTIONS

1. What is the minimum number of viruses you added to your cells? Why is this the minimum number?

2. Why was the plate used for plating the 10^{-6} dilution labeled 10^{-7}?

3. What was the concentration of viruses (virus/ml) in the original stock solution?

4. How is a viral plaque similar to a bacterial colony?

5. How does HSV I's life cycle differ from bacteriophage T_4's life cycle?

6. Samantha has a history of cold sores. She's been getting them periodically since she was a child. Should she have been surprised by her current outbreak? Explain.

WHAT KIND OF MICROBE IS IT?

Each of the previous seventeen exercises has introduced you to microorganisms of a eucaryotic, procaryotic, and viral nature. You learned new techniques that allowed you to microscopically and biochemically characterize microorganisms. In this exercise you will use these characteristics to identify two microbes. Good luck!

BACKGROUND INFORMATION

Identification of a microorganism includes determining if it belongs to an established taxon. But before it can be assigned to a **taxonomic** group, the organism must be named. **Nomenclature** is the assignment of names to organisms and putting them in taxonomic groups according to international rules. The assignment is based on similarities and differences between organisms. Sometimes this can be difficult because few anatomical or visual differences exist. Nevertheless, many identification schemes have been developed to separate and name microorganisms.

One such scheme is shown in **Table 18.1**. It is called a **dichotomous** identification scheme because it is repeatedly divided into two parts until a characteristic identifies a single member. This key works only for the microorganisms listed in it. To identify an unknown microorganisms at large, numerous characteristics and keys would be used.

Another approach many people use to identify a microorganism is to develop a flow chart. Flow charts can be made by taking the dichotomous key and using the same division to develop a "flow" of information about the microorganisms until an identification is made. Both of these keys are called "artificial keys" because there is no single correct way to write one.

Most schemes for classification already assume that you know the microorganism is procaryotic or eucaryotic. This one, however, assumes no such previous knowledge. Therefore, you must first determine whether your microorganism is a procaryote or eucaryote. One important characteristic that distinguishes procaryotes and eucaryotes is size. Procaryotes are almost always much smaller (1 to 10 micrometers) than eucaryotes, which vary greatly in size from 10 micrometers to 100 or greater. Of course, there are exceptions to this rule, but for the microbes you will identify in this exercise, a culture and microscopic examination of their size should quickly lead you down the right path. If you feel confirmation is needed, a Wright's stain or methylene blue stain can be done to detect nuclei of your microbes.

It is up to you to decide which tests are needed to identify your unknowns; you get two. Keep efficiency in mind and do not perform unnecessary tests. Choose tests that split all possible species into two groups. Observation of growth characteristics from cultures, wet mounts, and stains should give you clues about how to proceed. Avoid contamination of your unknowns by ascertaining the purity of your cultures and by using good aseptic technique. Also reduce confusion by recording the results of tests as soon as you observe them and by keeping an accurate log of your work.

You have performed most of the biochemical tests in previous exercises. However, there are a few tests you are not familiar with and they will be explained in the procedure of this exercise. Follow the key or flow chart you make to determine the identity of your unknown and *do not* perform unnecessary tests.

PURPOSE

- To learn about identification schemes and how these are used to identify organisms
- To identify two unknown microbes and report your results in a lab report

THE EXERCISE

MATERIALS:

Two unknown broth culture tubes per person, each containing any one of the nineteen microorganisms listed in **Table 18.1**.

Other media and reagents available on request:

Animal plasma (germ tube test)
Mannitol fermentation broth
0.3 ml saline in tubes
Malachite green solution (endospore stain)
Gram-stain reagents
LPCB stain
New methylene blue N solution
Potato dextrose agar plates
Trypticase soy agar plates
3% hydrogen peroxide
ONPG disks
Tryptone broth
Kovac's reagent (indole test)
Sudan black B (PHB stain)
Microscope slides
Coverslips
Pasteur pipets
Small test tubes

PROCEDURE:

1. Examine the tubes of the unknowns. Determine if each microbe is, or can be, uniformly dispersed throughout the medium. If not, describe the growth in the tube.
2. Prepare a wet mount of each unknown to begin your observations. **Note:** You may use either bright-field or phase microscopy to view your preparations.
3. To avoid the unnecessary "shotgun" approach of doing every stain and every biochemical test, develop a flow chart based on the dichotomous key shown in **Table 18.1**.
4. Have your instructor review this chart before proceeding with the identification of your unknowns.
5. Proceed with the identification of your unknowns following the flow chart or dichotomous key.

TABLE 18.1 Key to the Abbreviated Identification of Selected Microorganisms

I. Eucaryotes
  A. Chloroplast present—Algae
    1. Motile, unicellular: *Euglena* sp.
    2. Nonmotile, filamentous: *Spyrogyra* sp.
  B. Chloroplast absent
    1. Motile—Protozoa
      a. Ciliated: *Paramecium* sp.
      b. Flagellated: *Giardia lamblia*
    2. Nonmotile—Fungi
      a. Unicellular, budding—Yeast
        1. Makes germ tubes: *Candida albicans*
        2. Does not make germ tubes: *Saccharomyces cerevisiae*
      b. Hyphae formed—Moulds
        1. Long sporangiophore with dark, round sporangium containing sporangiospores, nonseptate hyphae, rhizoids present: *Rhizopus*
        2. Conidiophore terminates in swollen vesicle, phialides and conidiospores, septate hyphae, no rhizoids: *Aspergillus*

II. Procaryotes
  A. Gram-positive cells
    1. Rods
      a. Endospores present
        1. Acid from mannitol, no PHB[1] inclusions: *Bacillus subtilis*
        2. No acid from mannitol, produces PHB inclusions: *Bacillus cereus*
      b. No endospores present
        1. Catalase positive, club-shaped cells: *Corynebacterium* sp.
        2. Catalase negative: *Lactobacillus* sp.
    2. Cocci
      a. Cells in pairs and chains, catalase negative: *Streptococcus* sp.
      b. Cells in clusters, catalase positive: *Staphylococcus* sp.
  B. Gram-negative cells
    1. Rods
      a. Oxidase positive: *Pseudomonas* sp.
      b. Oxidase negative
        1. Indole positive: *Escherichia coli*
        2. Indole negative: *Klebsiella pneumoniae*
    2. Cocci, oxidase positive
      a. Acid from lactose (ONPG +): *Neisseria lactamica*
      b. No acid from lactose (ONPG −): *Moraxella catarrhalis*

[1]PHB is poly-β-hydroxybutyrate inclusion bodies (Sudan black B stain).

6. Request additional media or reagents after you have completed the preliminary observations of your microorganisms. If you must perform new additional tests, such as catalase, ONPG, or methylene blue stain, be sure to observe the test results with positive and negative controls set up by your instructor.

7. Your final task is to report the findings for each unknown in a different kind of laboratory report. This laboratory report will utilize a recording system that is similar to the ones used every day in clinical laboratories to identify and report culture results. The report should give your instructor a clear idea of the steps you took each day to identify your microbes. Use the REPORT forms to indicate these steps, including the identity of each of your unknowns. The tests, of course, should reflect the logical thinking from the flow chart you developed. Include the flow chart you developed for each microbe with your laboratory report. Alternatively, your instructor may ask you to write a formal lab report.

ADDITIONAL TESTS

Catalase Test

Organisms that possess the enzyme catalase are able to decompose hydrogen peroxide to water and oxygen. Normally, hydrogen peroxide is accumulated as a result of aerobic carbohydrate metabolism and can be lethal if not decomposed. In this test, microorganisms with catalase break down a 3% concentration of H_2O_2 and produce visible oxygen gas bubbles. Catalase is a hemoprotein which is also found in red blood cells. Therefore, when testing a microbe growing on a blood medium, care must be taken to avoid disturbing any red blood cells and falsely testing their catalase activity, too.

MATERIALS:

3% hydrogen peroxide and glass slides

PROCEDURE:

1. Put one drop of 3% H_2O_2 on a glass slide.
2. Transfer the top of a well-isolated colony with an applicator stick or needle to the H_2O_2 on the slide.
3. Look for the appearance of gas bubbles.

INTERPRETATION:

Positive: Formation of gas bubbles
Negative: No gas bubbles produced

CONTROLS:

A known catalase-positive and catalase-negative microorganism should be used to check the stability of the hydrogen peroxide.

ONPG Test

To utilize lactose, a microorganism must possess two distinct enzymes, **lactose permease**, which allows lactose to enter the bacterial cell, and β-**galactosidase**, which breaks down lactose to galactose and glucose. The ortho-nitrophenyl-beta-D-galactosidase (ONPG) test is a rapid test useful in determining whether a microorganism has the enzyme β-galactosidase and can hydrolyze lactose. Some microbes have β-galactosidase but not lactose permease. These microorganisms utilize lactose slowly (delayed lactose-fermenters) because even though they do not have lactose permease, lactose will slowly diffuse across the cell membrane. ONPG is an alternative substrate for the enzyme β-galactosidase. ONPG enters the cell without the aid of permease and is hydrolyzed by β-galactosidase (**Figure 18.1**). Therefore, ONPG is useful for detecting β-galactosidase in microorganisms that do not have lactose permease. Hydrolysis of ONPG by β-galactosidase yields o-nitrophenol, a yellow compound, and galactose. The development of a yellow color indicates the microorganism has β-galactosidase (hydrolyzes lactose) and is a lactose fermenter.

MATERIALS:

ONPG disks and small test tubes with 0.3 ml of saline

PROCEDURE:

1. Inoculate 0.3 ml of saline with enough microorganism to make a heavy suspension.
2. Aseptically add one ONPG disk to the tube.
3. Incubate the tube at 35°C for 2 hours.

INTERPRETATION:

Positive: A yellow color in the solution. A positive test can occur in as little as 10 minutes with a heavy inoculum
Negative: No color change within 2 hours

METHYLENE BLUE STAIN

This stain is used to stain the nuclei of cells. It should only be used if you are having a difficult time determining whether your unknown is a yeast. In yeast cells the nucleus will stain dark blue, distinguishing it from the much lighter background of the

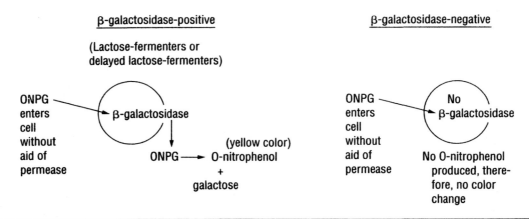

Figure 18.1   A diagram of β-galactosidase-positive and -negative reactions.

cytoplasm. Gram-positive cocci such as staphylococci and streptococci will stain a uniform dark blue color. Remember staphylococci and streptococci are much smaller than yeast, do not bud, and do not have a nucleus. This stain should only be performed as a backup to the Gram stain and only if you are unclear about having a yeast as an unknown.

MATERIALS:

New methylene blue N solution
Microscope slides
Small test tubes
Pasteur pipet

PROCEDURE:

1. Make a suspension of your microorganism in water.
2. Add 3 drops of the suspension to a small test tube.

3. Add 3 drops of the methylene blue solution to the tube.
4. Mix and allow the mixture to stand for 10 minutes at room temperature.
5. Mix the tube again and add 1 drop to a microscope slide.
6. Using another slide or your pipet, spread the solution over the slide.
7. Allow it to dry and view the smear under the microscope.

INTERPRETATION:

Yeast nuclei stain a dark blue and are distinguished easily from the clear or light blue cytoplasm. Procaryotic microbes are much smaller and will stain dark blue throughout the cell.

REPORT FORM   Name_____

List the dates you performed tests, along with their results, in consecutive order.

Date: _____

Wet mount:_____

Unknown #_____   Identification_____

REPORT FORM

Name_____ ●

List the dates you performed tests, along with their results, in consecutive order.

Date: _____

Wet mount:_____

Unknown #_____   Identification _____ ●

FLOW CHART(S) FOR IDENTIFICATION OF UNKNOWNS

SECTION III

MICROBIAL GROWTH AND REPRODUCTION

As you have learned in the previous exercises, microbes come in a variety of sizes and shapes. They are found in many different habitats and they vary with respect to their tolerance of environmental conditions. But all organisms share one common goal: reproduction. In order to reproduce, organisms obtain energy from their environment and use it for biosynthetic processes that ultimately lead to reproduction. In this section, you will learn how microbes obtain energy. You will also explore life cycles and population growth of microbes.

EXERCISE 19

THE QUEST FOR ENERGY

In previous exercises, you have explored some of the mechanisms used by microbes to obtain energy from their environments. You have examined the ability of microbes to use different sugars and amino acids as sources of energy. You have observed how bacteria can be identified using differential media that detect fermentative and respiratory activity. Thus far, your attention has been focused on organisms that use organic molecules as a source of energy. In this exercise, you will learn about other mechanisms for obtaining energy and also discover some of the common themes observed in metabolic processes.

Gil had worked hard to become a top-notch science writer. The effort had paid off—he was now writing for the leading popular science magazine published in the United States. Attaining that goal brought him great satisfaction, but the news he had just received was frosting on the cake. His editor had just told him about his next assignment. He was to join a team of scientists studying hydrothermal vents more than 2,000 meters below the surface of the Pacific Ocean. He was to observe first-hand an exotic ecosystem powered primarily by chemolithotrophic bacteria—bacteria that use inorganic molecules as a source of energy. What was also amazing about these bacteria is that they survive and flourish at extremely high temperatures and pressures. Gil would leave in a week, but it seemed like an eternity.

BACKGROUND INFORMATION

In 1977, scientists first observed the surprisingly rich ecosystems near hydrothermal vents. What was most interesting about these ecosystems was that they were *not* totally dependent on photosynthetic organisms as primary producers. Instead, the primary producers used inorganic molecules such as hydrogen sulfide (H_2S), hydrogen gas (H_2), and thiosulfate ($S_2O_3^{2-}$) as sources of energy.

Microbiologists have long been aware that microbes, bacteria in particular, exhibit great diversity in their ability to obtain energy from the environment. There are two major groups of organisms, **chemotrophs** and **phototrophs**. Chemotrophic organisms use chemical molecules as a source of energy and phototrophs use light as a source of energy. The chemotrophs can be further distinguished based on the type of molecule used. **Chemolithotrophs,** as already noted, use inorganic molecules, whereas **chemoorganotrophs** use organic molecules.

At first glance, processes that obtain energy from light, organic molecules, and inorganic molecules would seem to be very different. But in fact, these processes are united by certain unifying concepts. At the core of all metabolic processes that provide energy for organisms are **oxidation/reduction** reactions. In the case of chemotrophs, the molecule oxidized is the energy source. In the case of phototrophs, light-gathering molecules such as chlorophyll are oxidized after they absorb light. The electrons released by the oxidations are accepted by various molecules depending on the metabolic process (**Figure 19.1**). With the exception of fermentation, all electrons released from or by an energy source are passed down a chain of electron acceptors. These electron acceptors are components of large enzyme complexes and are embedded in membranes and called **electron transport systems** (ETS). The passage of electrons through an ETS is accompanied by movement of protons unidirectionally across the membrane. This establishes a proton gradient and a charge difference across the membrane which is referred to as the **proton motive force** (PMF).

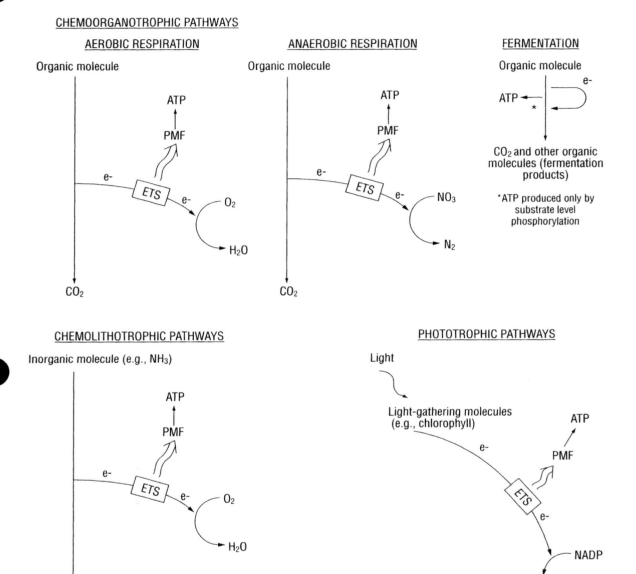

Figure 19.1 A comparison of various energy-providing metabolic processes. Movement of electrons through the ETS leads to formation of the PMF, which is used to synthesize ATP.

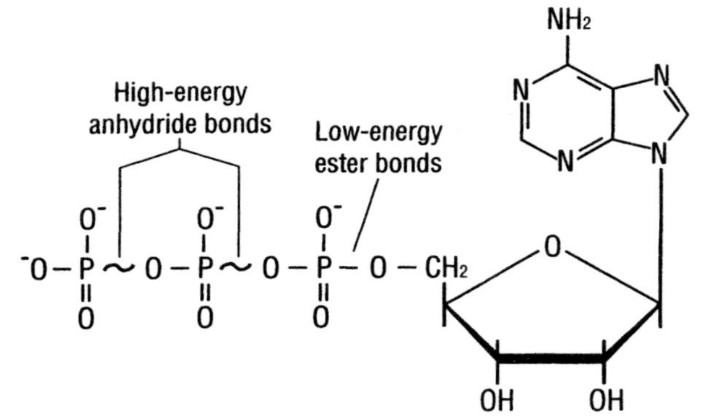

High-energy
anhydride bonds   Low-energy
                   ester bonds

Figure 19.2   Structure of ATP.

But how is the energy released by oxidation/reduction reactions conserved in a form easily used by organisms? The answer to that question brings us to another unifying concept—the use of a common energy currency, **adenosine triphosphate** (ATP). ATP conserves energy, for the most part, in two high-energy phosphate bonds (**Figure 19.2**). When one or both of these bonds are hydrolyzed, the energy released can be used to drive endergonic, or energy-consuming, processes (**Figure 19.3**) such as amino acid biosynthesis.

ATP is produced by three different processes: **substrate-level phosphorylation, oxidative phosphorylation** and **photophosphorylation**. Substrate-level phosphorylation occurs when high energy intermediates of a catabolic pathway (e.g., phosphoenolpyruvate, or PEP) are hydrolyzed. The hydrolysis is coupled to phosphorylation (addition of phosphate) of ADP, yielding ATP. The energy released by hydrolysis of PEP is transferred to the newly formed ATP molecule. Oxidative phosphorylation results from the coupling of electron transport through an ETS to generation of a PMF. When cells cause protons to move down the gradient (i.e., from an area of high concentration to an area of low concentration), ATP synthase (ATPase) phosphorylates ADP to ATP. Photophosphorylation results from light-driven electron transport through an ETS. Again a PMF is established and used for ATP synthesis.

During this exercise, you will observe and measure the respiratory activity and ATP levels of cells. In Part A, you will observe respiratory activity of bacterial cells. This is done by exposing cells to 2-(4-iodophenyl)-3-(4-nitrophenyl)-5-tetrazolium chloride, mercifully called INT. The typical ETS consists of specific enzymes involved in the transport of electrons to a terminal electron acceptor. Some of these enzymes will catalyze the transport of electrons to alternate electron acceptors such as INT. When INT is reduced, it produces dark red crystals that absorb light maximally at 485 nm (**Figure 19.4**). An increase in absorption at 485 nm after exposing cells to INT is a measure of the respiratory activity of that population.

In Part B, you will use the luciferin/luciferase assay to measure the amount of ATP in bacterial populations of different cell densities. This assay is based on the light-producing reaction that occurs in

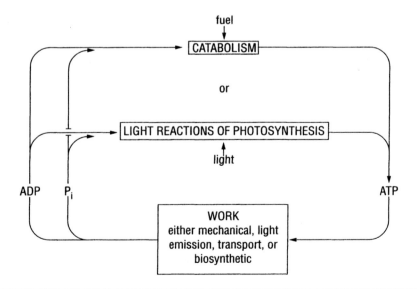

Figure 19.3   The ATP/ADP cycle in cells.

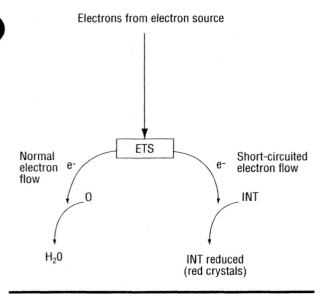

Figure 19.4 The "short-circuiting" of electron flow by INT. The production of the reduced form of INT (red crystals) indicates cells are respiring.

firefly tails. A similar reaction occurs in some bacteria. Light is emitted when luciferin is oxidized. This endergonic reaction is driven by the hydrolysis of ATP to AMP (**Figure 19.5**). The luciferin/luciferase assay is routinely used by microbiologists to measure the physiological state of microbial populations and to determine biomass, which is the size of a microbial population. In this exercise, the luciferin/luciferase assay serves the purpose of not only demonstrating the measurement of ATP, but also ATP's role in driving endergonic reactions in cells.

PURPOSE

- To explore the different mechanisms microbes use to obtain energy from their environments
- To observe respiratory activity in bacterial cells
- To measure the amount of ATP in bacterial cultures of different cell densities

THE EXERCISE

Part A: Measurement of Respiratory Activity

MATERIALS:

Escherichia coli strain K12 in 0.85% NaCl (pH 6.5) at a density of ~10^{10} cells/ml
1 M sodium malonate
Sterile water

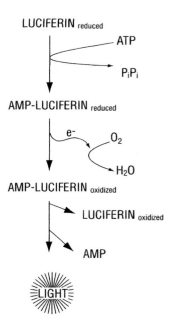

Figure 19.5 The light-generating oxidation reaction of luciferin.

Test tubes
Spectrophotometer and cuvette
10 mM INT
10× phosphate buffer (100 mM potassium phosphate buffer containing 8.5% NaCl and 50 mM $MgCl_2$ at pH 6.5)
Shaker
Formaldehyde

PROCEDURE: Work in groups of two or three

1. Obtain three test tubes and add the reagents shown below to each. **Note:** Sodium malonate inhibits electron transport.

	Tube 1	Tube 2	Tube 3
10× phosphate buffer	100 μl	100 μl	100 μl
E. coli cells	100 μl	—	100 μl
Water	700 μl	800 μl	600 μl
1 M sodium malonate	—	—	100 μl
10 mM INT	100 μl	100 μl	100 μl

2. Shake the tubes vigorously at 25°C for 2 hours. **Note:** If you are also doing Part B, then do so during this incubation period.
3. Add formaldehyde to each tube so that the final concentration is 3.7%. **Note:** Formaldehyde stops the reaction by killing the cells.

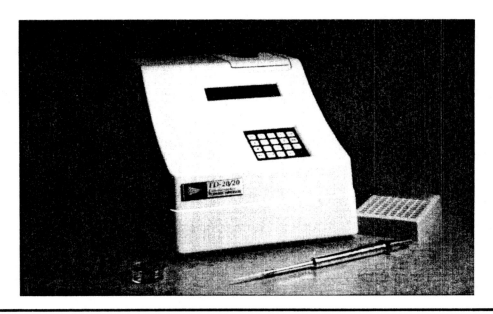

Figure 19.6 A luminometer. (Courtesy of Turner Designs.)

Caution: Formaldehyde is a potential carcinogen. It is also a skin and eye irritant, and is toxic if ingested. Wear gloves and handle with care.

4. Transfer the solution in Tube 1 to a cuvette and measure the absorbance of light at 485 nm. Record the reading in the RESULTS section.

5. Rinse the cuvette several times with water and repeat step 4 with Tubes 2 and 3.

Part B: Measurement of ATP

MATERIALS:

Serial dilutions of an overnight culture of *E. coli*
ATP releasing agent
Luciferin/luciferase reagent
Luminometer
Luminometer tubes
HEPES buffer
Water
ATP standard curve

PROCEDURES: Work in groups of two or three

1. Obtain a sample of *E. coli* cells and a luminometer tube. **Note**: Different groups will use samples of different cell densities so you can see the correlation between population size (biomass) and ATP levels. Data from all groups will be used to complete the table in the RESULTS section.

2. Prepare the following reaction mixture in the luminometer tube. **Note:** Your instructor will prepare the blank (no cells control).
   Blank: To be prepared by instructor
      50 µl water
      50 µl ATP releasing agent
      50 µl HEPES buffer
   Cells: To be prepared by students
      50 µl cell sample
      50 µl ATP releasing agent
      50 µl HEPES buffer

3. Place the tube in the luminometer and put the injector in place (**Figure 19.6**).

4. Add 100 µl of luciferin/luciferase. The amount of luciferin and luciferase added is in great excess to the amount of ATP in each sample. Therefore, the light emitted will be proportional to the amount of ATP in each sample.

5. Read the light output and record in the RESULTS section.

6. Use the ATP standard curve to determine the amount of ATP/ml in your sample.

REFERENCES

Brock, et al. *Biology of Microorganisms*, 7th ed., Englewood Cliffs, NJ: Prentice-Hall, 1994.

Nelson, W.H., ed. *Instrumental Methods for Rapid Microbiological Analysis*. Deerfield Beach, FL: VCH Publishers, 1985.

Smith, J.J., and McFeters, G.A. Effects of Substrates and Phosphate on INT (2-(4-iodophenyl)- 3-(4-nitrophenyl)-5-phenyl tetrazolium chloride) and CTC (5-cyano-2,3-ditolyl tetrazolium chloride) Reduction in *Escherichia coli. Journal of Applied Bacteriology* 80(1996):209-215.

Tunnicliffe, U. Hydrothermal Vent Communities of the Deep Sea. *American Scientist* 80:(1992)336-349.

RESULTS

Respiratory Activity of *E. coli* Strain 12:

	Absorbance 485 nm
Tube 1	
Tube 2	
Tube 3	

ATP Measurement of Different Cell Densities:

	Photon Units	ATP (µg/ml)
No cells		
10^{-6} Dilution of cells		
10^{-4} Dilution of cells		
10^{-2} Dilution of cells		
Undiluted cells		

REFLECTIONS

1. In Part A, three different tubes were prepared. What information does each tube provide? Why was it important to include all three to demonstrate respiratory activity of microbes?

2. Was the respiratory activity measured in Part A the result of aerobic or anaerobic electron transport? Explain. (Hint: You shook the reaction tubes vigorously during the 2-hour incubation period.)

3. There are a number of high-energy compounds generated by the metabolic reactions of cells. Using your textbook or another source, list three. What are the Gibb's free energy changes that occur when these molecules are hydrolyzed?

4. Consult your textbook or another source to find the Gibb's free energy change that occurs when glucose-6-phosphate is hydrolyzed. Compare this value to that of hydrolysis of ATP and the three molecules listed in Question 3. What can you say about ATP's role in metabolism based on these comparisons?

FIRST THERE WAS ONE, THEN THERE WERE TWO

The ultimate goal of the quest for energy is reproduction. In this exercise and the next, you will learn more about the reproduction of microbes. In this exercise, your focus will be on the growth of bacterial populations and how the size of a population can be measured.

The turkey was stuffed and in the oven, being cooked by the low, slow, sleep-in-the-next-morning method. By cooking the turkey at an oven temperature of 200°F overnight, the Gibson family could relax and enjoy their holiday. After placing the turkey in the oven, the cutting board, used for preparing and stuffing the turkey, was wiped dry with a paper towel and left on the kitchen counter. When the Gibsons awoke the next morning, the turkey was examined by all and then basted a few times. It looked juicy and tender and was well on its way to being done. Dinner would easily be ready by 2:00 P.M. At 10:30 A.M. the cutting board was used to prepare carrot sticks, celery sticks stuffed with cream cheese, and other vegetables to be served raw as part of the relish tray. The relish tray was assembled, covered loosely with plastic wrap, and placed on the counter. The cutting board was wiped clean with a damp cloth. At noon, the turkey was removed from the oven. The kitchen was warm enough to keep the turkey warm. At about 1:30 P.M., the turkey was transferred to the cutting board. About half of the meat was carved and enough stuffing to fill one serving bowl was removed. The rest was left in the warm turkey. The guests began arriving at 2:00 P.M. Dinner was delicious and everyone ate their fill. The children ran off to play while the adults relaxed around the table. No one felt like cleaning up. At about 6:00 P.M., a few people began nibbling again, so more meat and stuffing were removed from the turkey that had been left

sitting on the kitchen counter. Both were still somewhat warm, and pouring a little hot gravy on top made a tasty snack. At 8:00 P.M., the guests began to head home. The kitchen was eventually cleaned and the leftovers refrigerated. The remains of the turkey and the stuffing it contained were refrigerated intact. It had been a long day and none of the Gibsons had the energy to completely carve and empty the turkey. The next night, at about 10:00 P.M., one of the Gibson children awoke with severe stomach cramps and diarrhea. Within four hours, all the members of the Gibson family were suffering from similar symptoms. Fortunately, the hospital was nearby. The Gibsons quickly drove to the emergency room, where they were examined and fecal specimens obtained. The diagnosis was salmonellosis. The Gibsons were sent home with instructions to warn their guests that they may also become ill. Everyone, including several of the guests, recovered without treatment.

BACKGROUND INFORMATION

Unfortunately for the Gibson family and their guests, microbes such as *Salmonella* do not celebrate holidays by eating and relaxing. Whenever microbes have a ready food supply, they will do what they do so well: reproduce. Most bacteria reproduce by **binary fission.** This relatively simple reproductive process involves enlargement of the parent cell, followed by splitting into two progeny cells. The enlargement and division of one cell are not easily or conveniently observed. Therefore, when microbiologists study microbial growth, they are usually referring to the increase in numbers of microbes in a population that results from active reproduction.

Microbiologists have developed a variety of methods for measuring the number of cells in a population. The most obvious approach is to simply count

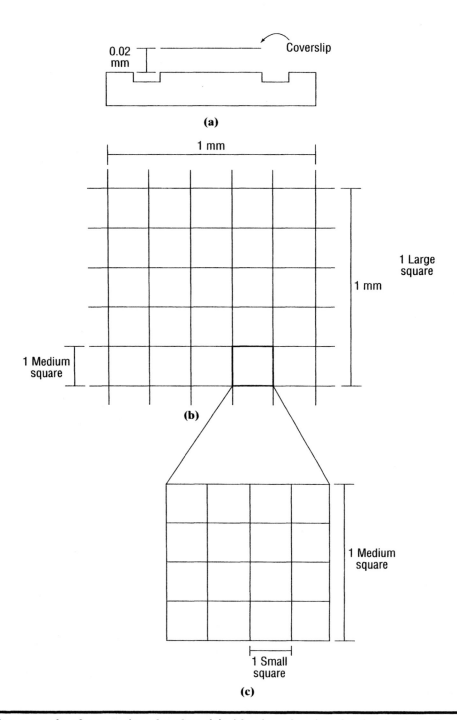

Figure 20.1   An example of a counting chamber: (a) side view showing the depth of the liquid between the coverslip and slide, (b) the grid observed when examined through the microscope, and (c) close-up of one medium square showing the small squares.

the number of cells by removing a sample of a culture, diluting it if necessary, and examining it microscopically. This approach is called a **direct count.** To make the counting easier and more precise, counting chambers can be used (**Figure 20.1**). The direct count quickly provides the number of cells in a population (usually expressed as cells/ml), but it does not distinguish living from dead cells. To enumerate the living cells in a culture, a **viable cell count** can be done. With this method, a sample of the culture is diluted and then plated onto a growth medium (**Figure 20.2**). One common method used to plate the samples is the spread plate method (**Figure 20.3**). When diluted sufficiently, each viable cell capable of reproducing gives rise to a single isolated colony. By counting the colonies, a measurement of the viable cells in the population is obtained. The measurement is expressed as **colony forming units (cfu)**, usually cfu/ml of culture. Colony forming units are used because single cells as well as clumps of two or three cells will form a colony. Both direct counts and viable cell counts require a variety of manipulations of a culture sample. These manipulations can be time-consuming and tedious. A much easier method of gauging population size is to use a turbidimetric method. This method is based on the observation that as a microbial population increases in size, the culture becomes more turbid, or cloudy. Turbidity can be measured using a spectrophotometer (**Figure 20.4**). The population size in this case is expressed as absorbance rather than as cells/ml or cfu/ml. However, by using a standard curve that relates absorbance to cells/ml (as measured by direct counts) or cfu/ml (as measured by viable cell counts), absorbance can be converted into a measure of cell density.

By using the methods described above, microbiologists can measure the number of microbes at one point in time, or they can follow the growth of a population over time. The former is useful in the food industry where microbial contamination of a foodstuff must be minimal. For instance, in a dairy, samples of milk are routinely collected and the number of microbes in the milk determined. Likewise, the microbial load in drinking water is monitored by municipal water treatment plants. Measuring the

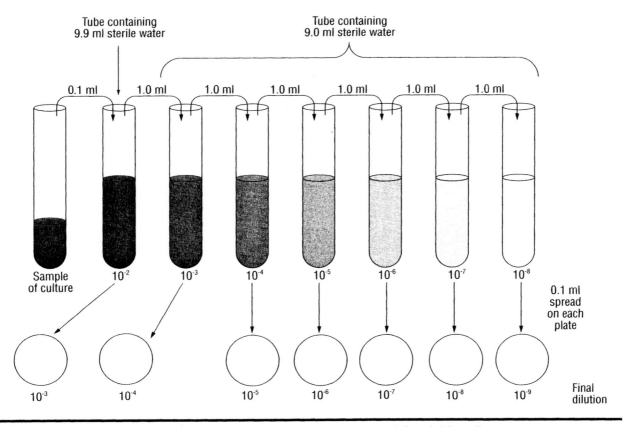

Figure 20.2 Serial dilutions and platings to be used for viable cell counts.

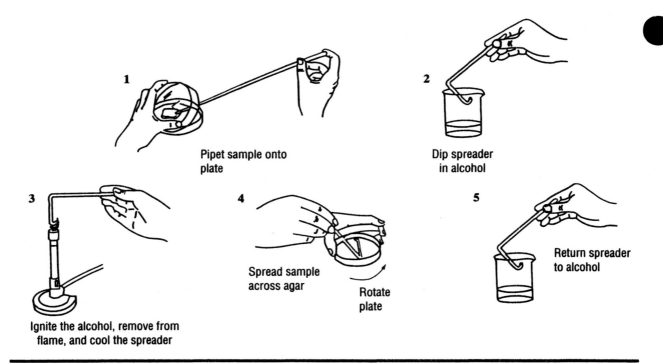

Figure 20.3   The spread plate method for inoculating plates. (Adapted from Atlas, Parks, and Brown. *Laboratory Manual of Experimental Microbiology.* St. Louis: Mosby–Year Book, 1995. With permission.)

Calculation of Generation Time

The relationship between the initial number of cells in a population and the number after some period of exponential growth is given by:

$$N = N_0 2^n$$

where,

   N = the cell number after a period of growth
   N_0 = the initial number of cells
   n = the number of generations

This formula can be reexpressed in terms of n

$$n = \frac{\log (N) - \log (N_0)}{\log 2} = \frac{\log (N) - \log (N_0)}{0.301}$$

Generation time is the time in hours taken to complete one generation. Or expressed mathematically,

$$t/n$$

For instance, if the initial cell density is 4×10^4 and after 2 hours the cell density is 1×10^6, then $t = 2$, and

$$n = \frac{\log (1 \times 10^6) - \log (4 \times 10^4)}{0.301} = 4.65$$

and $t/n = 2/4.65 = 0.43$ h

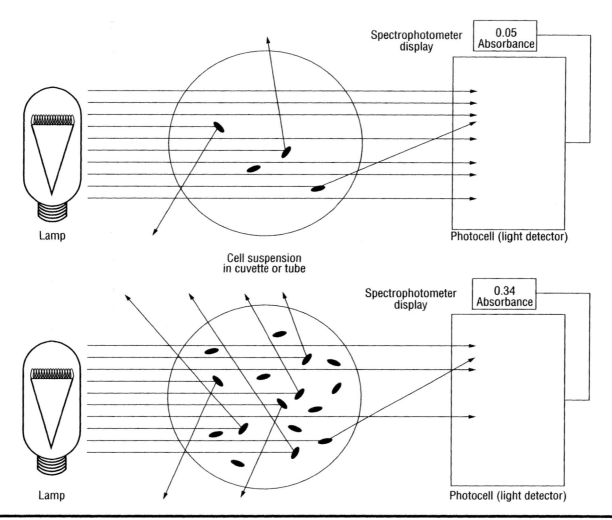

Figure 20.4 Turbidity measurements made by a spectrophotometer. In the upper cell suspension, there are relatively few cells. Most light passes through the suspension and is detected by the light detector. In the lower cell suspension, more cells are present. Light striking the cells is scattered and so does not strike the light detector. Therefore, the absorbance increases.

growth of a population over time is useful because the resulting growth curve can be used to determine the **generation time** characteristic of a particular microbe growing under certain conditions (see box on previous page). This is important both in industry and in setting up experiments where populations of a certain size or in a particular phase of growth are required.

In this exercise, you will use direct counts, the spread plate method for obtaining viable counts, and turbidity measurements to measure the growth of a bacterial population over time. The data for each method will be collected and analyzed. Standard curves relating absorbance to cells/ml and cfu/ml will also be con-

structed. Using the appropriate growth curves, the generation time of the population will be calculated.

PURPOSE

- To learn about the growth of microbial populations
- To use viable counts, direct counts, and turbidimetric methods for measuring the size of microbial populations
- To learn advantages and disadvantages of each measurement of population size
- To calculate the generation time of an exponentially growing culture

THE EXERCISE

MATERIALS:

Broth culture of *Saccharomyces cerevisiae*
Uninoculated YEPD
One test tube containing 9.9 ml of sterile water
Seven YEPD plates
Sterile 1 ml and 0.1 ml pipets (or micropipetters and sterile tips)
Counting chamber
Spectrophotometer
Cuvette
Six test tubes containing 9 ml sterile water
Culture spreader soaking in alcohol in a beaker
Bunsen burner
30°C shaker

PROCEDURE: Work in groups of three

The entire class, working together, will collect data on the growth of a population of cells. Sampling times at 20-minute intervals will be rotated through the class as described by your instructor (**Figure 20.5**). Every time your group is to sample the culture, it will obtain a 2 ml sample and transfer it to a sterile tube. You will use this sample to carry out Parts A, B, and C, which are described below.

Approximately 3 hours before the laboratory period began, your instructor inoculated 500 ml of YEPD with 5 ml of an overnight culture of *S. cerevisiae*. Your instructor immediately removed 1 ml and measured its absorbance at 550 nm (t = 0 minutes). The culture was then incubated at 30°C with shaking.

Time	Group
2:10 P.M.	1 and 2
2:30 P.M.	3 and 4
2:50 P.M.	5 and 6
3:10 P.M.	7 and 8
3:30 P.M.	9 and 10

Figure 20.5 Possible rotation of sampling through a class of thirty students working in groups of three. The laboratory period runs from 2:00 P.M. to 3:50 P.M. When Group 1 samples the culture at 2:10 P.M., it measures the size of the population by turbidity, direct counts, and plate counts.

Part A: Measuring the Size of a Population Turbidimetrically

1. Remove 1 ml of the sample and place it in a cuvette.
2. Determine absorbance at a wavelength of 550 nm. If using a dual-beam spectrophotometer, the reference cuvette will contain sterile YEPD. If using a single-beam spectrophotometer, also measure the absorbance of sterile YEPD and subtract that value from the absorbance of the sample.
3. Record your results in the RESULTS section. **Note:** At later time points, absorbance may reach levels not accurately measured by the spectrophotometer. It will then be necessary to dilute the sample in YEPD before measuring absorbance. To get the absorbance value of the undiluted sample, the absorbance of the dilution is multiplied by the inverse of the dilution. For instance, if the sample is diluted 1/10, and the absorbance of the dilution is 0.31, then the absorbance of the undiluted sample is calculated as $0.31 \times 10 = 3.1$. This is the value recorded in the RESULTS section.

Part B: Measuring the Size of a Population by Direct Counts

1. Use a Pasteur pipet to transfer some of the sample to a counting chamber. **Note:** Counting chambers differ with respect to how the sample is placed in the chamber. Your instructor will demonstrate the correct method for the counting chambers you will use.
2. Place the coverslip on the slide. **Note:** The coverslip is of a particular size and shape and can't be substituted for by a standard coverslip. When the coverslip is in position, the volume of liquid in the calibrated area of the slide is a constant value depending on the counting chamber. For the counting chamber shown in **Figure 20.1,** the volume is 0.02 mm³ (1 mm × 1 mm × 0.02 mm).
3. Examine the counting chamber with the 10× objective of a microscope. Center the counting grid then rotate the 40× objective into position.
4. Count the number of yeast cells. A minimum of 300 cells should be counted for the most accurate results. **Note:** It is important to develop a systematic approach to counting the cells. If the counting chamber is like that shown in **Figure 20.1,** then enough medium-sized

Calculation of Cells/ml Using the Counting Chamber Shown in Figure 20.1

- Suppose 5 medium squares were counted:

  Square 1 - 65 cells
  Square 2 - 57 cells
  Square 3 - 62 cells
  Square 4 - 59 cells
  Square 5 - 66 cells

- First calculate the average number of cells per medium square:

  309 cells/5 medium squares = 61.8 cells per medium square

- Next use the formula below to calculate the cells/ml:

$$\left(\frac{\text{Average \# cells}}{\text{Medium square}}\right)\left(\frac{25 \text{ medium squares}}{\text{Large square}}\right)\left(\frac{\text{Large square}}{0.02 \text{ mm}^3}\right)\left(\frac{10^3 \text{ mm}^3}{\text{cm}^3}\right)\left(\frac{1 \text{ cm}^3}{\text{ml}}\right) = \text{cells/ml}$$

or simplified:

$$(\text{Average \# cells/medium square}) \times 25 \times 50 \times 10^3 = \text{cells/ml}$$

Using this example:

$$61.8 \times 25 \times 50 \times 10^3 = 7.72 \times 10^7 \text{ cells/ml}$$

squares must be counted to give a total of more than or equal to 300 cells. It is best to record the number of cells per medium square. The small squares within each medium square can be used to establish a scanning pattern. For instance, first count the cells in the top row of small squares moving from left to right, then count the cells in the second row of small squares moving from right to left, the third row from left to right, and the final row from right to left (**Figure 20.6**).

5. Calculate the number of cells/ml and record your results in the RESULTS section. **Note:** The calculation of cells/ml differs depending on the counting chamber. Your instructor will describe the calculations you must use. The calculations of the chamber shown in **Figure 20.1** are illustrated above (see box).

Part C: Measuring the Size of a Population by the Plate Count Method

Day 1

1. Prepare the series of dilutions shown in **Figure 20.2.** **Note:** Review the steps for making serial dilutions

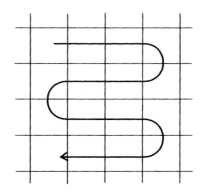

Figure 20.6 A suggested pattern for scanning a medium square.

in Exercise 17. Remember to change pipets or pipet tips with each dilution.

2. Label seven nutrient agar plates as shown in **Figure 20.2.**

3. Transfer 0.1 ml (100 µl) of the 10^{-2} dilution to the plate labeled 10^{-3}. **Note:** Remember

that eventually the cell density in the population will be expressed as cfu/ml. Since only 0.1 ml of the 10^{-2} dilution tube is being plated, this is the equivalent of diluting the solution in the tube 1/10, thus the final dilution plated is 10^{-3}.

4. Remove the spreader from the alcohol and pass it through the flame of the Bunsen burner (**Figure 20.3**). **Note:** As the alcohol burns off, the spreader is sterilized. Be careful not to bring the flame near the beaker of alcohol.
5. After cooling place the spreader on the surface of the nutrient agar and rotate the plate. **Note:** This spreads the cells over the surface of the agar. It is important to cover the entire surface. Therefore, depending on the size of the spreader, it may be necessary to move the spreader back and forth, or in an elliptical pattern across the agar as the plate is rotated.
6. Cover the Petri dish.
7. Return the spreader to the alcohol.
8. Repeat steps 3 through 7 for the remaining dilutions. **Note:** Change pipets or pipet tips and resterilize and cool the spreader for each plating.
9. Incubate the plates at 30°C for 1 to 2 days.

Day 2

1. Count the number of colonies on each of the plates from Day 1. Use only those plates with 30 to 300 colonies to calculate the cfu/ml. Record your results in the RESULTS section.
2. Give your data from the time points you sampled to your instructor. Your data will be combined with that from other groups and the class data will be given to you. Carry out the remaining steps using the class data.
3. Plot the results of the turbidimetric measurements. This is done by plotting absorbance (y-axis) versus time (x-axis). Use the semilog paper provided. **Note:** The relationship between population size and time is an exponential function (**Figure 20.7**). Therefore, in order to prepare a graph showing a linear relationship, semilog paper is needed.
4. Plot the results of the direct counts. This is done by plotting cells/ml (y-axis) versus time (x-axis). **Note:** Use the semilog paper provided.
5. Plot the results of the colony counts. This is done by plotting cfu/ml (y-axis) versus time (x-axis). Use the semilog paper provided.

Time (Hours)	Number of Cells
0	1
0.5	2
1	4
1.5	8
2	16
2.5	32
3	64
3.5	128
4	256
4.5	512
5	1024
5.5	2048
6	4096
.	.
.	.
10	1,048,576

(a)

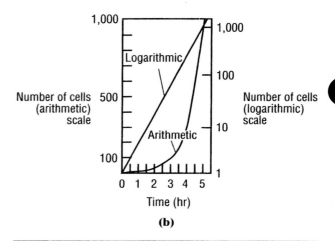

(b)

Figure 20.7 The relationship between time and the growth of a population of cells: (a) a set of sample data, and (b) the data plotted using an arithmetic scale and a logarithmic scale. The number of cells can be expressed as cells/ml, cfu/ml, or absorbance.

6. For each time point, plot the cfu/ml for that time point versus the absorbance for that time point. Use the standard graph paper provided.
7. For each time point, plot the cells/ml for that time point versus the absorbance for that time point. Use the standard graph paper provided.

RESULTS

Results of the plate counts for the samples you worked with.

Time Sampled	Number of Colonies for Each Dilution Plated						
	10^{-3}	10^{-4}	10^{-5}	10^{-6}	10^{-7}	10^{-8}	10^{-9}

Calculate the cfu/ml for each time sample you worked with in the space below and record those values in the table below.

Record the results for all measurements for the samples you worked with in the table below.

Time Sampled	Absorbance	Direct Counts (cells/ml)	Plate Counts (cfu/ml)

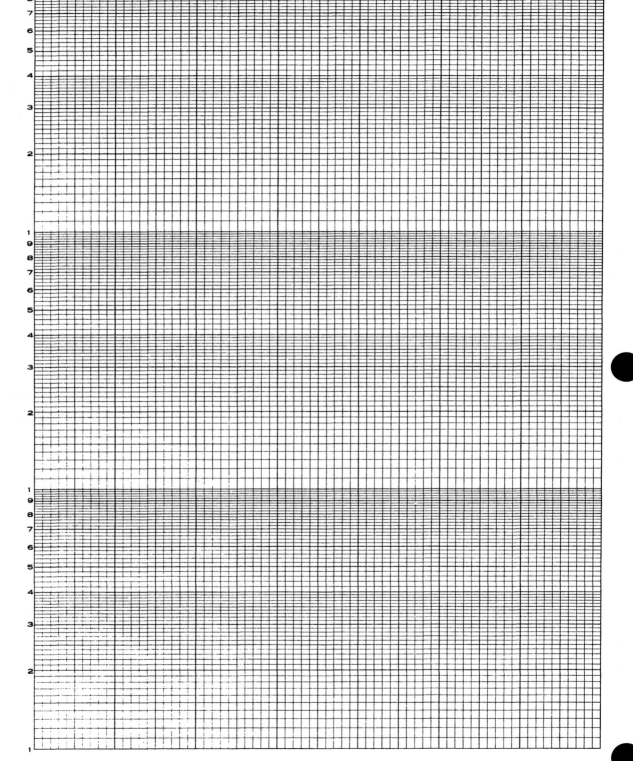

SEMI-LOGARITHMIC
3 CYCLES X 10 DIVISIONS PER INCH

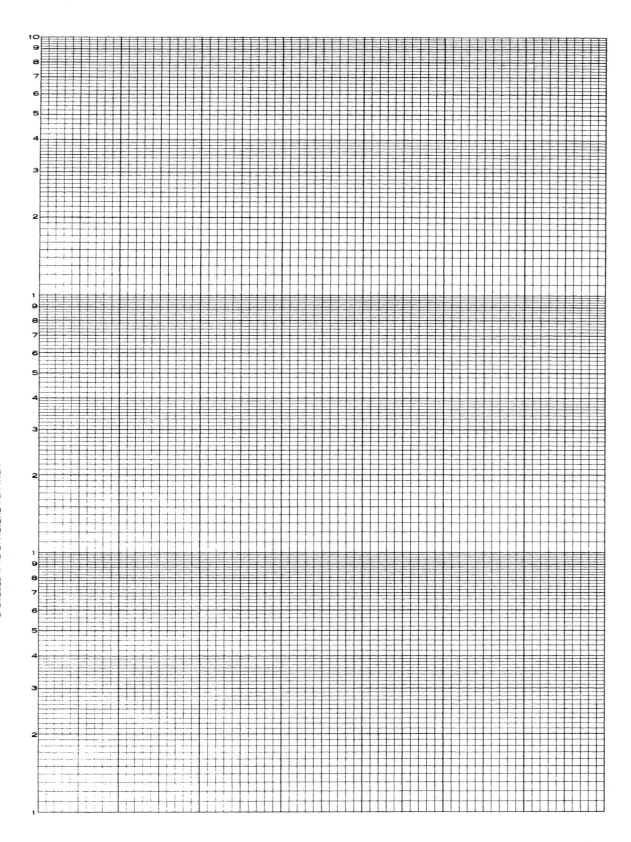

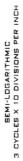

SEMI-LOGARITHMIC
3 CYCLES X 10 DIVISIONS PER INCH

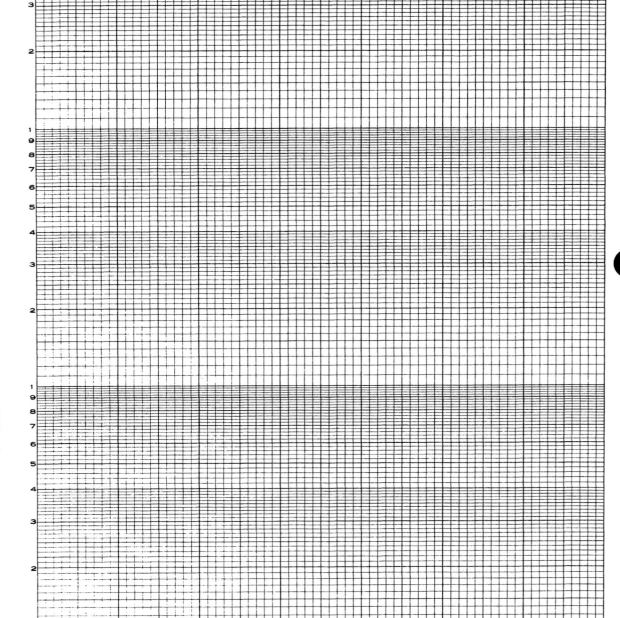

SEMI-LOGARITHMIC
3 CYCLES X 10 DIVISIONS PER INCH

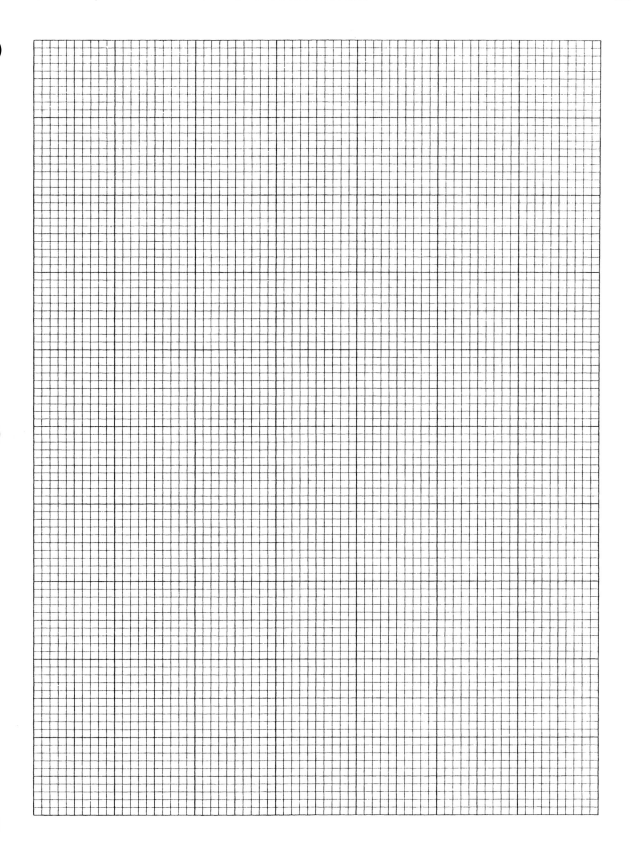

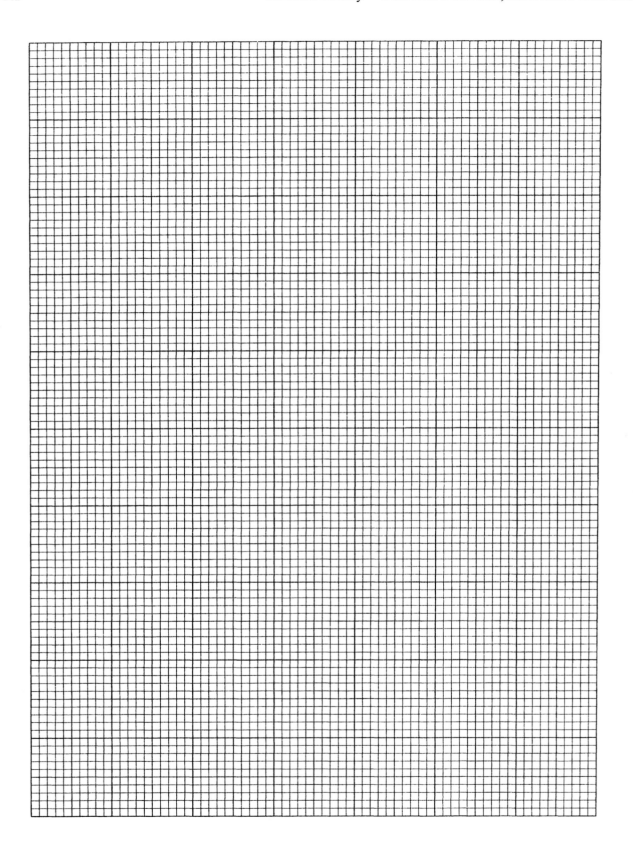

REFLECTIONS

1. Examine each of the graphs that plots cell density versus time. Most, if not all, of the graph should show a linear relationship between cell density and time. The linear portion of the data represents a phase of population growth called the exponential (or log) phase. In your own words, describe what is happening during this phase of growth.

2. Suppose you were following the growth of a population by measuring absorbance and at one point in time you measured an absorbance of 0.83. Use your graphs of absorbance versus cells/ml and absorbance versus cfu/ml to determine the cells/ml and the cfu/ml at that absorbance.

3. Examine the class data and look closely at the measurements for each time point. Are the cells/ml determined from direct counts the same as the cfu/ml determined from the plate counts? Explain why this is or is not so.

4. Use each graph (absorbance versus time, cells/ml versus time, cfu/ml versus time) or sets of data to determine the doubling time of the culture. Are these values the same? Explain why this is or is not so.

5. Suppose at noon, when the Gibsons removed their turkey from the oven, there was one *Salmonella* cell alive in the stuffing inside the turkey. If the doubling time of this species is 30 minutes, estimate the number of cells in the stuffing when the adults started nibbling again at 6:00 P.M. Consult a textbook or other source to determine if the resulting population of bacteria could have been the cause of the family's illness. Explain.

6. What errors did the Gibson family make in the preparation and storage of their food? How might these contribute to contracting salmonellosis?

7. In recent years, it has been noted that when bacteria are exposed to certain conditions (e.g., sublethal disinfectant), they are temporarily unable to reproduce. What impact would this have on the assessment of the quality of water leaving a water treatment plant? Answer this question three times. The first time, assume the technician at the plant uses direct counts to measure the number of microbes in the water. The second time, assume the technician uses viable plate counts, and the third time, assume the technician uses turbidimetric measures.

EUCARYOTIC REPRODUCTION

In the previous exercise, you measured the increase in the size of a population of microbes reproducing asexually. In this exercise you will observe examples of sexual life cycles in eucaryotic microbes.

The summer of 1994 was finally coming to an end and Sam, a 50-year-old laborer, was glad to see it go. Sam had lived his entire life in the Houston area, and this summer had been one of the hottest summers in memory. Unfortunately, the hot weather coincided with the demise of Sam's air conditioner and his landlord never fixed it. So Sam spent the summer tormented by mosquitos that squeezed through holes in the window screens. Sam never replaced the screens because he spent much of the summer ill. The illness began in late July with a fever and recurring headaches. Sam thought he had the flu until one day a friend found him dazed and confused—almost delirious. After two visits to the hospital emergency room, he was tentatively diagnosed with viral meningitis. A routine peripheral blood smear was examined and nothing unusual was noted. All other tests were negative as well. Then, almost as suddenly as it began, his illness waned and he recovered.

About 6 weeks later, the symptoms began again. Sam revisited his doctor. His physician ordered a routine peripheral blood smear and careful observation of the smear revealed Plasmodium vivax. *Sam had malaria! The doctor explained that Sam's current episode was probably a relapse. It was likely that the parasite had entered a dormant stage in the liver after the first episode. Sam was treated with chloroquine and recovered within a few days. He was also treated with a course of primaquine to prevent another relapse.*

BACKGROUND INFORMATION

Although malaria is rare in the United States, it is the leading cause of morbidity and mortality worldwide. *Plasmodium vivax*, a protozoan and one of the causative agents of malaria, has a complex life cycle that involves two different types of cell division, **mitosis** and **meiosis.** *P. vivax* reproduces sexually using mitosis and meiosis at different stages of its life cycle. Sexual reproduction is distinguished from asexual reproduction based on the number of "parents" involved. In asexual reproduction, there is only one parent, and the progeny "born" to that parent are identical to it. Asexual eucaryotic organisms are limited to mitosis for reproduction. In sexual reproduction, two parents are needed to produce progeny. The cells of sexual organisms can divide either by mitosis or meiosis, with meiosis being used to create gametes, gamete-like cells, or haploid stages of the life cycle.

The primary function of both mitosis and meiosis is to properly sort chromosomes during cell division so that the progeny cells have complete sets of chromosomes. This is important because cells that lack chromosomes or have extra chromosomes are often unable to function properly. Such cells are called **aneuploids.** Mitosis and meiosis differ, however, in terms of the end product. Mitosis yields two progeny cells identical to the parent cell, whereas meiosis produces four progeny cells with half the sets of chromosomes of the parent. Most typically, meiosis begins with a diploid cell and produces haploid progeny.

Some eucaryotic microbes are capable of only asexual (mitotic) reproduction. Most however, employ both mitosis and meiosis in their life cycles and are capable of sexual reproduction. Sexual microbes alternate between diploid and haploid states with fusion or fertilization restoring the diploid state and meiosis restoring the haploid. Mitosis occurs at one or more times during the life cycle, depending on the microbe. As a result, microbes that reproduce sexually can have quite amazing life cycles in which the various stages occur in different environments. Furthermore, the microorganism can look quite distinct at different times—so much so that it may not be recognized as the same microbe. As you will see, understanding the life cycle of a microbe can be of practical importance as some microbes are pathogenic at one stage of their life cycle but not another.

In this exercise, you will examine two different microbes and observe portions of their life cycles. The first to be examined is *P. vivax* whose life cycle is shown in **Figure 21.1.** Sam was infected by sporozoites

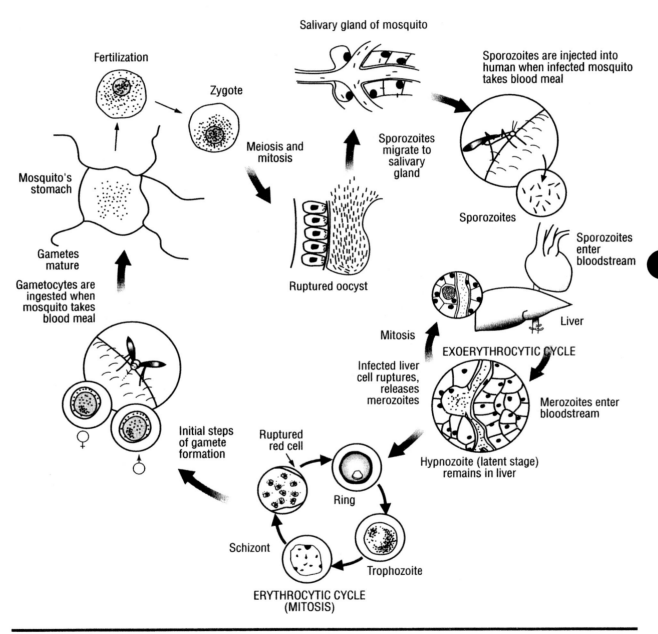

Figure 21.1 The life cycle of *P. vivax.*

present in the saliva of a mosquito that bit him. The haploid sporozoites were carried by Sam's blood to his liver, where they invaded his liver cells. Within the liver, the sporozoites underwent mitosis, increasing their numbers. Eventually the parasites were released into the bloodstream, this time in a different form called a merozoite. Merozoites infect red blood cells (RBC) and reproduce within them. As can be seen in **Figure 21.1,** merozoites released from an infected RBC can infect other RBC. When merozoites are released, the body defenses respond, resulting in the fever and chills observed in malarial episodes. Not all merozoites continue this RBC-infection cycle. Instead, some differentiate into immature gametes. If immature gametes are transmitted to a mosquito through a bite, they mature within the mosquito's stomach. Ultimately, fertilization occurs, forming a diploid zygote. Later, the zygote undergoes meiosis and differentiation to give rise to haploid sporozoites, and the cycle begins again. In this exercise, you will observe portions of the life cycle of *P. vivax* by examining prepared slides of the parasite at various stages of its life cycle.

The second organism you will work with is *Ustilago hordei,* a fungus that causes a plant disease called covered smut of barley (**Figure 21.2**). The life cycle of this fungus begins when moistened dormant diploid teliospores of *U. hordei* in soil or on barley seeds germinate and simultaneously undergo meiosis. The resultant haploids are yeast-like

sporidia that reproduce mitotically by budding. As yeast-like sporidia, the fungus is not pathogenic and the host plant is unharmed. However, if a haploid of one mating type (A or a) encounters another haploid of opposite mating type, cytoplasmic fusion occurs giving rise to a heterokaryon containing two haploid nuclei, one from each mating type. The heterokaryon does not maintain the yeast-like characteristics of its parents. Instead, it switches to filamentous growth, and it is the filamentous heterokaryon that is pathogenic. The mycelium grows through the barley plant to the flowers, where the fungal cells form spores as the seeds develop. The two nuclei in each spore fuse giving rise to teliospores, and the cycle begins again. In this exercise, you will observe the formation of conjugation tubes when *U. hordei* cells of opposite mating types are mixed. Formation of these tubes is an initial step in mating. You will also observe the switch from the yeast form to filamentous growth following mating.

PURPOSE

- To observe sexual reproduction in two different eucaryotic microbes
- To observe how mitosis, meiosis, and mating can be combined in various ways to give a variety of different life cycles

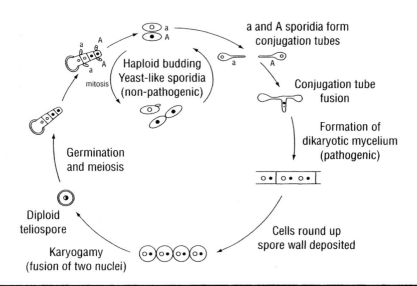

Figure 21.2   The life cycle of *U. hordei.* (Courtesy of John Sherwood.)

THE EXERCISE

Part A: Plasmodium vivax

MATERIALS:

Prepared slides of human blood or mosquito salivary glands showing different stages of *P. vivax* infection

PROCEDURE: Work in groups of three

1. Each member of your group should obtain and examine a slide prepared from a different stage of the *P. vivax* life cycle.
2. Each member should try to identify all possible stages observed in their slide (**Figure 21.3**).
3. Exchange slides. Help the other members of your group identify the stages you identified in your original slide.
4. Working as a group, order the different forms of the malaria parasite observed according to the information in **Figure 21.1** and **Figure 21.3**.
5. Record your observations in the RESULTS section.

Part B: Ustilago hordei *Conjugation Tubes*

MATERIALS:

1-week-old plate cultures of haploid *U. hordei* strains, one 8A the other 8a
Humid growth chamber with sterile microscope slide
70% alcohol
Sterile water
Micropipetter and sterile pipet tips
Microcentrifuge tube
Two small sterile test tubes containing 0.5 ml sterile distilled water
One plate of 1.5% water agar (about 10 ml per plate)
Bunsen burner
Microcentrifuge
Spatula

PROCEDURE: Work in groups of three

1. Aseptically transfer a large isolated colony of strain 8A into one tube of sterile water. Mix gently.
2. Aseptically transfer a large isolated colony of strain 8a into the second tube of sterile water. Mix gently.
3. Soak the spatula briefly in 70% alcohol. Then flame the spatula to sterilize it.
4. Use the sterile spatula to cut a 1 cm square piece of agar from the water agar plate. Place the square on the sterile microscope slide inside the humid growth chamber (see Exercise 13, **Figure 13.5**).
5. Add 6 μl of sterile water to a microcentrifuge tube.
6. Add 2 μl of each cell suspension (8A and 8a) to the water. Spin the tube for a few seconds in a microcentrifuge to mix the solutions.
7. Pipet all 10 μl of the mixture onto the water agar square in the humid growth chamber.
8. Incubate at room temperature (RT) for 2 to 24 hours.
9. While the conjugation tubes form, make a wet mount of 8A and 8a cells using cells from the plate cultures.
10. Record your observations of the morphology of each strain in the RESULTS section.
11. After 2 to 24 hours of incubating the cells in the humid growth chamber, remove the microscope slide from the chamber and examine the cells on the water agar square using both the 10× and 40× objectives. Identify conjugation tubes (**Figure 21.4**).
12. Record your observations in the RESULTS section.

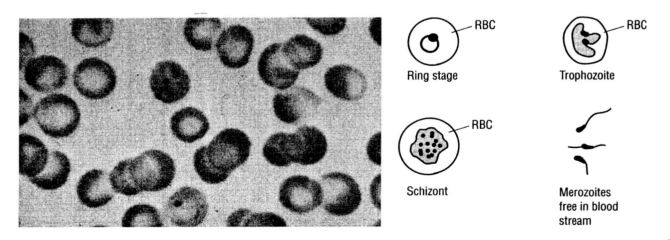

Figure 21.3   Various stages in the life cycle of *P. vivax* which may be observed in prepared slides.

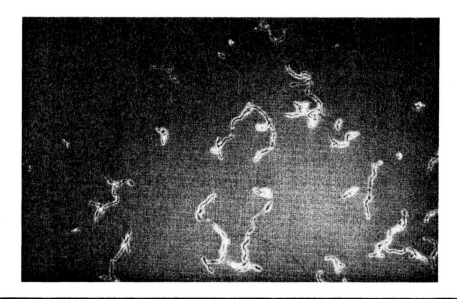

Figure 21.4 *U. hordei* conjugation tubes. (Courtesy of John Sherwood.)

Part C: Ustilago hordei *Mating Reaction*

MATERIALS:

Suspensions of strains 8A and 8a (from Part B)
Dissecting microscope
One YEPD + 1% charcoal agar plate
Micropipetters and sterile pipet tips

PROCEDURE: Work in groups of three

Day 1

1. Label a plate of YEPD + 1% charcoal agar as shown in **Figure 21.5.**
2. Spot inoculate 5 μl of the 8A suspension over the *A* and *A x a* labels.
3. Spot inoculate 5 μl of the 8a suspension over the *a* and *A x a* labels. Place the 8a suspension directly on top of the spot of the 8A suspension above the A x a label. This is the location where the two opposite mating types have been mated.
4. Allow plates to dry, then invert and incubate them at RT for 1 to 2 days.

Day 2

1. Describe the growth on the YEPD + 1% charcoal agar plate when viewed with the unaided eye.
2. If you have a dissecting microscope, use it to describe the growth in more detail.
3. Record your observations in the RESULTS section.

REFERENCES

Bell, R., et al. Local Transmission of *Plasmodium vivax* Malaria-Houston, Texas, 1994. *Morbidity and Mortality Weekly Report* 44(1995):295-303.

Diggs, L.W., et al. *The Morphology of Human Blood Cells*, 5th ed., Abbott Park, IL. Abbott Laboratories, 1985.

Katz, M., et al. *Parasitic Diseases*, 2nd ed., New York: Springer-Verlag, 1989.

Martinez-Espinoza, A.D., et al. Improved Media for Testing the Mating Reaction and Genetic Complementation of *Ustilago hordei. Canadian Journal of Botany* 70(1992):788-793.

Martinez-Espinoza, A.D., et al. Morphological and Mutational Analysis of Mating in *Ustilago hordei. Experimental Mycology* 17(1993):200-214.

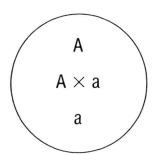

Figure 21.5 Labeling of YEPD + 1% charcoal agar plate.

RESULTS

P. vivax stages observed: Order your observations and label the drawings according to the stages in their life cycle.

U. hordei conjugation tubes:

Objective used: _____
Wet mount of 8A cells

Objective used: _____
Wet mount of 8a cells

Objective used: _____
Cells conjugating on water agar square

U. hordei mating reaction: Describe the growth on YEPD + 1% charcoal agar of each of the inocula below.

A

a

A x a

REFLECTIONS

1. Why were *a* and *A* spots included in the *U. hordei* mating experiment?

2. A number of important pathogenic fungi are dimorphic (i.e., exist in yeast forms and filamentous forms). Consult a textbook or other source and name one. Is the switch from one type of growth to another associated with the infectious process for this organism?

3. The ciliated protozoan *Paramecium caudatum* mates by a process called conjugation. Conjugation involves both meiosis and mitosis in an interesting way. Consult a biology textbook or other source and describe the mitotic and meiotic events observed during conjugation. How does *P. caudatum* mating compare to that observed for *U. hordei*?

4. Both mitosis and bacterial binary fission yield two progeny cells identical to the parent cell. How do these two types of cell division differ?

5. Procaryotes are asexual microbes that are incapable of true sexual reproduction. Explain why this is so.

EXERCISE 22

"SEX" LIVES OF BACTERIA

In Exercise 21, you observed microbes capable of sexual reproduction. All were eucaryotes because procaryotes are limited to asexual reproductive processes such as binary fission. The hallmark of sexual reproduction is that it allows for the maintenance of genetic variation in a population. This occurs because new combinations of genes are formed as the result of the gene-shuffling that occurs during meiosis and mating. Asexual reproduction does not shuffle genes. But, procaryotes have developed mechanisms for transferring DNA from one organism to another, and as a result, shuffling genes. In this exercise, you will observe one mechanism—bacterial conjugation.

The Fortino family had been growing grapes for nearly 100 years. In those years, they had learned and implemented progressive cost-effective techniques that had as little impact on the environment as possible. They also had seen the importance of developing new grape varieties with greater disease resistance. Developing new varieties was a slow process that involved standard plant-breeding techniques and other procedures such as grafting plants.

Jim, the eldest of the fourth generation of Fortinos, was enjoying the sun as he examined a group of young vines growing from a grafted variety. From a distance it was clear that the grafts had all taken, as the vines looked healthy. But Jim knew that closer examination might reveal abnormal growths near the juncture of the rootstock with the graft. These growths are called crown galls. The detection of crown gall disease would not only lead to the loss of the vine, but because it is easily spread, could cause the loss of an entire field. Once crown gall disease is detected in a field, it is

sometimes necessary to remove all susceptible plants and use the field to grow nonsusceptible plants (e.g., corn) for several years. Loss of the field for this long would be a great financial setback for the family. Fortunately for Jim, the warm sun was an omen. His new variety was free of galls.

BACKGROUND INFORMATION

Crown gall disease is caused by bacteria belonging to the genus *Agrobacterium*, the most well-known member being *Agrobacterium tumefaciens*. Several genes involved in pathogenesis have been identified and localized on a large plasmid called the Ti plasmid, which is short for tumor-inducing plasmid. Any *Agrobacterium* cell that contains the Ti plasmid can cause crown gall disease, while those without it do not. Unfortunately for fruit growers and nursery owners, the plasmid can be transferred to *Agrobacterium* cells not bearing the plasmid. This is accomplished by **bacterial conjugation.** As a result, more disease-causing *Agrobacterium* cells are generated.

Bacterial conjugation is a phenomenon in which DNA from a donor bacterium is transferred to a recipient. It is distinguished from other types of bacterial DNA transfer (**Table 22.1**) by the requirement for physical contact between the donor and recipient. The ability to establish such contact and effect transfer of DNA is encoded by genes on conjugative plasmids. Conjugative plasmids may also carry genes that confer antibiotic resistance. These plasmids are of particular concern in medicine because they can promote rapid development of antibiotic-resistant populations of bacterial pathogens.

Although Ti-mediated conjugation is of obvious practical importance in agriculture, it is not the best

TABLE 22.1 Mechanisms of DNA Transfer in Procaryotes

Type of DNA Transfer	Characteristics
Conjugation	Plasmid-mediated; cell-to-cell contact is required
Transduction	Virus-mediated; virus particle transfers DNA from donor to recipient
Transformation	Recipient takes up free DNA from dead donor cell

studied model of bacterial conjugation. That honor goes to Fertility-factor (F-factor)–mediated conjugation observed in *Escherichia coli.* This conjugation system was the first discovered. In this system, donor cells (F$^+$ or Hfr) contain the F-factor and recipient cells (F$^-$ cells) do not. Genes carried by the plasmid encode information for a sex-pilus (**Figure 22.1**). This pilus connects the donor to the recipient and thus allows for transfer of DNA. If the plasmid is free in the cytoplasm (F$^+$ cell), then only the plasmid is transferred from the donor to the recipient. However, if the F-factor is integrated into the donor cell's chromosome (Hfr cell), then chromosomal DNA is transferred to the recipient (**Figure 22.2**). As can be seen in **Figure 22.2b** and **Figure 22.2c,** the transfer of chromosomal DNA occurs from a fixed point and in a particular direction, depending on the site of insertion and the orientation of the plasmid in the chromosome. The DNA transferred by an Hfr strain is not capable of replication independent of the chromosome. Therefore, the only Hfr DNA maintained in the recipient is that which recombines into the F$^-$ cell's chromosome.

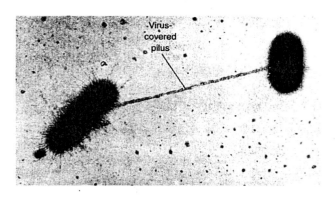

Figure 22.1 Two bacterial cells connected by a sex-pilus.

In this exercise, you will mix an Hfr *E. coli* strain with an F$^-$ strain and observe the transfer of DNA to the recipient over time. As the result of this transfer, recombinant cells will be formed. These recombinants will have characteristics of both parents. Based on your observations, you will be able to suggest the relative location of genes along the donor chromosome.

PURPOSE

- To observe the transfer of DNA from bacterium to bacterium by bacterial conjugation

THE EXERCISE

MATERIALS:

1 ml of a culture of *E. coli* genotype: Hfr Gal$^+$ Leu$^+$ Lac$^+$ Str^s

EMB/galactose plus streptomycin plates

Minimal plus streptomycin plates

Tubes containing 2 ml of 0.1 M phosphate buffer, pH 7.3

Vortex mixer

Alcohol in beaker

20 ml of a culture of *E. coli* genotype: F$^-$ Gal$^-$ Leu$^-$ Lac$^-$ Str^r

EMB/lactose plus streptomycin plates

50 ml of minimal broth in a 250-ml flask prewarmed to 37°C

37°C shaking water bath

Pipets

Culture spreaders

PROCEDURE: Work in groups of four or five

Day 1

1. Combine the Hfr culture with the F$^-$ culture. **Note:** The phenotypes of these two strains are given in abbreviated form above. The genetic shorthand means that the Hfr donor is able to ferment both galactose and lactose, is able to synthesize the amino acid leucine, and is sensitive to the antibiotic streptomycin. The recipient (F$^-$) is unable to ferment galactose and lactose, is incapable of synthesizing the amino acid leucine, and is resistant to streptomycin. The ratio of 20 F$^-$:1Hfr is used because there is higher efficiency of DNA transfer using this ratio.

2. Place the mixture in the 37°C shaking water bath and shake gently (~50 RPM) for 5 minutes. **Note:** This brief incubation permits the cells to establish mating pairs.

TRANSFER OF PLASMID ONLY

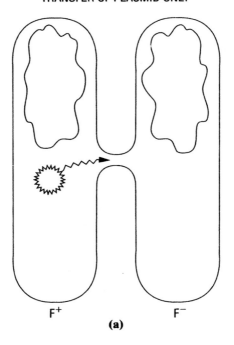

TRANSFER OF INTEGRATED PLASMID AND CHROMOSOMAL DNA

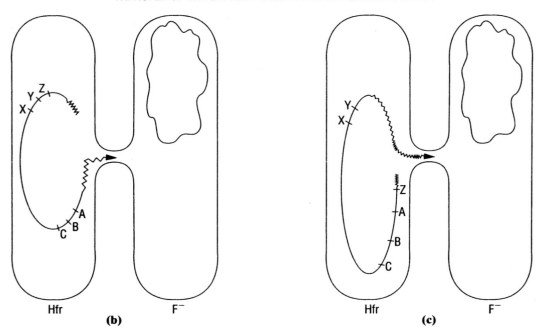

Figure 22.2   DNA transfer by conjugation: (a) $F^+ \times F^-$; (b) Hfr $\times$ F^-; and (c) Hfr $\times$ F^-. Note the difference in the site of integration and orientation of the plasmid.

3. Transfer 0.1 ml of the mated cells to the flask of minimal broth and mix gently. Record the time of this transfer in the RESULTS section. **Note:** A minimal growth medium is one that provides a source of carbon, usually a simple sugar, and inorganic sources of nitrogen, phosphorus, sulfur, and a few trace elements. Using these simple molecules, the microbe must synthesize all the carbohydrates, amino acids, nucleotides, and other growth factors it needs. The Hfr strain is able to synthesize all amino acids, including leucine, so it will grow on a minimal medium. The recipient (F^-) is incapable of leucine synthesis so is unable to grow on a minimal medium.

4. Immediately transfer 0.5 ml of the minimal broth culture to a tube containing 2 ml of phosphate buffer. **Note:** Work quickly and return the culture to the water bath as soon as possible, so that DNA transfer continues over the course of the experiment.

5. Vortex the sample at top speed. **Note:** Vortexing the cells disrupts the mating pairs.

6. Transfer 0.1 ml of the sample to the EMB/galactose plus streptomycin plate.

7. Flame sterilize the culture spreader, cool, and spread the cells over the surface of the agar. **Note:** See Exercise 20 for details of the spread plate method.

8. Repeat steps 6 and 7 for the EMB/lactose plus streptomycin plate.

9. Repeat steps 6 and 7 for the minimal plus streptomycin plate.

10. Repeat steps 4 through 9, every 5 minutes for 30 to 45 minutes. Remember to record the time of sampling throughout the experiment.

11. Invert all plates and incubate at 37°C.

Day 2

1. Examine the colonies growing on the EMB/galactose plates. Colonies of cells capable of fermenting galactose (Gal^+) will be dark red, whereas Gal^- colonies will be white. Count the number of both for each sampling time and record in the RESULTS section.

2. Examine the colonies growing on the EMB/lactose plates. Colonies of cells capable of fermenting lactose (Lac^+) will be dark red, whereas Lac^- colonies will be white. Count the number of both for each sampling time and record in the RESULTS section.

3. Count the number of colonies growing on the Minimal agar plates and record in the RESULTS section.

4. Plot the number of recombinants detected by each growth medium vs. time on a single graph. This is done by plotting time on the x-axis and the number of each type of recombinant on the y-axis. Since you are observing transfer of three genes, there will be three different curves.

REFERENCES

Agrios, G.N. *Plant Pathology.* San Diego: Academic Press, 1988.

Miller, J.H. *Experiments in Molecular Genetics.* Cold Spring Harbor, NY: Cold Spring Harbor Labs Press, 1972.

Miller, J.H. *A Short Course in Bacterial Genetics.* Cold Spring Harbor, NY: Cold Spring Harbor Labs Press, 1992.

Ream, W. *Agrobacterium tumefaciens* and Interkingdom Genetic Exchange. *Annual Reviews of Phytopathology* 27(1989):583-618.

RESULTS

Time	EMB/Galactose		EMB/Lactose		Minimal
	Red Colonies	White Colonies	Red Colonies	White Colonies	

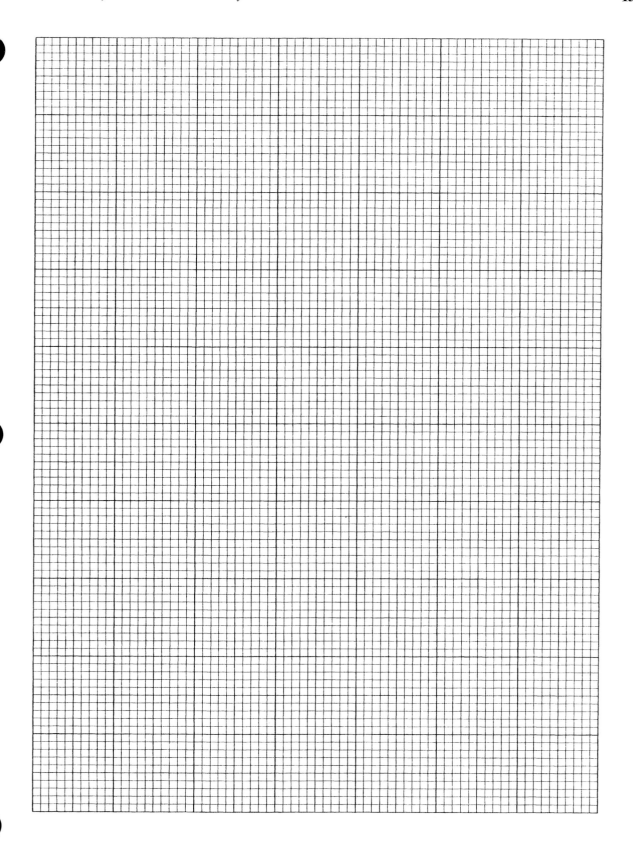

REFLECTIONS

1. Which colonies growing on the EMB/galactose plates are recombinants? Explain.

2. Which colonies growing on the EMB/lactose plates are recombinants? Explain.

3. Which colonies growing on the Minimal plates are recombinants? Explain.

4. Using the information from the graph and **Figure 22.2,** draw a map of the *E. coli* chromosome showing the relative location of the *lac, gal* and *leu* genes. **Note:** Genetic loci of *E. coli* are designated by three letter abbreviations, italicized, and written in lower case.

5. The gene for streptomycin sensitivity used in this experiment is not transferred within the time allotted for this experiment. What role(s) does this gene play in this experiment?

6. In the late 1970s, it was discovered that a large portion of the Ti plasmid of *Agrobacterium* is transferred to the infected plant. This DNA is called T-DNA, short for Transferred DNA. What role does this DNA play in the disease process?

7. Why did this discovery capture the attention of plant geneticists interested in genetically engineering important crop plants?

SECTION IV

MICROBIAL GENETICS

In previous sections, you have learned about the morphological, metabolic, and growth characteristics of different microorganisms. To a large extent, these characteristics are determined by the genes a microbe carries within its genome. Microbial genetics is the study of the genes of microorganisms. Like general genetics, microbial genetics employs classical approaches (e.g., mutagenesis and analysis of mutants) and molecular approaches (e.g., DNA isolation and DNA sequencing) to study gene structure and function. In this section, you will learn some of those techniques.

EXERCISE 23

THE SEARCH FOR MUTANTS

In order to understand gene structure and function, geneticists routinely make use of altered forms of genes. These mutant genes can be harbored by natural variants in a population, but many times geneticists must create mutations (mutagenize), then identify (screen) and isolate the mutants. In this exercise, you will mutagenize a culture and then screen the mutagenized cells for a particular type of mutation. In particular, you will screen a mutagenized culture of the yeast *Saccharomyces cerevisiae* for auxotrophic mutations.

Janine's life was tragically short. She was born in 1975, before acquired immunodeficiency syndrome (AIDS) was recognized. She grew up in a tough neighborhood in New York City. As a teenager she always seemed to be fighting with her parents. Finally, at the age of sixteen, she ran away. To survive on the streets, she turned to prostitution. That was how she contracted the human immunodeficiency virus (HIV). She continued to live on the street, in crowded apartments, and shelters. Her HIV infection quickly progressed to AIDS and in 1994, she contracted tuberculosis (TB). Janine's doctors stressed the importance of taking the prescribed medications for the several months needed to cure TB. Within a month, Janine started feeling better. Since it wasn't always convenient to go to the clinic and the medicine was expensive, she soon stopped taking it. Janine's condition quickly worsened. The TB was back with a vengeance. She went back on medication, but it didn't help; the population of TB bacteria infecting her had become resistant to the antibiotics most effective for treating TB. Janine died two months later.

BACKGROUND INFORMATION

Underlying the story of Janine's short life is another story—the story of a population of the bacterium *Mycobacterium tuberculosis*. This population, like all populations of organisms, contained individuals with unique genomes. Each individual had slightly different abilities for surviving and reproducing within its environment. Such genetic variants arise as the result of changes in the nucleotide sequence in the DNA. These changes are called **mutations.** Mutations impact organisms in various ways. Some are beneficial; however, most mutations are thought to be harmful, even lethal.

Janine's story describes a mutation that is extremely beneficial to the microbe carrying it, but disastrous to the microbe's human host—a mutation that confers antibiotic resistance. Unfortunately, the more antibiotics that are used, the more likely such resistant mutants will persist and increase in number within a population. This is because antibiotic-resistant mutants generally only have a growth advantage when the antibiotic is present. Under such conditions, the sensitive cells die, while the resistant cells survive to reproduce more resistant cells.

Geneticists view the study of mutations as a critical step toward understanding organisms at the genetic level. Among other things, mutations can be used to identify genes, to locate genes on chromosomes, to study the transmission of genes from one generation to the next, and to understand gene interactions. For these reasons, methods for increasing rates of mutations and identification of mutants were developed early in the history of genetics—even before it was known that DNA is the genetic material.

Although antibiotic and drug-resistant microbes are extremely important, they were not the first mutants isolated by early microbial geneticists. The earliest types of mutations isolated were mutations affecting the ability of a microbe to synthesize molecules required for its growth. Many microbes are able to synthesize all amino acids, purines, pyrimidines, and other complex organic molecules. Microbes produce these molecules when cultured on a growth medium containing a simple sugar and inorganic sources of nitrogen, phosphorus, sulfur, and a few trace elements. Such a medium is known as a **minimal medium.** They can do so because they have genes encoding enzymes that catalyze reactions in the biosynthetic pathways that produce these complex molecules. If one gene required for the synthesis of a molecule is mutated (e.g., the amino acid tryptophan), more often than not, the mutation is deleterious. Even one nucleotide change can significantly alter the structure of the resultant enzyme, such that the enzyme is no longer functional. Such mutations are called **auxotrophic mutations,** and the microorganism harboring them is called an **auxotroph.** Auxotrophs are unable to grow on minimal medium. Instead, they must be cultured on a growth medium containing, at a minimum, the growth factor (in this case, tryptophan) that the microbe can't synthesize. The non-mutant microbe, capable of growth in a minimal medium (e.g., without any tryptophan included), is called a **prototroph.**

Auxotrophic mutations are very useful in genetic studies. Initially, they were used to understand biochemical pathways; that is, to determine the number of enzymatic steps in a biosynthetic process, and intermediates in a pathway. They have since been useful as markers to follow chromosome segregation, and for mapping other mutations. They have also been extremely useful in understanding complex processes such as recombination and regulation of gene expression.

Although mutations occur spontaneously, the rate at which they occur is quite low in most organisms. Therefore, when one wishes to isolate mutations of any type, the first step is to increase the number of mutants present in a population. This is done by exposing a population of microbes to physical or chemical agents that interact in some fashion with DNA and as a result, alter the sequence of nucleotides. This process is called **mutagenesis.** In this exercise, you will use ultraviolet (UV) light as a mutagen. UV light is nonionizing radiation (wavelength 100 to 320 nm) that is absorbed by the nitrogenous bases of DNA. As a result, the DNA is damaged. When the cell attempts to repair the damage,

changes in the nucleotide sequence occur. A common wavelength used for UV mutagenesis is 260 nm, which is highly lethal. Typically, cells are exposed to UV light for a length of time known to kill about 90% of the cells in the population. The surviving 10% are then examined for the presence of a mutation. Detection of the mutant is dependent on our ability to observe a phenotype. In this exercise, we will compare growth of the survivors on a **complete medium** (one containing all possible growth factors) and on a minimal medium. Those that grow on the complete medium but not the minimal medium are auxotrophic mutants.

Even though UV light increases the number of mutants in a population, the mutants are still the minority. In order to find the rare mutants, many individuals must be examined. Imagine a plate of complete medium (e.g., YEPD) with 300 colonies of which only one or two are auxotrophs. Now imagine streaking each of those 300 colonies onto minimal medium to find those one or two auxotrophs. If you are also imagining a pain in your wrist resulting from all the streaking, then you understand a major problem in genetics—how to screen large numbers of organisms to find the uncommon mutants.

Fortunately, a solution for screening microbial populations was found quite early in the history of microbial genetics. In 1952, Joshua and Esther Lederberg developed a technique that is still an important tool in microbial genetics. This technique is called replica plating (**Figure 23.1**). In this procedure, colonies on one medium can be transferred to a "virgin" medium using a replica velvet. Replica velvets are simply squares of velvet material that are sterilized. The transfer is accomplished by gently pressing a master plate (the plate with colonies) on to a velvet. Cells from each colony on the master plate stick to the fabric. When the "virgin medium" is pressed to the velvet, the cells are transferred to that medium. Thus, growth on the master plate has been duplicated exactly to the replica plate. In this exercise, you will mutagenize cells on a complete medium that serves as the master plate. When the cells grow into colonies, they will be replica plated to a minimal medium and auxotrophs can then be identified.

PURPOSE

- To learn about mutations and their use to geneticists
- To use standard techniques (UV mutagenesis and replica plating) for isolating mutant microbes

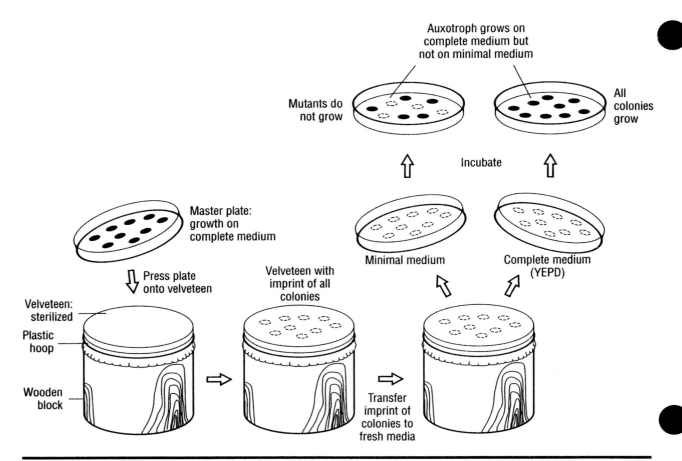

Figure 23.1   The replica plating method.

THE EXERCISE

Day 1

MATERIALS:

A tube containing a haploid, prototrophic strain of
  S. cerevisiae at a cell density of ~2.5 × 10⁴ cells/ml
Bunsen burner
Four YEPD plates
Micropipetters and sterile pipet tips
Culture spreader soaking in 70% ethanol

PROCEDURE: Work in groups of four

1. Label the YEPD plates M1, M2, M3, and M4,
    respectively (**Figure 23.2**). **Note:** YEPD is a com-
    plete medium used for growing *S. cerevisiae*. It
    contains *y*east *e*xtract, *p*eptone and *d*extrose (glu-
    cose). The yeast extract and peptone are excellent
    sources of amino acids, purines, pyrimidines, and

vitamins. These four plates will serve as master
plates (M = master) in the replica plating you will
do during Day 2 of the exercise.

2. Pipet 10 μl of the yeast culture on the plate
    labeled M1.

3. Remove the culture spreader from the alcohol.
    Flame it to sterilize and cool briefly.

4. Use the culture spreader to spread the inoculum
    over the surface of the medium. **Note:** See Exer-
    cise 20 for details of the spread plate method.

5. Repeat steps 2 through 4 for the M2 plate.

6. Repeat steps 2 through 4 using 100 μl of inoculum
    and the plates labeled M3 and M4.

7. Remove the lids of all your plates and expose
    the plates to UV light for the time indicated by
    your instructor. **Note:** Each group will expose
    their plates to UV light for a set time. The times
    used by different groups in the class will vary

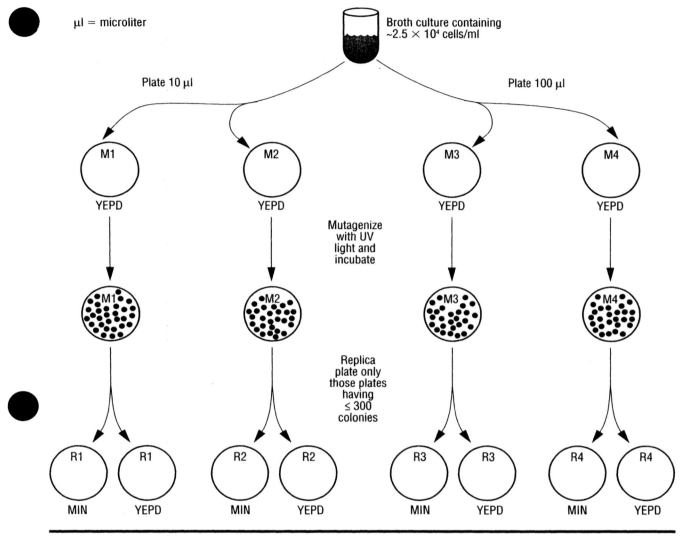

Figure 23.2   An overview of the mutagenesis and screening procedure to be used in this exercise.

from 0 seconds (s) to 60 s. Data from the class will be collected and used to analyze the outcome of the mutagenesis.

8. Immediately place the plates in the dark and incubate at 30°C. **Note:** Incubation in the dark is required because *S. cerevisiae* has a photo repair system which, if functioning, will decrease the number of mutations generated.

Day 2

MATERIALS:

Plates from Day 1
Replica plating blocks with hoops for securing velvets
Sterile replica velvets

One to four minimal media plates (MIN plates)
One to four YEPD plates

PROCEDURE:

1. Count the number of colonies on the master plates.
2. Report your results to your instructor. Your instructor will post the results of all groups in your class. Record your data and the class data in the RESULTS section. **Note:** Only those plates with less than 300 colonies will be used in the remainder of the exercise.
3. Put an X or some other mark on the edge of the bottom of any master plates having less than 300 colonies. **Note:** In order to identify

colonies on a master plate and its replica plate, the plates must be properly oriented with respect to each other. The X or other mark serves as a point of reference for orientation of the plates. Alternatively, use the M1, etc., label for orientation.

Before proceeding, examine Figure 23.2 carefully. This outlines the replicating procedure. Note that M1 plates serve as master plates for R1 plates (both MIN and YEPD), which are the replica plates. M2 plates serve as master plates for R2 plates and so on. It is unlikely that you will have more than two master plates to replicate. Some of you may have none to replicate.

4. Label a MIN and a YEPD plate R1 (**Figure 23.2**). **Note:** These two plates will have the colonies from the master plate (M1) replicated to them. The MIN replica plate (R1) will be compared to the master plate (M1) to identify auxotrophs. The YEPD replica plate is a control used to determine if all colonies on the master plate were transferred.

5. Repeat step 4 for the remaining MIN and YEPD plates, labeling one set R2, another R3, and the last R4 (**Figure 23.2**). **Note:** Some of the master plates will have more than 300 colonies, and some will have no colonies. Therefore, you will only need as many sets of replica plates as you have master plates with less than 300 colonies.

6. Make an X or other mark on the edge of the bottom of the replica plates (R1, R2, etc.) (see step 3).

7. Place a sterile replica velvet, rough side up, on a replica block. Use the hoop to secure the velvet to the block (**Figure 23.1**) As you look down on the block, the upper edge will be used as an orientation reference. You will align the X or other mark on the plates with the upper edge of the block. **Note:** Use aseptic technique to keep the velvet sterile. Open the package so that the rough side of the velvet is not exposed. Only touch one corner of the velvet as you lift and position it on the block. Do not leave the velvet on the block for longer than needed to replica plate the master plates.

8. Remove the lid from a master plate and invert the bottom of the plate over the replica velvet. Orient the plate so the X or mark is at the upper edge of the velvet (**Figure 23.1**). **Note:** The orientation is done before placing the plate on the velvet. If the plate is moved after coming in contact with the velvet, the colonies will be smeared around the plate and the velvet.

9. *Gently* press the plate against the velvet. Then lift and replace the lid. **Note:** If you look at the velvet you may see where cells from the colonies have been transferred to the velvet.

10. Remove the lid from the corresponding MIN replica plate and invert the bottom of the plate over the replica velvet. Orient the plate so the X or other mark is at the upper edge of the velvet (see step 8).

11. *Gently* press the replica plate against the velvet. Then lift and replace the lid. **Note:** You have just replicated the colonies from the master plate to the MIN replica plate.

12. Replicate the colonies from the master plate (if less than 300 colonies) to the corresponding YEPD plate by repeating steps 10 and 11 with the appropriate YEPD plate. **Note:** You have just replicated the colonies from the master plate onto the YEPD replica plate.

13. Repeat steps 7 through 12 for all the other master plates. Always do the corresponding MIN replica plate first, then the corresponding YEPD replica plate.

14. Incubate the replica plates at 30°C.

15. Store the master plates in the cold for the next laboratory period.

Day 3

1. Examine the MIN replica plates by orienting each over its master plate. This is best done by placing the master plate above a light source (e.g., colony counter) so that light shines through the two plates. Your instructor will demonstrate how to do this.

2. Determine if any colonies on the master plate did not grow on the MIN replica plate. Those colonies are auxotrophic colonies. Count the number of auxotrophic colonies and record them in the results section.

3. Also check to see if there are any "missing" colonies on the YEPD replica plates.

4. Report to your instructor the number of auxotrophs you identified on each plate, and the UV exposure time you used to mutagenize the cells. Your instructor will post the class data. Record your data and the class data in the RESULTS section.

5. Using the "10 µl" plate counts, graph the number of colonies on the master plates versus UV exposure

time. This is done by plotting UV exposure time on the x-axis and number of colonies on the y-axis. You will need to use semilog paper. Determine the exposure time that killed approximately 90% of the cells.

6. Also graph the total number of auxotrophic colonies versus UV exposure time. This is done by plotting UV exposure time on the x-axis and the total number of auxotrophic colonies on the y-axis. Plot this graph on standard graph paper.

REFERENCES

Sherman, F., et al. *Laboratory Course Manual for Methods in Yeast Genetics.* Cold Spring Harbor, NY: Cold Spring Harbor Laboratory Press, 1986.

RESULTS

Colony counts on the master plates:

Plate	Inoculum Size	Exposure Time					
		0 s	5 s	15 s	30 s	45 s	60 s
M1	10 µl						
M2	10 µl						
M3	100 µl						
M4	100 µl						

Number of auxotrophic mutants (colonies that grew on master plate but not on MIN replica plate):

MIN Replica Plate	Exposure Time					
	0 s	5 s	15 s	30 s	45 s	60 s
R1						
R2						
R3						
R4						
Total						

*If you did not replicate all master plates, place ND (not done) in the appropriate cell(s) in the table.

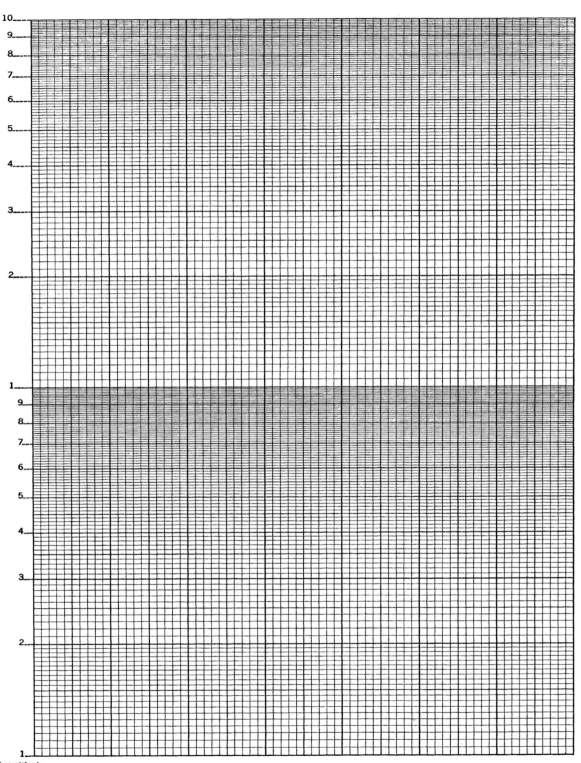

Semi-Logarithmic
2 Cycles x 10 to the inch

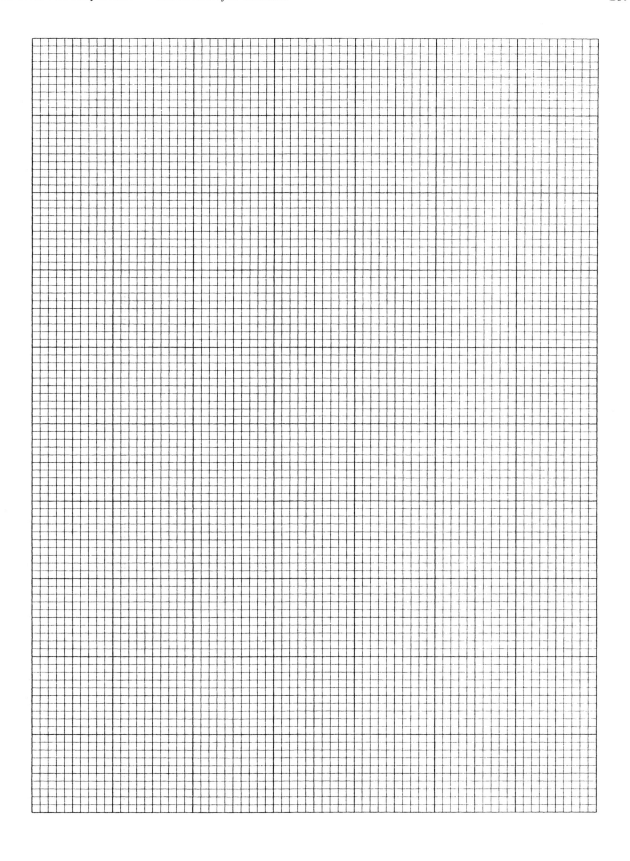

REFLECTIONS

1. Examine the graph of number of auxotrophs versus UV exposure time. In a sentence or two, describe the relationship between these two variables. Why do you think geneticists typically look for auxotrophic mutations after exposing cells to a UV dosage that kills 90% of the cells?

2. It is possible to make solutions of individual amino acids, and other growth factors. These can be incorporated into a growth medium. Describe how you might determine the nature of the defects in the auxotrophic mutants your class isolated. That is, how could you determine which growth factor an auxotroph is unable to synthesize?

3. It is possible to select for antibiotic-resistant bacteria. Describe how you might isolate bacteria resistant to ampicillin, starting with a culture of sensitive bacteria.

4. Suppose you observed a colony on a master plate that did not grow on the MIN replica plate or on the YEPD replica plate. How could you explain this observation?

ISOLATION OF PLASMIDS

Late 1990, a small girl went down in medical history as the first to be treated by gene therapy to correct a genetic disorder. Such an event had been almost impossible to conceive 20 years earlier when the tools for genetic engineering and gene therapy were first being discovered. Today the possibilities for genetically engineering crop plants and for treating disease seem limited only by concerns about the safety of engineered organisms and ethical questions. We have the methods and tools for genetic engineering. Now the question is, should we use them. In this and the next two exercises, you will gain experience using some of those tools.

Certain varieties of wheat are resistant to a disease called stripe rust. But what enables those varieties to resist the attack of the fungal pathogen Puccinia *while others are susceptible? After weeks spent creating a genomic library from a resistant variety of wheat and several more weeks screening that library, Jeff finally identified a clone that contained the resistance gene. With the clone in hand, a better understanding of the interaction between the fungal pathogen and its plant host was possible. Such information was vital to the understanding of disease processes in plants, and could lead to the development of strategies for protecting crops without the use of pesticides.*

Jeff had a long way to go, however, before he could engineer plants to be resistant to pathogens. His next step was to determine which recombinant cloning vector carried the disease-resistance gene. After that he needed to identify the portion of the wheat DNA insert responsible for resistance to stripe rust disease. That portion of the insert would then be cloned into another

cloning vector and studied further. In the next two exercises, you will continue to follow Jeff's story.

BACKGROUND INFORMATION

Jeff is reaping the benefits of approximately 100 years of research by many scientists in a variety of scientific disciplines. This work led to an understanding of the chemical nature of cellular genetic material (DNA), the function of DNA, and the discovery of tools and techniques that allow investigators to manipulate DNA outside cells. To a large extent, DNA encodes instructions for the synthesis of proteins. In many cases, these proteins serve as enzymes that catalyze reactions necessary for cells to survive, grow, and reproduce. The information in DNA is divided into units called **genes.** Each gene consists of a sequence of nucleotides that specifies the order of amino acids in a particular protein.

In their attempts to better understand how organisms function and reproduce, scientists sometimes turn for answers to the proteins involved, or to the genes that encode those proteins. To study a gene at the molecular level, scientists often **clone** the gene. Cloning involves isolating DNA from an appropriate population of cells or tissue, breaking or cutting the DNA into smaller pieces and inserting those pieces into a **cloning vector.** The cloning vector is a DNA molecule that is used to make millions of copies of the gene of interest, and to move that gene from one cell to another. The cloning process typically results in the production of thousands of **recombinant DNA** molecules (vectors with foreign DNA inserts), but often only one of the recombinant molecules contains the gene of interest. The critical step in the cloning procedure is to identify the cloning vector that contains the gene of interest. Once that clone has been identified, the gene can be manipulated in a variety of ways to further understand its structure and function.

In the time since the first gene was cloned, numerous cloning vectors have been constructed using naturally occurring DNA molecules such as plasmids and viral genomes. Each cloning vector has features that make it better suited for cloning certain genes, or for studying a gene once it has been cloned. Despite the diversity of cloning vectors now available, all share the characteristic of being able to replicate separately from chromosomes. This characteristic is a defining feature of **bacterial plasmids,** which were among the first molecules to be used as cloning vectors. Furthermore, many plasmids have the additional characteristic of carrying antibiotic-resistance genes. These genes are very useful when screening for bacteria containing recombinant plasmids.

In this exercise, you will isolate a plasmid from *Escherichia coli*. Recall that most of the DNA found in a bacterium is in the single, large, circular bacterial chromosome. Plasmids are considerably smaller than the chromosome, and it is this difference that is largely the basis for their separation from the chromosome. Isolation of plasmids involves breaking open cells, then using a number of reagents and steps to remove cellular components while leaving the plasmid in a solution. This procedure is not completely effective, however. An additional step, **agarose gel electrophoresis,** is necessary to further purify the plasmid.

Electrophoresis is a technique used to separate molecules by moving them in an electrical field. We will use agarose gel electrophoresis to move DNA through a gel made from an extract of agar (agarose). DNA is negatively charged and moves toward the positive electrode in an electrophoresis chamber. The distance it moves depends on the amount of time the DNA is exposed to the electrical field and on the size and shape of the DNA (e.g., linear, open circle, supercoiled circle). In general, smaller, more compact DNA molecules move more quickly than large molecules. After DNA molecules are separated by agarose gel electrophoresis, they can be visualized by staining the gel with dyes that bind DNA. One routinely used stain is **ethidium bromide.** Ethidium bromide is a flat (planar) molecule that squeezes into the spaces between nucleotides adjacent to each other in a single DNA strand. When ethidium bromide is illuminated with ultraviolet light (UV), it fluoresces. Thus the DNA–ethidium bromide complexes can be seen. Because ethidium bromide is a

suspected carcinogen,[1] you will not stain and photograph the DNA in the gel. This task will be carried out by your instructor.

PURPOSE

- To isolate and visualize plasmid DNA using agarose gel electrophoresis and ethidium bromide staining

THE EXERCISE

Day 1
MATERIALS:
Pelleted, plasmid-containing *E. coli* cells in a microcentrifuge tube

GTE (25 mM Tris-chloride, pH 7.5, containing 50 mM glucose and 10 mM disodium ethylene diamine tetraacetate [EDTA])

Gel electrophoresis running dye

Microcentrifuge

Micropipetters and sterile pipet tips

TE (10 mM Tris-chloride, pH 8 containing 1 mM EDTA)

KOAc (5 M potassium acetate), on ice[2]

95% ethanol, on ice

70% ethanol

NaOH/SDS (0.2 N sodium hydroxide containing 1% sodium dodecyl sulfate)

Molten agarose

*Hin*dIII cut bacteriophage lambda (λ) DNA

Electrophoresis chamber and power source

1X TAE buffer (40 mM Tris-acetate buffer containing 1 mM EDTA)

55°C water bath

Isolation of Plasmid

Yesterday, an *E. coli* strain containing a plasmid was inoculated into a very rich growth medium. The medium contained an antibiotic at a concentration that kills bacteria that do not harbor the plasmid. Thus, the only bacteria that grew were plasmid-containing bacteria. This morning, 1 ml aliquots of cells were dispensed into microcentrifuge

---

[1]Ethidium bromide can cause changes (mutations) in genetic material. Therefore, it has also been hypothesized to be a carcinogen.

[2]Although designated as 5 M KOAc, this solution is actually 3 M with respect to potassium and 5 M with respect to acetate.

tubes. The cells were spun in the microcentrifuge for about 1 minute. This step pelleted the cells in the bottom of the tube. The supernatant fluid was decanted, or poured out, leaving the pellet in the bottom of the tube.

PROCEDURE: Work in groups of two to five as directed by your instructor

1. Obtain a microcentrifuge tube of pelleted, plasmid-containing *E. coli* cells.
2. Add 100 μl of GTE. Resuspend the cells by mixing with a vortex.
3. Add 200 μl of NaOH/SDS. Mix gently, but thoroughly. **Note:** This step lyses the cells, releasing the cytoplasm into the buffer. NaOH/SDS also selectively denatures, or separates the strands of the chromosomal DNA and complexes with cellular proteins.
4. Incubate the cells on ice for 5 minutes.
5. Add 150 μl KOAc. Mix gently but thoroughly. **Note:** This step causes proteins, chromosomal DNA, and large RNA molecules to precipitate.
6. Incubate the cells on ice for 5 minutes.
7. Spin the microcentrifuge tube in a microcentrifuge for 5 minutes. Your instructor will help you place the tube in the microcentrifuge so that it is properly balanced. **Note:** This step pellets much of the cell debris and organic molecules that were precipitated in earlier steps.
8. Decant the supernatant fluid into a new microcentrifuge tube. **Note:** The plasmid remains intact and in solution in all earlier steps, and it is present in the supernatant fluid. The pellet and the original tube can be discarded.
9. Add 1 ml ice cold 95% ethanol to the supernatant fluid in the new microcentrifuge tube. **Note:** The ethanol precipitates the plasmid.
10. Incubate the plasmid at −20°C for 15 minutes. **Note:** This time can be used to prepare the agarose gel (see below).
11. Spin the tube for 15 minutes. **Note:** This step pellets the precipitated plasmid.
12. Decant and discard the supernatant fluid. **Note:** Do not shake the tube before or after decanting or the pellet may be lost. Even if you do not see a pellet in the bottom of the tube, it is probably still there as long as you decanted carefully.
13. Add 500 μl of 70% ethanol to the pellet in the tube. Resuspend the plasmid pellet by gently rocking the tube. **Note:** This step washes the plasmid, removing excess salts that can interfere

with subsequent procedures. The plasmid does not dissolve in the ethanol.

14. Spin the microcentrifuge tube for 5 minutes.
15. Decant and discard the supernatant fluid.
16. Air dry the pellet for about 15 minutes.
17. Resuspend the DNA in 100 μl TE. Save this tube. You are now ready to load the gel if the agarose gel is already prepared. **Note:** The plasmid dissolves in TE.

Preparation of Agarose Gel

Earlier today, agarose was added to TAE buffer, a buffer routinely used for electrophoresis. The concentration of agarose is 0.8% (w/v) or 0.8 grams of agarose per 100 ml of buffer. This concentration of agarose allows free movement of DNA and RNA in the range of 0.5 to 10 kilobases (kb), and therefore is effective for separating the plasmid molecules from contaminating chromosomal DNA and RNA. The agarose/buffer solution was heated in a microwave to melt the agarose. It is being kept as a liquid in a 55°C water bath.

1. Your instructor will demonstrate how to prepare the gel mold (**Figure 24.1**). The well-former, or comb, creates depressions in the gel that are called wells. Aliquots of your plasmid solution will eventually be placed in these wells. **Note:** Some gel molds are set up within the electrophoresis chamber, whereas others are set up outside the chamber.
2. Pour the gel, and let it solidify for about 25 minutes. If you are still isolating the plasmid, continue with that while the gel solidifies. **Note:** If you have completed the plasmid isolation, you can prepare the plasmid for electrophoresis (see Electrophoresis of Plasmid, steps 1 through 3) while the gel solidifies.
3. Remove the comb from the gel. The gel is now ready for use if it was formed in the chamber. For gels formed outside the chamber, dismantle the gel mold and place the gel in the electrophoresis

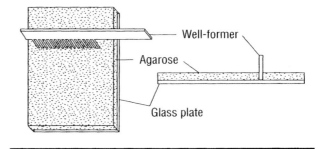

Figure 24.1 Preparation of an agarose gel.

chamber. **Note:** Sometimes gels formed in the electrophoresis chamber need to be reoriented in the chamber after the gel has solidified. On occasion, wells collapse when the comb is removed. If possible, immerse the gel in buffer in the chamber before removing the comb.

4. Fill the chamber with TAE buffer so that the buffer just covers the gel. **Note:** The buffer contains ions which promote current flow through the chamber.

Electrophoresis of Plasmid

1. Obtain a microcentrifuge tube.
2. Transfer 10 µl of the plasmid solution to the tube.
3. Add 2 µl of gel electrophoresis running dye to the tube. **Note:** The running dye has two functions. First, it keeps DNA from floating out of the wells as the well is loaded. Second, the running dye, like DNA and RNA, is negatively charged and moves toward the positive electrode during electrophoresis. However, the running dye is a very small molecule and moves much faster through the gel than does the DNA. By following the dye's migration, we can determine when to stop the electrophoresis.
4. When the gel is solidified, complete steps 3 and 4 in Preparation of Agarose Gel and proceed to the next step, loading the gel.
5. Load samples of plasmid from all groups in your class into the gel using the following suggested scheme. Your instructor will provide details of the loading scheme based on the size of your class, the number of samples, and the electrophoresis equipment available for use.

   First Lane: *Hin*dIII cut λ DNA. **Note:** This is purified λ DNA that has been cut into linear fragments by the restriction endonuclease *Hin*dIII *(see* Exercise 25). The sizes of the fragments are known. The solution loaded in the well was made using 5 µl of a preparation of λ DNA at a concentration of 61 ng λ DNA/µl and 2 µl gel running dye.

   Center Lanes: Plasmid samples from each group in the class (**Figure 24.2**). **Note:** Each member of the class should make a drawing of the gel, recording what sample is in each lane.

   Last Lane: *Hin*dIII cut λ DNA (as in First Lane).

6. Cover the electrophoresis chamber, attach electrodes from the power source, and turn on the power source (**Figure 24.3**). The gel will run at 50 to 80 volts for 2 to 3 hours. Be sure the electrodes are attached to the power source so that the wells are closest to the negative pole and farthest from the positive pole.

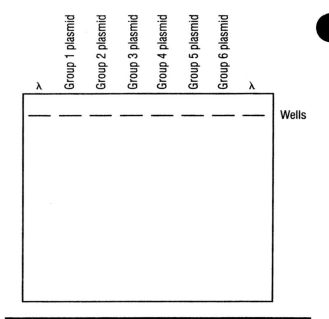

Figure 24.2 An example of a gel-loading scheme using an eight-lane gel. Your gel may have fewer or more lanes.

Day 2

Your instructor ran the power source at 50 to 80 volts until the gel running dye had migrated from 2/3 to 3/4 the distance of the gel. The power was then turned off and the gel removed. The gel was stained in an ethidium bromide solution for about 15 minutes. Your instructor wore gloves and other protective clothing while staining the gel because ethidium bromide is a suspected carcinogen. After staining, the gel was placed on a UV light source (transilluminator) and viewed (**Figure 24.4**). The ethidium bromide fluoresces when exposed to UV light. A photograph of each gel was taken.

1. Obtain a photograph of your gel.
2. Find the lane that contains your group's plasmid. Below each well, you will observe one or more bright bands against a dark background. Plasmids exist in several different forms in cells and in plasmid preparations. These include open (relaxed) circles, supercoiled circles, and catenanes (two circles linked together, which are supercoiled or relaxed).
3. Locate a lane with *Hin*dIII cut λ DNA. You should observe six bands in this lane. The uppermost band was formed by linear DNA fragments 23 kb in length. The lengths of the fragments, moving down the lane, are 9.4 kb, 6.6 kb, 4.4 kb, 2.3 kb, and 2.0 kb (**Figure 24.5**).

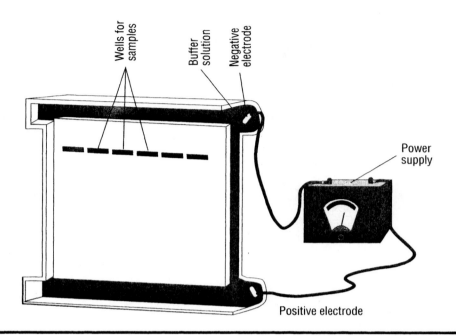

Figure 24.3 Set up of electrophoresis equipment.

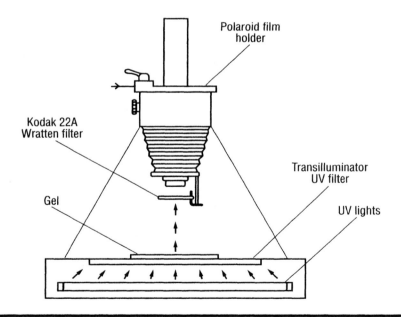

Figure 24.4 Ultraviolet light transilluminator and Polaroid camera setup.

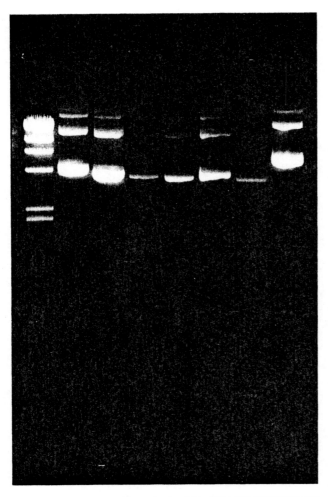

4. Use a ruler to measure the distance of each band in the λ DNA lane from the well. This is the distance migrated by the fragments in each band. Record the distances migrated in the RESULTS section.

5. Graph distance migrated (x-axis) versus size of fragment (y-axis) using semilog paper. You should observe a linear relationship for all fragments except the 23 kb fragment. Draw the best fit line using all points except the 23 kb fragment point. The line you have drawn is called a **standard curve.** Since the concentration of agarose used in this gel allows free movement of nucleic acids in the range of 0.5 to 10 kb, a linear relationship between the log of the size of the DNA and its mobility in the gel is observed only within this size range.

6. Use a ruler to measure the distance traveled by the plasmid bands. Record the distances in the RESULTS section.

7. Use the standard curve to determine the size of a linear DNA molecule which would migrate the same distance as the various forms of the plasmid. Record the results in the RESULTS section.

REFERENCES

Birnboim, H.C., and Doly, J. A Rapid Alkaline Extraction Procedure for Screening Recombinant Plasmid DNA. *Nucleic Acids Research* 7:(1979) 1513-1523.

Crosa, J.H., et al. Plasmids. In *Methods for General and Molecular Bacteriology.* Washington, DC: American Association for Microbiology Press, 1994.

Sambrook, J., et al. *Molecular Cloning: A Laboratory Manual,* 2nd ed. Cold Spring Harbor, NY: Cold Spring Harbor Laboratory Press, 1989.

Figure 24.5 An example of an agarose gel after staining with ethidium bromide and illumination with UV light.

RESULTS

Distances migrated by λ DNA fragments:

| 23 kb _____ | 6.6 kb _____ | 2.3 kb _____ |
| 9.4 kb _____ | 4.4 kb _____ | 2.0 kb _____ |

Distances migrated by various plasmid forms:

Sizes of linear DNA which would migrate the same distance as the various forms of the plasmid:

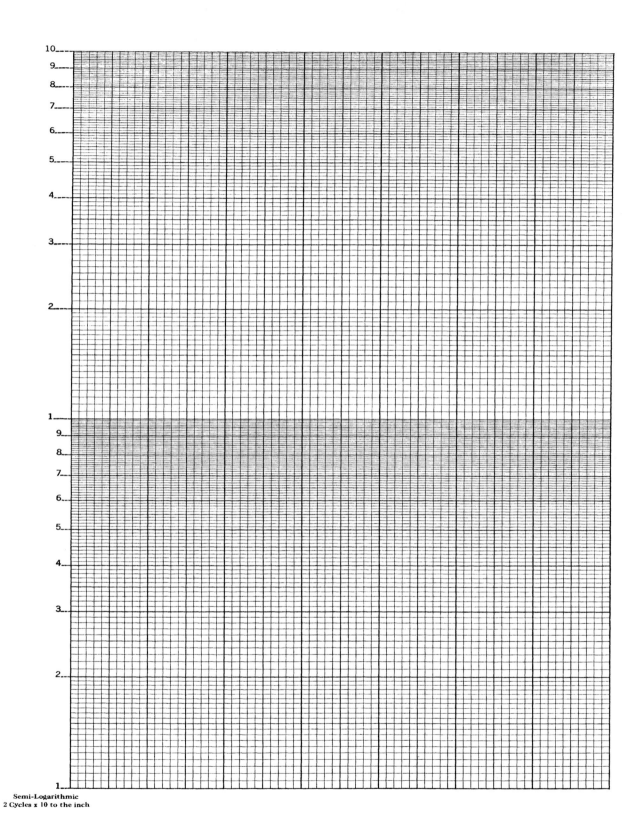

Semi-Logarithmic
2 Cycles x 10 to the inch

REFLECTIONS

1. Assume the density of plasmid-containing cells you had when you began this exercise was 10^8 cells/ ml. How many copies of the *E. coli* chromosome were in the microcentrifuge tube after lysing the cells? Remember your tube contained 1 ml of cells which had been pelleted.

2. If each *E. coli* cell contained fifty copies of the plasmid, how many copies of the plasmid were in the microcentrifuge tube after lysing the cells?

3. In your own words, explain what a band on a gel is, and how it is visualized.

4. The stripe rust resistance gene is part of a recombinant DNA molecule consisting of cloning vector linked to wheat DNA. What is a cloning vector? Give two examples of specific DNA molecules routinely used as cloning vectors.

5. Describe how Jeff could use agarose gel electrophoresis to confirm that a plasmid is recombinant.

6. You were *not* instructed to use the standard curve to calculate the *size of the plasmid*. Why not?

7. The plasmid in your preparation exists in a number of different forms. Which form do you think will migrate the fastest? Is your intuition correct? To answer this question will require some research into the theory and mathematics underlying electrophoretic procedures.

EXERCISE 25

AT THE CUTTING EDGE

In the previous exercise, you gained experience isolating plasmids and using agarose gel electrophoresis. Procedures for purification of DNA and electrophoresis are routinely used by genetic engineers to isolate and manipulate a gene of interest. In this exercise, you will use a restriction endonuclease to cut a recombinant DNA molecule. As a result, foreign DNA will be removed from a plasmid cloning vector.

Jeff had successfully isolated the recombinant plasmid that contained the gene for resistance to stripe rust disease (see Exercise 24). Jeff's task now was to remove the large insert of wheat DNA, which probably contained more than one wheat gene, and determine the boundaries of the resistance gene. Jeff thought this would take about a month, and then he should be able to clone a smaller fragment of wheat DNA containing just the resistance gene into an appropriate m13-derived cloning vector. He would then determine the sequence of nucleotides in the gene. Using the nucleotide sequence and the genetic code, Jeff could predict the sequence of amino acids in the protein encoded by the resistance gene. He would then compare the resistance protein to other proteins in the hope that it would help him learn the function of the protein. This would be the first step in understanding how this gene conferred resistance to disease.

BACKGROUND INFORMATION

In 1978, the Nobel Prize in Physiology or Medicine was awarded to Daniel Nathans, Hamilton Smith, and Werner Arber for their work

on enzymes that cut DNA at specific sites. These enzymes, called **restriction endonucleases,** were critical to the work Jeff had already done to clone, or make many identical copies of, the stripe rust resistance gene. They are also critical to the work he was about to do, which was to determine the boundaries of the gene and subclone it, or clone smaller portions of a gene or foreign DNA into another cloning vector.

Restriction endonucleases have the ability to recognize specific sequences of nucleotides in DNA and cut the sugar-phosphate backbone within or near those sequences (**Figure 25.1**). When scientists use a restriction endonuclease to cut DNA, they refer to the process as a "restriction digestion." Restriction digests are done in an aqueous solution and upon completion of digestion, all fragments are in the same solution. In order to physically separate the fragments, electrophoresis is done and the separated DNA fragments are visualized by staining with ethidium bromide (see Exercise 24). In this exercise you will use a restriction endonuclease to cut a **recombinant plasmid;** that is, a plasmid with foreign DNA inserted into it. As a result, the foreign DNA will be cut out of the plasmid. Plasmid and foreign DNA will then be separated by agarose gel electrophoresis.

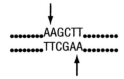

Figure 25.1 The sequence of nitrogenous bases in double-stranded DNA recognized by the restriction endonuclease *Hin*dIII. The arrows indicate where the sugar-phosphate backbone is cut by the enzyme.

PURPOSE

- To cut a recombinant plasmid with a restriction endonuclease
- To separate DNA fragments by agarose gel electrophoresis and then visualize the fragments with the fluorescent stain ethidium bromide
- To calculate the size in kilobases of DNA fragments using DNA fragments of known length

THE EXERCISE

Day 1

MATERIALS:

Isolated recombinant plasmid
Microcentrifuge tubes
10× restriction buffer
Gel electrophoresis running dye
Molten agarose
Microcentrifuge
Electrophoresis chamber and power source
Micropipetters and sterile pipet tips
Sterile distilled water
Restriction endonuclease
*Hind*III cut bacteriophage lambda (λ) DNA
1× TAE buffer
37°C and 55°C water baths

PROCEDURE: Work in groups of two to five, as directed by your instructor

Restriction Digestion of Plasmid

1. Label a microcentrifuge tube "restriction digest" or RD.
2. Use micropipetters to add the following reagents to the tube.
   - 30 μl recombinant plasmid
   - 14 μl sterile distilled water
   - 5 μl 10× restriction digest buffer
   - 1 μl restriction endonuclease

   Note: Touch the pipet tip to the side of the tube to release the small quantities of liquid into the tube. You must also remember to change pipet tips after each addition so that you do not cross-contaminate any of the solutions. Your instructor may want to add the restriction endonuclease to the digest mixture to prevent accidental contamination or pipetting errors.
3. Place the microcentrifuge tube in a microcentrifuge and pulse briefly to mix the reagents and bring the liquid to the bottom of the tube.

4. Incubate the reaction mixture at 37°C for 1 hour.
5. Save the undigested plasmid preparation for Electrophoresis of Digested Plasmid. Proceed to Preparation of Agarose Gel while the plasmid is being digested.

Preparation of Agarose Gel

Earlier today, agarose was added to TAE buffer, a buffer routinely used for electrophoresis. The concentration of agarose is 0.8% (w/v) or 0.8 grams per 100 ml of buffer. This concentration of agarose allows free movement of DNA and RNA in the range of 0.5 to 10 kilobases (kb). Therefore, it is effective for separating the DNA fragments produced by the digestion. The agarose/buffer solution was heated in a microwave to melt the agarose. It is kept as a liquid in a 55°C water bath.

1. Your instructor will demonstrate how to prepare the gel mold (see Exercise 24, **Figure 24.1**). The comb creates depressions in the gel which are called wells. Aliquots of the uncut plasmid and the restriction digests will eventually be placed in these wells. **Note:** Some gel molds are set up within the electrophoresis chamber, whereas others are set up outside the chamber.
2. Pour the gel and let it solidify for about 25 minutes. **Note:** Continue to Electrophoresis of Digested Plasmid while the gel solidifies.
3. Remove the comb from the gel. The gel is now ready for use if it was formed in the chamber. For gels formed outside the chamber, dismantle the gel mold and place the gel in the electrophoresis chamber. **Note:** Sometimes gels formed in the electrophoresis chamber need to be reoriented in the chamber after they have solidified. On occasion, wells collapse when the comb is removed. If possible, immerse the gel in buffer in the chamber before removing the comb.
4. Fill the chamber with TAE buffer so that the buffer just covers the gel.

Electophoresis of Digested Plasmid

1. Obtain a microcentrifuge tube and label it "cut."
2. Transfer 23 μl of the digest mixture into the tube labeled "cut."
3. Add 2 μl of gel electrophoresis running dye and set aside. **Note:** The running dye serves two functions. First, it keeps DNA from floating out of the wells when being loaded in the gel. Second, the running dye, like the DNA and RNA, is negatively

charged and moves toward the positive pole. However, the dye is a very small molecule and moves much faster through the gel. By following the dye's movement, we can decide when to stop the electrophoresis.

4. Your instructor (or one group) will prepare two tubes of a solution containing 10 μl of the undigested plasmid and 2 μl of the gel electrophoresis running dye. **Note:** By comparing the digested DNA to the undigested DNA, you can tell how successful the restriction digestion was.

5. Load the samples of DNA into the gel using the following suggested scheme (**Figure 25.2**). If each group is using plasmid isolated from Exercise 24, then the center lanes should be loaded with undigested and cut plasmid from each group. Be sure to appoint at least one person to record the order of samples loaded in the gel.

*First Lane: Hin*dIII cut λ DNA; **Note:** This is purified λ DNA that has been cut into linear fragments by the restriction endonuclease *Hin*dIII. The sizes of the λ fragments are known and can be used to calculate the size of the plasmid fragments. The solution loaded into the well

was made using 5 μl λ DNA at a concentration of 61 ng λ DNA/μl, and 2 μl running dye
Second Lane: Undigested plasmid (see step 4)
Center Lanes: Cut DNA samples prepared by class
Next to Last Lane: Undigested plasmid
*Last Lane: Hin*dIII λ DNA

6. Cover the electrophoresis chamber, attach electrodes from the power source, and turn on the power source, (see Exercise 24, **Figure 24.3**). The gel will run at about 50 to 80 volts for 2 to 3 hours. **Note:** Be sure the electrodes are attached so that the wells are closest to the negative pole and farthest from the positive pole.

Day 2

Your instructor ran the power source at 50 to 80 volts until the running dye had migrated from 2/3 to 3/4 the distance of the gel. The power was then turned off and the gel removed. The gel was stained in ethidium bromide for about 15 minutes. Your instructor wore gloves and other protective clothing while staining the gel because ethidium bromide is a suspected carcinogen. Then the gel was placed on a UV light source (transilluminator) and viewed (see Exercise 24, **Figure 24.4**). A photograph of each gel was taken.

1. Obtain a photograph of your gel.
2. Find the lanes that contain your group's cut plasmid. Below each well, you will observe two or more bright bands against the dark background (**Figure 24.5**). Each band represents a position where DNA fragments of the same length migrated. Check with your instructor to determine which bands represent the bands produced when all plasmids in your reaction mixture are completely cut. **Note:** The plasmid preparations you are using may contain contaminating molecules (e.g., salts) that interfere with the digestion. Therefore, some of the bands you observe may represent uncut plasmid or partially cut plasmid.
3. Examine a lane with *Hin*dIII cut λ DNA. You should observe six bands in this lane. The uppermost band was formed by fragments 23 kb in length. The length of the fragments, moving down the lane, are 9.4 kb, 6.6 kb, 4.4 kb, 2.3 kb, and 2.0 kb (see Exercise 24, **Figure 24.5**).
4. Use a ruler to measure the distance of each band in the λ DNA lane from the well. This is the distance migrated by the fragments in each band. Record the distances in the RESULTS section.

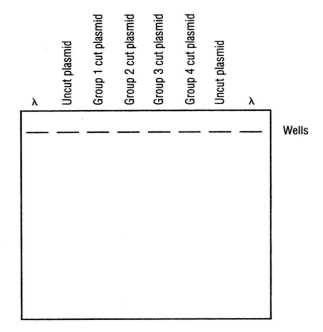

Figure 25.2 An example of a gel-loading scheme using an eight-lane gel. Your gel may have fewer or more lanes.

5. Graph distance migrated (x-axis) versus size of fragments (y-axis) using semilog paper. You should observe a linear relationship for all fragments except the 23 kb fragment. Draw the best fit line using all points except the 23 kb fragment point. The line you have drawn is called a **standard curve.** **Note:** Since the concentration of agarose used in this gel allows free movement of nucleic acids in the range of 0.5 to 10 kb, a linear relationship between the log of the size of the DNA and its mobility in the gel is observed only within this size range.
6. Use a ruler to measure the distance traveled by the bands in the "cut" lane and record the distances in the RESULTS section.

7. Use the standard curve to determine the size of the plasmid fragments. Only use those bands produced when the plasmid is digested to completion.

REFERENCES

Brock, et al. *Biology of Microorganisms,* 7th ed., Englewood Cliffs, NJ: Prentice-Hall, 1994.

Cosa, J.H., et al. Plasmids, in *Methods for General and Molecular Bacteriology.* Washington, DC: American Society for Microbiology Press, 1994.

Sambrook, J., et al. *Molecular Cloning: A Laboratory Manual,* 2nd ed. Cold Spring Harbor, NY: Cold Spring Harbor Laboratory Press, 1989.

RESULTS

Distances migrated by λ DNA fragments:

23 kb _____

9.4 kb_____

6.6 kb_____

4.4 kb_____

2.3 kb_____

2.0 kb_____

Distances migrated by plasmid fragments:

Sizes of plasmid fragments:

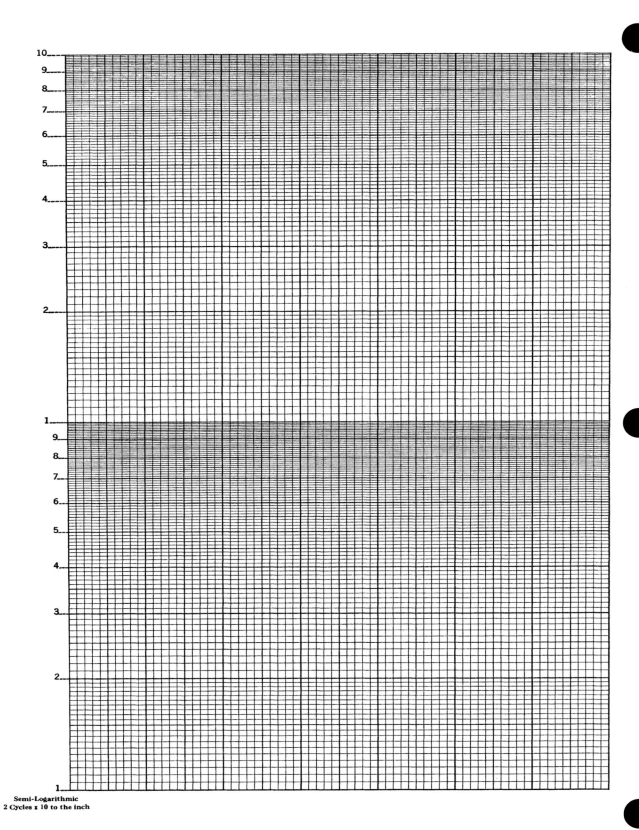

Semi-Logarithmic
2 Cycles x 10 to the inch

REFLECTIONS

1. What is the total size of the plasmid you digested? Explain how you reached this answer.

2. The recombinant plasmid you used in this exercise is composed of cloning vector DNA plus the foreign DNA. It was constructed for the purpose of cloning a particular gene (gene of interest) located on the inserted foreign DNA; your instructor will tell you what that gene is. Describe how the gene of interest might have been cloned starting with vector DNA (a plasmid from *E. coli*) and chromosomal DNA from the organism that was the source of the gene of interest. Drawings would be helpful. Remember that the foreign insert can be removed from the recombinant plasmid by cutting the plasmid with the restriction endonuclease you used in this exercise.

3. Draw a picture of what you think the recombinant plasmid looks like. In your drawing, show the approximate location of:
   a. Any antibiotic resistance gene
   b. The gene of interest
   c. The restriction endonuclease cutting sites

4. Jeff began his search for the stripe rust resistance gene by creating a genomic library. What is a genomic library and what steps might Jeff have taken to create the library?

5. Jeff plans to cut the stripe rust resistance gene from the original plasmid and insert it into an m13-derived cloning vector. For what purpose are m13-derived vectors especially useful? What feature(s) of the m13 life cycle makes it particularly useful for this purpose?

EXERCISE 26

TRANSFORMATION OF *ESCHERICHIA COLI* WITH PLASMID DNA

Molecular biologists employ a variety of procedures to isolate genes, manipulate the genes *in vitro*, and introduce genes into target cells. In this exercise, you will gain experience in transforming *Escherichia coli* with plasmid DNA. This technique, along with those you learned in the previous two exercises, constitute some of the tools most routinely used by the molecular biologist and genetic engineer.

Jeff was poised to start the next important phase of his research (see Exercises 24 and 25)—determining the sequence of nucleotides in the gene from wheat that confers resistance to stripe rust disease (srd^r). About a month earlier, Jeff had jumped the first hurdle when he identified the recombinant plasmid containing the srd^r gene. The gene was one of several located on the large fragment of wheat DNA that had been inserted into the plasmid cloning vector. To make the next steps easier, Jeff had to whittle the wheat DNA down to a fragment containing only the resistance gene. He accomplished this by using a restriction endonuclease to cut the wheat DNA out of the vector. He then separated the wheat DNA from the cloning vector, purified it, and cut it into smaller pieces with another restriction endonuclease. He then identified and isolated the fragment carrying the resistance gene. Two days earlier he had mixed the resistance gene with a linearized m13-derived vector and added the

enzyme DNA ligase. This enzyme catalyzes the joining of DNA molecules together to form recombinant molecules. He now had in his hand the ligation mixture that he hoped contained the new recombinant vector. Because there were relatively few of the desired recombinant molecules in the mixture, Jeff needed to introduce the recombinant DNA into E. coli so he could increase the number of recombinant molecules. As the E. coli cells reproduced, the recombinant molecules would be replicated and Jeff would have a ready supply of the srd^r-recombinant molecule. In just a few days, Jeff hoped he could begin sequencing the resistance gene.

BACKGROUND INFORMATION

In the late 1920s, Dr. F. Griffith began a series of experiments designed to elucidate the characteristics of *Streptococcus pneumoniae* responsible for its ability to cause disease. Working with virulent strains—those that cause disease—and non-virulent strains—those that do not cause disease—Griffith discovered that when he mixed living non-virulent cells with heat-killed virulent cells, the non-virulent cells became virulent. Griffith referred to this phenomenon as **transformation.** About 15 years later, an historic experiment was done by O.T. Avery, C.M. MacLeod, and M.J. McCarty. They demonstrated that DNA was the chemical component of the heat-killed cells responsible for transforming non-virulent cells to virulence. This meant that in Griffith's original experiments, the free DNA from dead virulent cells had been taken up and incorporated into the DNA of the living non-virulent cells. The Avery, MacLeod, and McCarty experiments were the first to demonstrate that DNA is the genetic material of cells; they are among the most important experiments in the history of genetics and molecular biology.

The discovery of transformation is a good example of the importance of serendipity in science. Had Griffith been studying the determination of virulence of another bacterium, he might not have discovered transformation. This is because many bacteria are not **transformation-competent.** *E. coli* is one such bacterium. Yet, for Jeff to succeed with his research project, he must mix *E. coli* cells with the recombinant DNA he had created in a test tube and hope that some of the cells would take up that DNA into their cytoplasm. Fortunately for Jeff, procedures have been developed for making *E. coli* cells temporarily transformation-competent.

In this exercise, you will use the calcium chloride procedure for transformation. This is a relatively simple method for tricking *E. coli* cells into taking up DNA from their environment. In this procedure, cells in the logarithmic phase of growth are harvested and placed in an ice-cold solution containing calcium chloride. The cells are then mixed with DNA, incubated on ice, and briefly heat shocked. The calcium chloride, cold shock, and heat shock render the *E. coli* membrane more permeable to DNA. You will be given cells of an ampicillin-sensitive *E. coli* strain that have already been exposed to calcium chloride. You will introduce a plasmid carrying a gene that confers resistance to ampicillin into those cells.

PURPOSE

- To transform *E. coli* with a plasmid conferring resistance to the antibiotic ampicillin
- To determine the transformation efficiency of the transformation experiment

THE EXERCISE

MATERIALS:

Two microcentrifuge tubes containing *E. coli* cells suspended in 0.2 ml sterile 10 mM Tris-chloride (pH 8) containing 50 mM calcium chloride
42°C water bath
TE (Tris-Cl, pH 8.0, containing 1 mM ethylene diamine tetraacetate [EDTA])
Sterile microcentrifuge tubes
Four LB plates

Culture spreader
Pipets (or micropipetters and sterile tips)
Ice
Solution of a plasmid conferring ampicillin-resistance (concentration = 1 ng/µl)
Luria Bertani (LB) broth
37°C water bath
Four LB-ampicillin (50 µg ampicillin/ml) plates
Alcohol in a beaker
Bunsen burner

PROCEDURE: Work in groups of two or three
Day 1

1. Obtain two tubes of calcium chloride–treated *E. coli* cells.
2. Place the cells on ice.
3. Label one tube of *E. coli* cells "plus (+) DNA" and the other tube "minus (−) DNA."
4. To the "+ DNA" tube, add 5 µl of the plasmid solution.
5. To the "− DNA" tube, add 5 µl TE.
6. Incubate both tubes on ice for 30 minutes.
7. Place both tubes in the 42°C water bath for 2 minutes.
8. Add 1 ml LB to each tube.
9. Incubate each tube at 37°C for 1 hour. **Note:** This step allows the cells to recover from their "shocking experience" and to begin expressing the ampicillin-resistance gene. As the cells incubate, continue with steps 10 through 13.
10. Label a sterile microcentrifuge tube "1/100 + DNA" (1/100 +).
11. Add 990 µl LB to this tube.
12. Label a second sterile microcentrifuge tube "1/100 − DNA" (1/100−).
13. Add 990 µl LB to this tube.
14. Label the LB-amp plates 1, 2, 3, and 4.
15. Label the LB plates 5, 6, 7, and 8. **Note:** When the 1 hour recovery period has ended, proceed to the next step.
16. Transfer 10 µl of the "+ DNA" solution to the "1/100 + DNA" tube. **Note:** You have just made a 10/1000 or 1/100 dilution of the transformation solution. This dilution will be plated on LB plates. All cells, transformed and non-transformed, will grow on these plates. Using the 1/100 dilution ensures there will be less than 300 colonies per plate.
17. Repeat step 16 for the "− DNA" solution.
18. Transfer 100 µl of the "+ DNA" solution to plate 1 (**Table 26.1**). Use the spread plate method (**see**

TABLE 26.1   Summary of Inoculations to be Made to LB-ampicillin Plates (Plates 1 to 4) and LB Plates (Plates 5 to 8)

Plate	+ DNA	− DNA	1/100 + DNA	1/100 − DNA
1	100 μl	−	−	−
2	10 μl	−	−	−
3	−	100 μl	−	−
4	−	10 μl	−	−
5	−	−	100 μl	−
6	−	−	10 μl	−
7	−	−	−	100 μl
8	−	−	−	10 μl

Exercise 20) to spread the inoculum over the surface of the medium, then set the plate aside so the liquid can be absorbed into the medium.

19. Transfer 10 μl of the "+ DNA" solution to plate 2. Spread the inoculum into the medium and set it aside.

20. Repeat steps 18 and 19 with the "− DNA" solution and plates 3 and 4.

21. Repeat steps 18 and 19 with the "1/100 + DNA" solution and plates 5 and 6.

22. Repeat steps 18 and 19 with the "1/100 − DNA" solution and plates 7 and 8.

23. Invert and incubate all plates at 37°C.

24. After 16 to 24 hours incubation, place plates at 4°C until the next laboratory period.

Day 2

1. Obtain your LB and LB-amp plates.
2. Count the number of colonies on each. Record the results in the RESULTS section.
3. Calculate the transformation efficiency of your experiment, using the following formula.

Transformation efficiency is expressed as number of transformants/μg DNA.

$$\frac{\text{\# transformants/fraction of total mixture plated}}{\text{Total amount of DNA added}}$$

In order to calculate transformation efficiency you must answer the following questions:

- Which set of plates gives you the number of transformants in the aliquot plated?
- What is that number?
- Which set of plates gives you the total number of viable cells in the aliquot plated?
- What is that number?
- What was the total volume of the mixture after adding LB?
- What fraction of the total volume of the "+ DNA" mixture was plated when 100 μl was spread onto the LB-amp plate? What about the 10 μl plate?
- What was the total amount of DNA in the "+ DNA" mixture?

REFERENCES

Hanahan, D. Techniques of Transformation of *E. coli.* In Glover, D.M. *DNA Cloning,* Vol. 1. Oxford: IRL Press, 1985.

Maniatis, T., et al. *Molecular Cloning: A Laboratory Manual.* Cold Spring Harbor, NY: Cold Spring Harbor Laboratory Press, 1982.

Provence, D.L., and Curtiss, R.C., III. Gene transfer in Gram-negative bacteria. In Gerhardt, P. *Methods for General and Molecular Bacteriology.* Washington, DC: American Society for Microbiology Press, 1994.

Stent, G.S. *Molecular Genetics: An Introductory Narrative.* San Francisco: W.H. Freeman Co., 1971.

RESULTS

Record the number of colonies on the LB-ampicillin and LB plates in the table below.

	Number of Colonies			
	+ DNA		− DNA	
	100 μl (Plate 1)	10 μl (Plate 2)	100 μl (Plate 3)	10 μl (Plate 4)
LB-ampicillin Plates				
	1/100 + DNA		1/100 − DNA	
	100 μl (Plate 5)	10 μl (Plate 6)	100 μl (Plate 7)	10 μl (Plate 8)
LB Plates				

REFLECTIONS

1. Why were both "+ DNA" and "− DNA" mixtures prepared and plated?

2. Assume the amount of plasmid molecules in the transformation mixture was in great excess to the number of cells in the transformation mixture. What fraction of the cells were transformation competent?

3. It is good practice to autoclave all cultures before disposal, even if the culture is of a non-pathogenic organism. Autoclaving not only kills the cells in the culture, but denatures and destroys proteins and nucleic acids. Based on what you have learned in this laboratory exercise, why is it especially important to autoclave genetically engineered organisms before disposal?

4. Since the development of the calcium chloride transformation procedure, other procedures have been developed. One is called electroporation. Using your textbook or other sources, describe this procedure for transformation.

SECTION V

MICROBIAL ECOLOGY

In the previous sections, you learned much about the basic biology of microorganisms. Now we turn our attention to the interactions of microbes with each other and with other organisms in an ecosystem. It is in the study of microbial ecology that the diversity, both metabolic and structural, of microbes becomes clear. For instance, microbes are exclusively responsible for certain biological transformations of the nitrogen cycle (e.g., denitrification, nitrification, and nitrogen fixation) and sulfur cycle (e.g., dissimilatory sulfate and S_0 reduction). In many ways, the functioning of Earth is dependent on microbial activity.

EXERCISE 27

TOWER OF MICROBES

> To understand basic cell processes, microbiologists work with pure cultures of microbes. However, microbial ecology focuses on the interactions of microbes. These interactions cannot be studied in pure culture. In this exercise, you will make a Winogradsky column. This miniature ecosystem will allow you to begin to understand the interdependence of all life forms.

It was June 1993. The sun was shining and the floodwaters were finally receding. Jim and his wife Ann stood silently looking at one of the fields of their productive Missouri farm. In a normal year this field would be full of young soybean plants. Instead, they only saw a wide expanse of muck-like soil that resulted from the field being underwater for nearly a month. When the levee broke, not only was their farm almost completely flooded, but their home was lost as well. They would build again on higher ground, but as they looked at the field, they wondered what had happened to the rich soil that had supported large yields before the flood. What had happened to the nutrients—were they washed away with the floodwaters? It seemed hard to imagine that this water-logged soil could ever be productive again.

BACKGROUND INFORMATION

Jim and Ann probably lost money in 1993 because it is unlikely they were able to harvest a crop that season. However, in the long run, they need not despair. Even as they assessed their water-logged fields, organisms in the soil, especially microorganisms, were beginning to carry out activities that would ultimately restore the fertility of the soil.

Soil is a complex habitat. Each soil particle is composed of organic material, minerals, and microbes living on and in the particle. In addition, a number of large organisms live either completely in the soil (e.g., certain insects and worms) or partially in soil (e.g., plants). The interactions of all the organisms in soil are critical to its structure and fertility. Although these soil-dwelling organisms are merely going about the business of providing for their own needs, in the process they contribute to nutrient cycling in this important habitat.

The biogeochemical cycles of major importance in soil are the carbon cycle and the nitrogen cycle, and to a lesser extent the sulfur and phosphorous cycles. This is because these elements are constituents of the biologically important molecules (proteins, nucleic acids, carbohydrates, and lipids). To Jim and Ann, the carbon and nitrogen cycles are most important. The carbon cycle is important because it provides carbon as CO_2 for plants and as organic carbon for the myriad of microbes inhabiting soil. Nitrogen is of concern because nitrogen is readily lost from soil due to denitrification, as well as nitrate loss in water runoff from fields.

In June 1993, the field Jim and Ann were observing was in some ways less like the typical soil habitat and more like the habitat that exists in the sediments of a lake. **Figure 27.1** shows a "cross section" of a lake. Imagine looking down at the surface of the water at either point A or point B and seeing a circle 10 cm in diameter. Now imagine the circle is the top of a cylinder that extends from the surface down into the sediments of the lake bottom. This cylinder, then, delineates a column. If oxygen levels, available nutrients, light intensity, and other parameters were measured at various depths of the column, gradients would be observed. These gradients are established, in part, by physical processes such as diffusion, but also by the activities of the organisms present in the column. As a result, the populations of

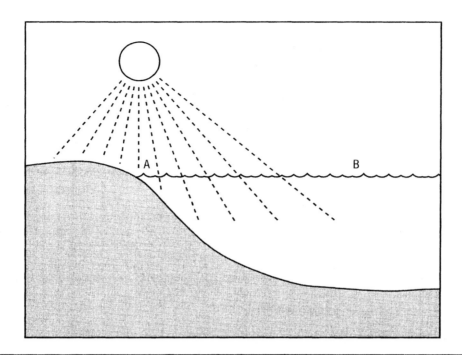

Figure 27.1 A typical lake habitat. Points A and B are reference points for hypothetical columns considered in the text and in a REFLECTIONS question.

microbes in the column can be described as occurring in layers. Each layer is composed of organisms occupying a niche; that is, each layer has a set of environmental parameters to which the organisms dwelling there are adapted. The column as a whole, then, is composed of interacting populations and is, in ecological terms, a **community.**

Studying the ecology of microbes is complicated by several factors. One factor is that microbial interactions can not be observed in pure culture. Another problem is that the microbes in a community are not easily identified by looking at them. You have already experienced this dilemma in earlier exercises where you microscopically examined microbes. The problem of identifying microbes in a microbial community still plagues microbial ecologists, although new techniques may help solve that problem (see Exercise 16). A solution for culturing microbes in a manner that allows observation of their interactions was developed in the 1880s by Sergei Winogradsky. Winogradsky was studying soil microbes and their role in nutrient cycling when he developed columns, now called Winogradsky columns, to observe the interactions of microbes. In this exercise, you will make a Winogradsky column, and in so doing, will

learn about the interactions of microbes within this model microbial community.

PURPOSE

- To prepare a Winogradsky column
- To discern the interactions of microbes in a model microbial community

THE EXERCISE

MATERIALS:

Clear glass or plastic tubes at least 15 cm in length
Incandescent lights
Glass rod or similar instrument for tamping down materials in the column

PROCEDURE: Work in groups of two or three
Part A: Getting Started
1. Begin by brainstorming in your group about the materials needed to make your Winogradsky column. The materials should include an inoculum from nature, such as soil or lake sediments; sources of fermentable molecules—in particular, a long-term supply of sugars (e.g. cellulose) and

amino acids (e.g. protein); as well as a supply of calcium carbonate, nitrogen, phosphorus and sulfur; and pond or river water. The materials you use can be obtained from home, local gardening or hardware stores, nearby lakes or other sites, and from refined chemicals in your department's stock room. Begin by thinking about the nutritional value of foods you regularly eat. Eggs, for instance, are excellent sources of proteins. The egg shells are rich in calcium. Gardening supplies are also good materials to consider. Gardeners regularly amend their soil with bone meal, gypsum, and other materials that add needed elements and nutrients and improve soil texture.

2. Finalize the list of materials needed, and assign responsibility for obtaining these different materials to the members of your group. Examine the tube in which you will build your Winogradsky column before leaving laboratory. Most of the tube will be filled with the inoculum, so plan accordingly.

Part B: Building the Column

1. If the materials you have chosen are rather large, break, cut, or tear them into smaller pieces.
2. Mix the inoculum and other materials together, and add enough water to make a mud-like slurry. Make a detailed record of the materials and amounts added in a notebook. You will use this notebook to record your observations of your column and the columns of other students in your class for the next 4 to 8 weeks.
3. Pour a few centimeters of the mixture into the tube.
4. Tamp the mixture down so there are no air bubbles trapped in it.
5. Repeat steps 3 and 4 until just a few centimeters are left in the tube.
6. Pour a layer of water in the remaining space.
7. Cover the tube loosely with foil or parafilm.
8. Illuminate the tube with the incandescent lights.

Part C

1. On a weekly basis, for the next 8 weeks examine your column and the columns of other students in the class. Make the following observations:
   • Describe and draw your column, noting appearance of color or other features.
   • Remove the lid of the column. Record and describe any distinctive odors.
   • Note any differences in the appearance of your column and the columns of others in the class.
2. Compare your observations to those made by others in your group. Are you seeing and smelling the same things? Are all columns developing in the same way and in the same time frame?
3. Use the time while your column develops to answer questions 1 and 2 in the REFLECTIONS section. These questions will help you predict the conditions in the column and reach conclusions about the interactions occurring in it.

REFLECTIONS

1. Imagine you are able to measure the oxygen levels in the Winogradsky column. Draw a picture of the column showing the relative amount of oxygen going from top to bottom.

2. A typical Winogradsky column contains a variety of microbes. **Table 27.1** lists some of them. Use your text and other resources to learn more about these organisms, especially with respect to their metabolic capabilities and oxygen requirements. Using this information, draw a Winogradsky column showing the relative locations of these microbes in the column.

TABLE 27.1 Microbes Commonly Found in a Winogradsky Column

Rhodospirillum sp.	*Thiobacillus* sp.
Cyanobacteria	*Desulfovibrio* sp.
Chromatium sp.	*Beggiatoa* sp.
Chlorobium sp.	*Thiothrix* sp.
Clostridium sp.	Algae

3. Two biogeochemical cycles are of particular importance in a Winogradsky column: the sulfur cycle and the carbon cycle. Using the information gathered to answer the first two questions, draw a figure that clearly demonstrates the interactions, at the biochemical level, of the microbes in a typical Winogradsky column. In other words, show how these two cycles are interconnected. Also show which microbes are responsible for the various transformations observed in each cycle.

4. Did you make any observations during this experiment that supported the predictions you made in answering question 2? Explain.

5. The cycling of nitrogen is of particular concern to Jim and Ann. How did an extended period of anaero-
   biosis in the soil impact its cycling?

6. The Winogradsky column best models the interactions of microbes in lake sediments. It is less accurate at
   modeling the interactions of microbes in the water. What natural phenomena occurring in a lake would
   make the water in a lake a much different environment than the water in the Winogradsky column?

7. Examine **Figure 27.1**. Label the littoral zone, limnetic zone, and profundal zone. How would a column
   starting at point A differ from a column starting at point B?

ENRICHING FOR AEROBIC, NITROGEN-FIXING BACTERIA

> The Winogradsky column (see Exercise 27) is an excellent way to explore the interactions of microbes and nutrient cycling. This exercise focuses on one cycle of particular concern to farmers and gardeners—the nitrogen cycle. This exercise also introduces an important tool used by microbial ecologists—enrichment cultures.

Don had been a serious gardener for years, and his many successes and failures had taught him a lot. He had learned, for instance, many of the "hows," "whens," and "whats" of fertilizing his garden. How to best fertilize was of major concern to Don now. He had just moved to a new area that had very different soil and weather patterns. His new yard had a great garden site, but he had moved in too late to get any crops this year. He did have plenty of time to prepare for next spring, however, so that fall, he worked compost into the soil and sowed Austrian winter peas. This legume would begin to grow and then be plowed into the soil next spring. By plowing the legume into the soil, Don would replenish the nitrogen. This would go a long way to ensuring a great harvest of fresh vegetables next summer.

BACKGROUND INFORMATION

Don knows from experience that one of the most important aspects of gardening is the provision of an adequate and suitable supply of nitrogen for his vegetable plants. Although the predominant molecule in the atmosphere is nitrogen gas (N_2) this form of nitrogen is not utilizable by plants as a source of nitrogen. The peas Don is planting will not be harvested, but rather used to replenish nitrogen in his garden plot by converting N_2 in the atmosphere into ammonia. The ammonia is then incorporated into plant protein and other nitrogen-containing molecules. What Don may not know is that it is not the plant responsible for this conversion, but a Gram-negative rod-shaped bacterium, *Rhizobium leguminosarum*. Although *R. leguminosarum* produces the enzyme that catalyzes nitrogen fixation, it only does so in the roots of its host legume. The plant and bacterium have an intimate and intricate relationship that has long been the focus of intense study. This **mutualistic** relationship begins when the bacterium invades the roots of the pea plant. There the bacterium differentiates into cells called **bacteroids.** Bacteroids have a swollen, misshapen appearance, and are sometimes branched. Thus, they are morphologically distinct from the free-living, rod-shaped bacterium. The plant and bacterium work together to create a habitat, the root nodule, which provides environmental conditions conducive to nitrogen fixation. Over the fall and in the spring, the bacteroids in the roots of Don's Austrian pea plants will fix nitrogen. The ammonia produced will be used by the plant and microbe to make amino acids, proteins, nucleotides, and nucleic acids. When Don plows the peas into the soil in the spring, the plant material will decompose and release nitrogen into the soil.

The bacterial enzyme that catalyzes nitrogen fixation is called **nitrogenase.** It is a large, multisubunit enzyme that uses molybdenum and iron as cofactors. The molybdenum and iron form centers which participate in electron transfer to N_2, and are required for enzyme activity. Another important characteristic of nitrogenase is that it is extremely sensitive to oxygen and is nonfunctional if oxygen levels are too high. This creates a dilemma for the bacterium. *Rhizobium* is aerobic and needs oxygen for respiration, yet it can not carry out nitrogen fixation if oxygen is abundant. The plant and bacterium work together to solve this problem. Both participate in the synthesis of an interesting protein called **leghemoglobin.** Leghemoglobin, like the related animal protein hemoglobin, binds oxygen and releases it to cells in the tissues of an animal's body. The function of leghemoglobin is similar. It binds oxygen and transfers the oxygen to the bacteroids, but it does so at a slow rate. The oxygen that enters the bacteroid is used immediately for respiration, so does not reach concentrations high enough to inhibit nitrogenase activity. Thus, a delicate balance is maintained between the requirement of oxygen for catabolic processes and the oxygen sensitivity of nitrogenase.

Because nitrogenase is so oxygen sensitive, it was initially thought that nitrogen-fixing bacteria must be anaerobes. And indeed, the first nitrogen fixers identified were. But in 1901, Martinus Beijerinck, a microbiologist whose role in the history of microbiology rivals Koch and Pasteur, decided to see if he could isolate a free-living, aerobic, nitrogen-fixing bacterium. He used a simple medium containing mineral salts, nitrogen, and a respirable carbon source (e.g., mannitol) which is not fermented by most bacteria. This simple medium put severe metabolic constraints on the microorganisms inoculated into it. When Beijerinck added a soil inoculum to the medium, he successfully isolated microbes in the soil capable of aerobic nitrogen fixation (e.g., *Azotobacter*). Beijerinck's experiment is a classic example of an **enrichment culture.** It clearly demonstrates the use of selective conditions to promote the growth of some microbes, while inhibiting the growth of others.

Beijerinck's successful enrichment for *Azotobacter* and other aerobic, nitrogen-fixing bacteria settled the question of their existence. However, it did little to explain how aerobic bacteria can fix nitrogen. We now know that aerobic, nitrogen-fixing bacteria protect their nitrogenase in a variety of ways. For instance, it is known that *Azotobacter* has one of the highest respiratory rates of all bacteria. It is thought that any oxygen entering the cell is immediately used for respiratory electron transport. This high respiratory activity, then, uses up the oxygen quickly so intracellular oxygen levels are low.

This exercise is divided into two parts. In Part A, you will enrich for aerobic, nitrogen-fixing bacteria. They will be examined microscopically and their cellular morphology and Gram reaction determined. In Part B, you will devise an experiment to isolate in pure culture the bacterium enriched for in Part A. To successfully complete Part B, you should review earlier exercises in the manual (e.g., Exercise 3).

PURPOSE

- To enrich for aerobic, nitrogen-fixing bacteria from soil
- To gain experience in the development and use of culture media

THE EXERCISE

Part A

MATERIALS:

Fresh soil
250 ml flask (with loose-fitting lid) containing 50 ml nitrogen-free broth (**Table 28.1**)
Shaker

PROCEDURES: Work in groups of two or three

1. Place approximately 0.5 g of soil in the flask and shake at room temperature for 5 to 7 days.
2. When growth is apparent, prepare a smear, Gram stain and examine it. Record your observations of cellular morphology and Gram reaction in the RESULTS section.

Part B

1. Enrichment cultures are not pure cultures. Brainstorm with your group to devise a procedure to

TABLE 28.1   Ingredients in Nitrogen-free Broth

K_2HPO_4	0.8 g
KH_2PO_4	0.2 g
$MgSO_4$	0.2 g
$CaSO_4$	0.1 g
$FeSO_4 \cdot 7H_2O$	0.003 g
MoO_3	0.001 g
Mannitol	5.0 g
Distilled H_2O	1000 ml
pH 7.6	

isolate in pure culture an aerobic, nitrogen-fixing bacterium, using your enrichment culture as an inoculum. **Note:** In order to achieve your goal, review the selective conditions used to develop your enrichment culture. Also review earlier exercises (e.g., Exercise 3) in this manual.

2. Carry out your procedure after consulting with your instructor. **Note:** Your procedure may involve the preparation of a growth medium. Your instructor will determine if you will do this, or if the medium will be prepared for you.

3. If you successfully obtain a pure culture, prepare a smear, Gram stain and examine it. Record your observations in the RESULTS section.

REFERENCES

Brock, T.D., et al. *Biology of Microorganisms*, 7th ed., Englewood Cliffs, NJ: Prentice-Hall, 1994.

Stacey, G., et al. *Biological Nitrogen Fixation*. New York: Chapman and Hall, 1992.

RESULTS

Record your observations of bacteria in the enrichment culture below.

Record your observations of cells in the pure culture below.

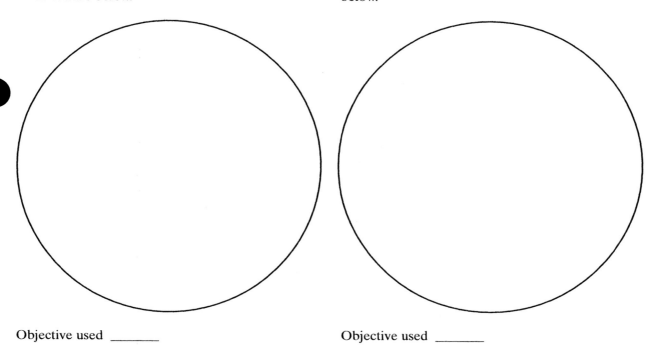

Objective used _____

Objective used _____

REFLECTIONS

1. **Table 28.1** lists the ingredients in nitrogen-free broth. Why would these ingredients be essential to the growth of an aerobic, nitrogen-fixing bacterium? Why was nitrogen (in any form) excluded from the medium?

2. Do you think all the microbes growing in your enrichment culture are nitrogen fixers? Explain.

3. How did you isolate a pure culture of the nitrogen-fixing bacteria in your enrichment culture (Part B)?

4. What evidence makes you feel confident that you did, indeed, obtain a pure culture of nitrogen fixers (Part B)?

5. When Don plows the Austrian pea plants into the soil in the spring, nitrogen will be released into the soil in the form of organic-nitrogen compounds. What form(s) does nitrogen have to be in to be taken up by plants? Describe the processes that occur to convert the organic nitrogen to the form(s) of nitrogen most accessible to plants.

6. Use what you have learned from this exercise and question 5 to draw the transformations of nitrogen that will occur in Don's garden beginning in the fall when he plants the peas, and next spring and summer when his vegetable crops are sown.

WATER, WATER, EVERYWHERE

In the previous two exercises, you have learned about biogeochemical cycles, primarily as they occur in soil or sediments. Aquatic environments also contribute to these cycles, though sometimes in much more complex ways. In this exercise, you will learn about the evaluation of water quality. As you will see, high-quality water is of importance to the functioning of many cycles on this planet, but it is also critical for maintaining public health. This exercise will introduce you to one way ecology impacts humans.

The plane began taxiing toward the runway. Greg leaned back in his seat, determined to get as much sleep as possible while he still had relatively comfortable conditions. His ultimate destination was a small village in Africa. There his living conditions would be considerably more Spartan. The village was in desperate need of someone with Greg's expertise. Its only water supply, a small lake, was seriously polluted. Diarrheal diseases were rampant in the village and were responsible for many deaths. Greg had 20 years of experience as a civil engineer and his goal was to help the village build a well that would provide safe drinking water. He would also assist in building a simple sewage collection and treatment system to lessen the village's impact on the lake. These relatively simple steps would greatly improve both the length and quality of life for the villagers.

BACKGROUND INFORMATION

On the surface, the small African village that is Greg's destination is quite different from the cities of many developed countries. However, it does share significant features with them. One is its location near a body of water. Humans have a tendency to locate their permanent communities along bodies of water, in part because we need water for drinking, cooking, and cleaning. Today, we are also attracted to water for its pleasing esthetic qualities and for the opportunities it may offer for relaxation and recreation.

When human populations were small and more nomadic, our impact on surface waters was imperceptible. Although humans introduced their wastes to surface waters, the incoming organic matter did not significantly alter the communities of aquatic organisms. The surface waters seemed unchanged because microbiological, chemical, and physical processes acted on the incoming wastes to degrade them and to purify the water. Microbiological processes include degradation of the organic matter by microbes in the water, usually by aerobic respiration. Chemical and physical processes include chemical oxidations and sedimentation, respectively.

But as human populations grow and permanent settlements are established, the ability of surface waters to self-purify is outpaced by the influx of human wastes. When this occurs, a sequence of events begins which, if unchecked, ultimately leads to a polluted body of water that is not potable. When a large influx of waste enters water, aerobic microbes degrade it and respire more rapidly, decreasing dissolved oxygen in the water. If organic matter continues to enter the water, the dissolved oxygen continues to decrease, and the water may even become anaerobic. If the dissolved oxygen is too low, aerobic aquatic organisms die, thus introducing even more organic material into the water. Furthermore, catabolism of the organic matter by microbes begins to occur by much slower, anaerobic processes such as fermentation. Over time, microbial waste products and decaying organisms render the water unpalatable to all except those with the strongest stomachs and poorest olfactory systems.

Surprisingly, it was not the poor taste and odor of polluted waters that propelled the development of procedures to lessen human impact on water. Rather, it was the realization that disease can be transmitted by water. A London physician, John Snow, was instrumental in this discovery. His studies on an epidemic of cholera in the 1840s demonstrated that the disease was transmitted by water contaminated with sewage. By preventing the use of the contaminated water, the cholera epidemic was brought under control. John Snow is often referred to as the "father of epidemiology" because of this investigation.

As can be seen in the above discussion, the concept "water quality" has at least two aspects. One is that good quality water has a pleasing taste and appearance. This indicates the water comes from a source where self-purification is occurring and the water is not polluted. The other aspect is that water is safe to drink; that is, it does not carry pathogenic microbes. Likewise, our attempts to ensure water quality are two-fold. We treat wastewater before releasing it into surface waters in an attempt to decrease the organic matter and the number of microbes, especially pathogens. We also treat drinking water to kill pathogens and to provide desirable taste, odor, and appearance qualities. Interestingly, both wastewater and drinking water treatment facilities employ processes that are observed in nature when a body of water self-purifies. However, the processes used in a treatment facility (e.g., filtration, sedimentation, and aeration) are much more controlled, rapid, and efficient.

In this exercise, you will perform two tests that are routinely used to monitor water safety and quality. The first test, the **coliform test** is based on the fact that many waterborne diseases are transmitted by the fecal-oral route. That is, the pathogen leaves its host in feces, and enters the new host by mouth, that is, by ingestion of water contaminated by feces. Therefore, if water is free of fecal contamination, it is considered safe to drink.[1] Fecal contamination is detected by testing for the presence of intestinal bacteria in the water. The microorganisms routinely tested for are called **coliforms.** Coliform bacteria are Gram-negative rods that do not form endospores but ferment lactose with gas formation within 24 hours when incubated at 35°C.

The second test you will perform is the **BOD test.** It is used to indirectly measure the amount of organic material present in water. Thus, it measures the amount of pollution. The BOD test is based on the fact that when organic material is present in water, microbes in the water oxidize it aerobically. If this occurs in a sealed container so that no additional oxygen can be dissolved in the water, then the oxygen level decreases over time. Thus, by measuring the concentration of dissolved oxygen (**DO**) before incubation and again after incubation, the biochemical oxygen demand (**BOD**) is determined. The more organic matter in the water (i.e., the more polluted), the greater the BOD; the less organic matter in the water (i.e., the less polluted), the lower the BOD. Dissolved oxygen can be measured in one of two ways, by an iodometric method or using membrane electrodes. In this exercise, DO will be measured by the Azide Modification of the Winkler (Iodometric) Method. In this method, a series of oxidation/reduction reactions occur after reagents containing manganese and iodide are added to the sample. The amount of DO in the sample determines the amount of manganese oxidized when the reagents are added. The amount of oxidized manganese, in turn, determines the amount of iodide oxidized to iodine (I_2). To complete the assay, the I_2 is quantified and expressed in terms of DO.

In this exercise, you will determine the number of coliforms and the BOD from a sample taken from flowing water being impacted by a **point source effluent** (PSE). The classic example of a PSE is the effluent released from a sewage treatment plant. The sample you test could be one taken upstream or downstream from the PSE, or the effluent itself. The results you obtain from your sample will be shared with other groups in the class. The class data will be used to draw conclusions about the stream's ability to neutralize the impact of the effluent.

PURPOSE

- To learn about the impact of humans on bodies of water
- To learn about self-purification of bodies of water

---

[1]Note that the concept of water safety in this case is defined by the absence of pathogenic microbes. There has been increasing concern about toxic, carcinogenic, and other harmful chemicals in drinking water. Although this is a serious concern, most standards of water safety are still based on whether or not the water tests positive for fecal microbes.

- To assay the quality of water samples from the local environment using two tests—one to quantify the number of coliforms in the samples, and the other to indirectly measure the organic matter in the samples

THE EXERCISE

Part A: Quantifying Coliforms

MATERIALS:

10 ml of one of the following samples:
 Point source effluent (PSE)
 A sample taken upstream of PSE
 A sample taken downstream of PSE
Sterile, 1 ml and 0.1 ml pipets (or micropipetters and sterile tips)
Seven m-Endo agar plates
70% alcohol in a beaker
Culture spreader
Bunsen burner
35°C incubator
Four tubes containing 9 ml of sterile water or saline

PROCEDURE: Work in groups of five or six

Day 1

1. Obtain one of the samples. Other groups in your lab will test the other samples. Data from all groups will be recorded in the table in the RESULTS section.
2. Using the sterile water in tubes, prepare a set of serial dilutions for each sample, as shown in Figure 29.1. (See Exercise 17 for a more detailed discussion of this procedure.) **Note:** There is space in **Figure 29.1** to calculate the final dilution to be plated. Fill in the blanks, then check your figures with your instructor. If they are correct, label the m-Endo agar plates accordingly and fill in the blanks in the table in the RESULTS section.
3. Working with one plate at a time, transfer the amounts indicated in **Figure 29.1** from the sample and each dilution to an m-Endo agar plate and spread the inoculum into the plate using the culture spreader. (See Exercise 20 for a more detailed description of this procedure.)
4. Allow the plates to dry, invert and incubate at 35°C for 24 hours.

Day 2

1. Examine the plates for colonies that are red with a metallic sheen. These are coliform colonies. All others are not coliforms. **Note:** The metallic sheen results from the interaction of basic fuschin in the medium with aldehydes produced by coliform bacteria as they ferment lactose.
2. Count the number of coliform colonies on each plate and record in the RESULTS section. **Note:** Be careful *not* to count the colonies that lack the metallic sheen as they are not coliforms.
3. Report the number of coliform colonies on each plate to your instructor. Your instructor will gather data from all groups and report it to the class.

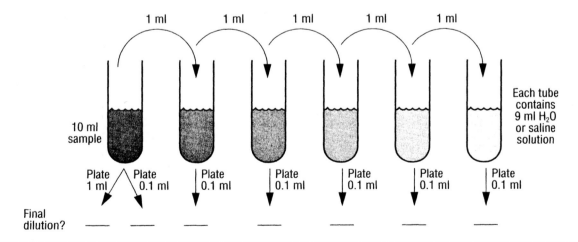

Transfer and mix, etc.

1 ml   1 ml   1 ml   1 ml   1 ml

10 ml sample

Each tube contains 9 ml H₂0 or saline solution

Plate 1 ml   Plate 0.1 ml   Plate 0.1 ml   Plate 0.1 ml   Plate 0.1 ml   Plate 0.1 ml   Plate 0.1 ml

Final dilution?

Figure 29.1 Dilutions and plating scheme for determining number of coliform bacteria in water samples. Calculate the final dilution plated from each tube.

4. Using plates with 30 to 300 coliform colonies calculate the number of coliform colony forming
units (cfu)/ml for each sample and record the
results in the RESULTS section.

Part B: BOD Determinations

Day 1

MATERIALS:

750 ml of one of the following samples:
    Point source effluent (PSE)
    A sample taken upstream of PSE
    A sample taken downstream of PSE
Manganous sulfate solution
Concentrated sulfuric acid
Sodium thiosulfate titrant (0.025 M $Na_2S_2O_3$) in buret
300 ml BOD bottles
Dilution water[2]
Graduated cylinders
1, 5 and 10 ml pipets
Alkali-iodide-azide reagent
Starch solution
Gloves
250 ml flask

PROCEDURE: Work in groups of five or six

**CAUTION: This procedure involves the use of dan-
gerous chemicals. Wear safety goggles and work in a
chemical safety hood.**

1. Obtain four pairs of BOD bottles and one of the
stream water or effluent samples. **Note:** Other
groups in your lab will determine the BOD for

_____

[2]Dilution water is not tap water. It is a special solution used
for BOD determinations.

the other samples. All data will be combined and
reported in the RESULTS section.
2. Label one bottle of each pair T_0 (Time zero).
Note: You will prepare dilutions of the sample
in these bottles and then determine the DO
immediately.
3. Label the second bottle of each pair of bottles T_5
(Time 5 days). **Note:** You will prepare dilutions
of the sample in these bottles but not determine
the DO for 5 days.
4. Prepare *duplicate* dilutions of the sample. Suggested dilutions are outlined in **Table 29.1**. Prepare
one set of dilutions in the T_0 bottles and the other
set in the T_5 bottles. This is best accomplished by
measuring the appropriate amount of dilution
water into the BOD bottle, then adding the corresponding amount of the sample. **Note:** If you have
the upstream or a downstream sample, use the dilutions suggested for stream water. If you have the
effluent sample, your instructor will indicate which
dilutions to use, depending on whether the effluent
is expected to have a high or moderate BOD.
5. The BOD bottles should be completely filled so
there are no air bubbles at the top. Place the caps
on the bottles and invert once or twice to mix.
Note: The cap should give an airtight seal. Sometimes this is accomplished using an additional
inner cap. Your instructor will demonstrate how
to obtain an airtight seal with the BOD bottles
you are using.
6. Place the T_5 bottles in a 20°C incubator and incubate for 5 days.
7. To the T_0 samples add (well below the surface) 1
ml of the manganous sulfate solution and 1 ml of
the alkali-iodide-azide reagent. **Note:** When

TABLE 29.1 Suggested Dilutions of Samples for BOD Determinations

Stream Water[a]		Effluent with Expected High BOD[b]		Effluent with Expected Moderate BOD[c]	
Volume of Sample (ml)[d]	**Volume of Dilution Water (ml)**	**Volume of Sample (ml)**	**Volume of Dilution Water (ml)**	**Volume of Sample (ml)**	**Volume of Dilution Water (ml)**
75	225	3	297	12	288
150	150	8	292	30	270
225	75	12	288	60	240
300	0	30	270	75	225

[a]The upstream, near-downstream and far-downstream samples should be diluted this way.
[b]Examples of samples with expected high BOD values include settled wastewater and runoff from a feedlot.
[c]Examples of samples with expected moderate to low BOD values include biologically treated wastewater.
[d]All volumes are calculated for 300 ml BOD bottles.

manganous sulfate (manganese is in the Mn^{2+} oxidation state) is added to water under alkali conditions (the alkali-iodide-azide solution contains 12.5 N NaOH), it reacts with water to form manganous hydroxide ($Mn[OH]_2$). The dissolved oxygen in the water then oxidizes the manganous hydroxide to manganic oxide (also called manganese dioxide–MnO_2) and related compounds. In these compounds, manganese is at a higher oxidation state (e.g., Mn^{4+}) (see box). The Mn^{4+} compounds are insoluble and form a brown precipitate.

8. Allow the bottles to sit until the precipitate fills about half the bottle.

9. Carefully obtain 1 ml of concentrated sulfuric acid and add it well below the surface of the fluid in the bottle. Replace the cap and invert to mix. **Note:** The sulfuric acid lowers the pH of the solution. Under these conditions, the Mn^{4+} is reduced back to Mn^{2+} and the iodide (added in the alkali-iodide-azide reagent) is oxidized to iodine (I_2). Since the amount of Mn^{4+} reflects the DO and the amount of I_2 formed depends on the amount of Mn^{4+}, the

amount of I_2 is equivalent to the DO of the water sample. The I_2 gives the water a yellow color.

10. Transfer 200 ml of the sample to an Erlenmeyer flask.

11. Obtain a buret containing sodium thiosulfate ($Na_2S_2O_3$). **Note:** The $Na_2S_2O_3$ should be at the zero mark on the buret.

12. Slowly add $Na_2S_2O_3$ to the sample in the Erlenmeyer flask. **Note:** The $Na_2S_2O_3$ reduces the I_2 back to iodide. As it does so, the yellow color of the water decreases. When the yellow color is completely gone, all the I_2 has been reduced.

13. When the solution turns a *pale* straw color, add a few drops of the starch solution. **Note:** It is difficult to tell exactly when the yellow color disappears (i.e., when all I_2 is converted back into iodide). When starch is added, it turns blue because of the presence of I_2. The disappearance of the blue color is more easily detected than the disappearance of yellow.

14. Continue until the blue disappears. **Note:** This process is called **titration**; it is the method of determining the amount of a substance in a

---

The Chemistry Behind the Winkler (Iodometric) Method for Determining Dissolved Oxygen (DO) in Water

The equations are not balanced because a complex mixture of Mn^{4+} compounds is formed.

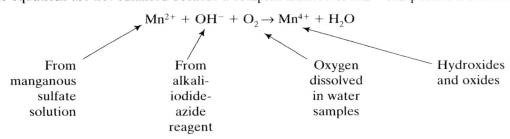

$$Mn^{2+} + OH^- + O_2 \rightarrow Mn^{4+} + H_2O$$

From manganous sulfate solution   From alkali-iodide-azide reagent   Oxygen dissolved in water samples   Hydroxides and oxides

The amount of Mn^{4+} produced depends on the amount of oxygen dissolved in water.

$$Mn^{4+} + I^- + H^+ \rightarrow Mn^{2+} + I_2 + H_2O$$

From alkali-iodide-azide reagent   From concentrated sulfuric acid

The acidic conditions drive the oxidation-reduction reaction. However, the amount of iodide oxidized is dependent on the amount of Mn^{4+} present. Since the amount of I_2 produced is dependent on the Mn^{4+} present, and the amount of Mn^{4+} is dependent on the amount of oxygen dissolved in the water, the I_2 produced is equivalent to the DO.

solution in terms of a reagent required to bring about an effect.

15. Note the volume of $Na_2S_2O_3$ required to titrate the I_2. Record this volume in the RESULTS section. **Note:** The volume of $Na_2S_2O_3$ required to reduce all the I_2, is used to calculate the amount of I_2 in the solution. We say the I_2 was titrated by $Na_2S_2O_3$, the titrant. Since the amount of I_2 in the solution is equivalent to the DO in the sample, determining the amount of I_2 tells us the DO.

16. Calculate the DO of each dilution tested using the following relationship: 1 ml $Na_2S_2O_3$ = 1 mg DO/l. Record this value in the RESULTS section.

Day 2

1. After 5 days of incubation of the T_5 BOD bottles, determine the DO in each, using the same procedure you used in Day 1 with the T_0 BOD bottles.

2. Record your results in the RESULTS section.

3. Calculate the BOD_5 using the following equation. (Use the paired dilution bottles where $DO_5 \geqslant 1$ mg/l and $DO_0 - DO_5 \geqslant 2$ mg/l. This dilution produces the most reliable result.)

$$BOD_5 = \frac{DO_0 - DO_5}{P}$$

Where,

BOD_5 = the BOD after 5 day incubation

DO_0 = DO in the T_0 bottle

DO_5 = DO in the T_5 bottle

P = decimal volumetric fraction of sample used (In a dilution containing a total volume of 300 ml, 75 ml of which is the sample, P = 75/300, or 0.25)

REFERENCES

Atlas, R.M., and Bartha, R. *Microbial Ecology*, 3rd ed., Redwood City, CA: Benjamin/Cummings Publishing Company, Inc., 1993.

Eaton, A.D., et al. *Standard Methods for the Examination of Water and Wastewater.* Baltimore: United Book Press, 1995.

Sawyer, C.N., and McCarty, P.L. *Chemistry for Environmental Engineering,* 3rd ed., New York: McGraw-Hill Book Co., 1978.

RESULTS

Record the number of coliform colonies from your samples and samples tested by other groups. Then calculate coliform cfu/ml for each sample, and record them in the table below.

	Final Dilution Plated	Number of Coliform Colonies	Coliform cfu/ml
Upstream Sample			
Effluent			
Near-Downstream Sample			
Far-Downstream Sample			

Record DO_0 and DO_5 for your sample and the samples tested by other groups in the table below.

	P	T_0 Bottles Volume of $Na_2S_2O_3$ Used in Titration	DO_0	T_5 Bottles Volume of $Na_2S_2O_3$ Used in Titration	DO_5
Upstream Sample					
Effluent					
Near-Downstream Sample					
Far-Downstream Sample					

Calculate the BOD_5 for each sample and record in the table below.

Sample	BOD_5
Upstream Sample	
Effluent	
Near-Downstream Sample	
Far-Downstream Sample	

REFLECTIONS

1. Did the PSE you were studying have an impact on the stream you sampled? Explain.

2. Suppose the body of water being studied in this experiment was a lake or small pond rather than a stream or river. How do you think this might have affected the impact of the PSE on the water?

3. Describe how a septic tank for a private home functions to decrease the BOD and number of pathogens in household wastewater.

4. Suppose you were Greg, on your way to help a small, African village deal with its wastewater. Taking into consideration the limited financial resources of the village, what type of treatment for wastewater would you suggest?

EXERCISE 30

GROWING MICROBES ON ROCKS

We have known for centuries that microbes in water can cause disease. Water can also harbor toxic chemicals that disrupt the marine ecosystem and kill most organisms. The clean up of toxic waters is also of concern to scientists. This exercise will focus on how organisms can facilitate this clean up through biological processes, known as bioremediation. It will also allow you to observe how bacteria such as *Thiobacillus ferroxidans* are used in mining, and how they can contribute to toxic waste sites such as acid mine drainages (acid- and iron-laden waters).

Using microbes as industrial tools is not new. They are used to make drugs, pesticides, solvents, plastics, food (such as cheese, yogurt, and bread), and to separate gold and copper from other rock. However, their use in the full-scale bioremediation of toxic materials is relatively new. A monumental success story in environmental circles is the clean up of Whitewood Creek in Lead, South Dakota. This is the site of Homestake Mine, which has been processing gold for over 100 years. In recent years, Homestake Mine began utilizing cyanide to process gold. This resulted in cyanide-contaminated water. The wastewaters from this process drain into Whitewood Creek and, before 1984, rendered it sterile from the mine site, throughout the Black Hills and beyond. Today, however, fisherman are regularly catching rainbow trout from this once polluted river.

The story of the recovery of Whitewood Creek began with research done by chemists, microbiologists,

and engineers. Their challenge was to design the most efficient, sustainable and cost-effective means of cleaning up the wastewater from the mine. Seven years later, they had developed a full-scale treatment facility that treats a maximum of 21,000 m^3 of wastewater per day. The scientists began by isolating cyanide-degrading bacteria from the water and mutating them so that they could degrade higher concentrations of cyanide. The bacteria were added to forty-eight rotating bioreactors through which the wastewater slowly passes. In these reactors, degradation occurs via biological pathways of cyanide, thiocyanate, and ammonia metabolism (a cyanide degradation by-product). In addition, the biofilms created in these reactors adsorb heavy metals and other suspended solids. The metals of concern are nickel, copper, lead, and zinc. A key in the development of the plant was the bioassay testing facility that monitors the toxicity of the water and evaluates treatment efficiency. As part of the testing process, effluent, which is eventually discharged into the river, is passed through holding tanks containing trout and small insects. If the fish and insects survive and reproduce, the "clean" wastewater is compatible with the dynamic ecosystem into which it is discharged.

BACKGROUND INFORMATION

The Homestake Mining Company story is one of several successful projects in the United States that have used microbes to clean up polluted water and soils. Despite these success stories, we are only beginning to explore the use of microbes and technology to treat contaminated sites because bioremediation is a complex and relatively new process. In addition, because developing successful treatment methods takes time, money, and the cooperative work of teams of scientists and engineers, it may be not be the cure for all contamination problems.

As indicated in the story above, microbes are used to clean up polluted wastes from mines. However, they are also involved in the mining industry in two other ways—one beneficial and the other detrimental. Microbes benefit the mining industry by speeding up the extraction of certain metals from ore. Many metals form highly insoluble minerals with sulfur. Some bacteria, **chemolithotrophs,** use these minerals as an energy source. (To review the metabolism of chemolithotrophs, refer to Exercise 19 or your textbook.) By sprinkling acid over iron sulfide (pyrhotite—FeS) or copper sulfide (covellite—CuS) ores, acidophilic aerobic, autotrophic chemolithotrophic bacteria solubilize the copper and iron, leaching them out of the ore. This is called **microbial leaching.** Microbial leaching is accomplished by piling up the ore in a heap and adding dilute sulfuric acid to the top of the pile. The acid percolates down through the rock, enabling chemolithotrophic bacteria to solubilize copper and iron. The liquid laden with the desired metal is drained from the bottom of the pile (**Figure 30.1**). It is then transported to a plant where the metal is reprecipitated and purified.

Microbes are detrimental to the mining industry because they are involved in the production of acid mine drainages. The drainage of acid from mine sites is the result of bacterial oxidation of sulfur-containing rock. One of these rocks is pyrite (FeS_2), one of the most common ores found at coal, iron, and copper mines. A bacterium that lives on pyrite and contributes to acid mine drainage is *Thiobacillus ferroxidans*. This unique microbe grows best in acid conditions where the pH is 2.5 or lower. It also has the ability to oxidize ferrous iron and use it as a primary

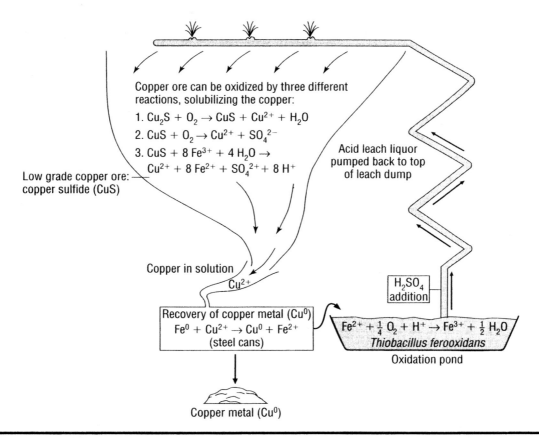

Copper ore can be oxidized by three different reactions, solubilizing the copper:

1. $Cu_2S + O_2 \rightarrow CuS + Cu^{2+} + H_2O$
2. $CuS + O_2 \rightarrow Cu^{2+} + SO_4^{2-}$
3. $CuS + 8\,Fe^{3+} + 4\,H_2O \rightarrow Cu^{2+} + 8\,Fe^{2+} + SO_4^{2+} + 8\,H^+$

Low grade copper ore: copper sulfide (CuS)

Acid leach liquor pumped back to top of leach dump

Copper in solution Cu^{2+}

Recovery of copper metal (Cu^0)
$Fe^0 + Cu^{2+} \rightarrow Cu^0 + Fe^{2+}$
(steel cans)

H_2SO_4 addition

$Fe^{2+} + \frac{1}{4}O_2 + H^+ \rightarrow Fe^{3+} + \frac{1}{2}H_2O$
Thiobacillus ferooxidans
Oxidation pond

Copper metal (Cu^0)

Figure 30.1 The process and reactions involved in the microbial leaching of low-grade copper ores yielding Cu^0 (copper metal).

source of energy. Because of this, *T. ferroxidans* is called an acidophilic chemolithotroph. *T. ferroxidans* prefers sulfur-rich habitats, especially those where sulfuric acid is present. With this in mind, it is easy to see why pyrite might be a logical place to find this microorganism. When pyrite is exposed to oxygen during the mining process, a slow chemical reaction occurs as follows:

$$FeS_2 + 3\tfrac{1}{2}O_2 + H_2O \rightarrow Fe^{2+} + 2SO_4^{2-} + 2H^+$$

This sets up acidic conditions under which *T. ferroxidans* takes residence and catalyzes the oxidation of ferrous (Fe^{2+}) to ferric (Fe^{3+}) ions at a faster rate. However, under the acidic conditions the ferric ions are soluble and can oxidize more pyrite to ferrous and sulfate ions:

$$14Fe^{3+} + FeS_2 + 8H_2O \rightarrow 15Fe^{2+} + 2SO_4^{2-} + 16H^+$$

The cycle continues as ferrous ions are oxidized by the bacteria to ferric ions that react with more pyrite (**Figure 30.2**). This attack of *T. ferroxidans* on pyrite contributes to acid mine drainage and the yellow outflows from the mining sites. In addition, when the water drainage becomes less acidic as it moves farther from the mine site, ferric ions become insoluble and form a red-brown precipitate called "yellow boy" by U.S. miners. The ferric iron complexes with sulfate minerals and forms a mineral called jarosite (usually found as $HFe_3[SO_4]_2[OH]_6$), which forms the unsightly yellow stain.

Oxygen plays an important role in acid mine drainage. It is used by *T. ferroxidans* as a terminal electron acceptor when electrons are released from ferrous iron. Therefore, remediation at many mine sites is accomplished by covering the mine tailings with soil, nutrients, and vegetation to limit oxygen supply and neutralize the soil. This has slowed and sometimes stopped acid drainage at some sites.

During this exercise you will observe the action of *T. ferroxidans* on pyrite. The pyrite will be placed in a minimal medium that supplies inorganic nutrients to better jump-start the reactions and ensure growth. The nutrients also better simulate environmental conditions under which acid mine drainage occurs. You will also be asked to design an experiment that demonstrates the microbe's requirement for oxygen.

PURPOSE

- To learn about the metabolism of an acidophilic chemolithotroph, *T. ferroxidans*
- To observe the oxidization of iron and sulfur in pyrite rock by *T. ferroxidans*

THE EXERCISE

MATERIALS:

Three 250 ml flasks, each containing 150 ml of sterile minimal medium (a 1:10 solution of modified 9-K medium)
Shaker
An overnight culture of *T. ferroxidans* grown in 9-K medium
Sterile pyrite crystals
Pipets

Modified 9-K Medium

3.0 g $(NH_4)_2SO_4$—Ammonium sulfate
0.1 g KCl—Potassium chloride
0.5 g K_2HPO_4—Potassium phosphate, dibasic,
0.5 g $MgSO_4 \cdot 7\ H_2O$—Magnesium sulfate, heptahydrate
0.01 g $Ca(NO_3)_2$—Calcium nitrate
1.0 ml 10N H_2SO_4—Sulfuric acid
700 ml distilled H_2O

Mix thoroughly to dissolve.
Autoclave and make a 1:10 dilution of the solution.

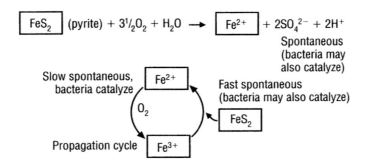

Figure 30.2   The oxidation of pyrite rock and the role bacteria play.

PROCEDURE: Work in groups of two to three

Part A

1. Label flask 1 and add approximately 10 to 15 grams of sterile pyrite rock to the flask. The greater the surface area on the pyrite, the faster the growth of the organism will proceed. Therefore, if possible, obtain small pyrite crystals (mesh) or grind the rock with a mortar and pestle.

2. Add 1 ml of an overnight culture of *T. ferroxidans*. This gives an initial cell density of approximately 10^8 bacteria/ml.

3. Flask 2 is a control flask. To it add approximately 10 to 15 grams of sterile pyrite rock but do not inoculate with *T. ferroxidans*.

4. Place both flasks on a shaker and rotate slowly (50 to 60 RPM) for 7 to 14 days at room temperature until an orange-brown color appears. The development of a rust-colored precipitate is indicative of growth.

5. Record your results in the RESULTS section.

Part B

1. Using the third flask containing modified 9-K medium, design an experiment which shows that *T. ferroxidans* needs oxygen to grow. Begin by thinking about ways to decrease the O_2 environment in the flask or medium. (Hint: Refer to Exercise 15 and the lysine decarboxylase procedure.) Also, think about ways of controlling O_2 levels without limiting CO_2. (*T. ferroxidans* grows autotrophically in 9-K medium and needs CO_2 as a source of carbon.)

2. Discuss your experimental design with your instructor and get approval before proceeding. Obtain any needed materials from your instructor.

3. Record your procedure and results in the RESULTS section.

4. Compare your results with the two treatments in flasks 1 and 2. Record your results in the RESULTS section.

REFERENCES

Brock, T. D., et al. *Biology of Microorganisms*, 7th ed., Englewood Cliffs, NJ: Prentice-Hall, 1994.

Silvermann, M.P., and Lundgren, D.G. Studies on the Chemoautotrophic Iron Bacterium *Ferrobacillus ferroxidans*. *Journal of Bacteriology*, 77(1959):642.

Whitlock, J.L., and Mudder, T.I. Report on the Homestake Wastewater Treatment Process: Biological Removal of Toxic Parameters from Cyanidation Wastewaters and Bioassay Effluent Evaluation, 1986.

RESULTS

Part A:

Color in flask 1: _____

Color in flask 2: _____

Part B:

Procedure

Results

REFLECTIONS

1. Which two factors important for the growth of the chemolithotroph *T. ferroxidans* have you eliminated if you created a completely anaerobic environment?

2. Do chemolithotrophs get their energy sources from organic or inorganic sources? Explain.

3. Why did we put flasks 1 and 2 on the shaker?

4. Besides the O_2 and CO_2 environment, what other condition does *T. ferroxidans* require that you could test? How would you design an experiment to test this?

5. The normal 9-K medium is made by adding $FeSO_4$ to the other ingredients. Why wasn't $FeSO_4$ included in the medium for the experiment you performed?

HUMANS AS HABITATS

We don't often think of ourselves as habitats, but in fact we are. Many different species of microbes colonize our skin, respiratory tract, intestinal tract, and genital sites. This exercise focuses on microbes that are part of our normal microbiota and lets you explore a microbial habitat we don't often think about—our skin.

Jim, a 69-year-old retired professor, just had cardiac bypass surgery. While in the hospital, he contracted a urinary tract infection and was treated with cephalosporin, an antibiotic. About 2 weeks later, he started to have periodic episodes of diarrhea, which became increasingly more frequent over a 3-day period. Jim finally sought help from his physician. By the time he was examined, he had a fever of 100.5°F. He was instructed to give the laboratory a stool specimen and was sent home with some antidiarrheal medication. The next day the laboratory reported a positive test for Clostridium difficile *toxin.*

Jim had never heard of this bacterium before, so he had many questions. From conversations with his doctor, he learned that he may have acquired C. difficile while in the hospital, but that he might also have acquired it from contact with soil or his dog's feces. Jim was informed that C. difficile is a major cause of diarrhea associated with antimicrobial drugs. It is also an important cause of nosocomial infections in hospitals and nursing homes. Hospitalized adults frequently become colonized with the bacterium and carry it asymptomatically. C. difficile produces endospores resistant to many antibiotics. Because of this, C. difficile often takes over the intestine when the normal microbial flora has been suppressed by antibiotics. At

some time during the antibiotic treatment, the endospores of C. difficile germinate and vegetative cells begin to multiply. The vegetative cells produce two toxins, toxin A, an enterotoxin, and toxin B, a cytotoxin. When the toxins, particularly toxin A, reach critical levels, they render the epithelial cells in the large intestine nonfunctional. This results in diarrhea. If the infection is untreated, a severe ulcerating bowel disease called pseudomembranous colitis can develop. Jim was lucky because after several days of treatment with vancomycin (the drug of choice for C. difficile), the organism was eradicated and his diarrhea ceased.

BACKGROUND INFORMATION

Jim's large intestine is a hospitable environment for the community of microbes that live there. Most are harmless and we happily share our bodies with them. Others are even beneficial, producing vitamins and aiding us nutritionally in other ways. The **normal microbiota,** or normal flora, of the large intestine are well adapted to life there. When nonresident microbes enter the large intestine, they generally compete unsuccessfully with the normal microbiota for the available nutrients. Thus, an extra benefit provided by our normal intestinal flora is their assistance in fighting nonresident microbes that may do us harm. But just like a forest or lake ecosystem, when a disturbance occurs (e.g., forest fire in the case of a forest ecosystem, or antibiotics passing through the digestive tract in the case of the intestinal habitat), the normal community structure is disrupted and new communities are established. In the case of the large intestine, such disturbances can lead to colonization by pathogens and disease results.

The large intestine is not the only part of the body normally inhabited by microbes (see **Table 31.1**). In general, any site in the body that is accessible to

TABLE 31.1   The More Common Members of the Normal Microbiota of the Human Body

| Location | Gram-positive Bacteria | | Gram-negative Bacteria | | Others[c] |
	Cocci	Rods	Cocci	Rods	
Skin	Staphylococci	*Propionibacterium acnes* Lactobacilli *Clostridium perfringens*[a]		Enteric bacilli[b]	
Mouth and oro-pharynx	Staphylococci Streptococci Anaerobic micrococci	Lactobacilli Corynebacteria	*Neisseria*	*Bacteroides Actinomyces Haemophilus*	*Mycoplasma* Spirochetes
Nose and naso-pharynx	Staphylococci	Aerobic corynebacteria			
Large intestine	Micrococci Streptococci	Lactobacilli		Enteric bacilli Clostridia *Bacteroides Pseudomonas*	
Vagina	Streptococci Staphylococci	Lactobacilli Aerobic corynebacteria		*Bacteroides*	*Candida albicans*

[a]Primarily on lower extremities.
[b]Primarily in perianal region.
[c]Not rods or cocci.

microbes, has sufficient moisture, and provides nutrients can serve as an excellent habitat for a wide variety of microorganisms. The skin is a prime example and it has several distinctive habitats for microbes. The outer layers of the skin, the epidermis, (**Figure 31.1**) is too dry for most microbes. However, microbes are commonly found associated with apocrine glands (in underarms, genital regions, nipples, and umbilicus) and sebaceous glands (hair follicles). These areas of our body provide plenty of moisture and nutrients. Most microbes that live on the skin must tolerate somewhat salty, acidic conditions characteristic of the skin. Interestingly, the acidic conditions are due in part to hydrolysis of lipids in sebum (the oily secretions of the sebaceous glands) by the bacteria associated with the gland.

Another factor that has an impact on the exact niche occupied by microbes indigenous to humans is their oxygen requirement. It makes sense that the large intestine is home to a large number of anaerobic microbes, but anaerobes are also important members of the normal microbiota of the mouth and skin. It must be remembered that certain areas in the mouth (e.g., gingival crevices and the deep layers of

dental plaque) and skin (e.g., deep in sebaceous gland pockets) are anaerobic.

In this exercise, you will characterize an isolate from the skin in terms of its cellular morphology and tolerance of certain environmental conditions. Before beginning your experiment, think carefully about the various regions of the skin. Then try to correlate the environmental conditions prevalent at a particular site to the microbe isolated.

PURPOSE

- To learn about and observe microorganisms that make up our normal microbiota
- To isolate and characterize bacteria from different places on our skin

THE EXERCISE

MATERIALS:

Sterile swabs
Nutrient agar plates
Nutrient agar plates with 5% NaCl, 10% NaCl, and 15% NaCl

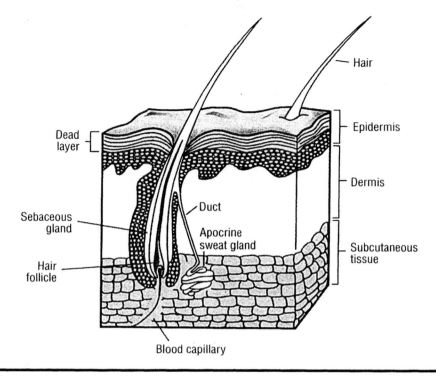

Figure 31.1 Anatomy of the human skin.

Gram stain reagents
Incubators at 30°C, 37°C, and 40°C
Tubes with sterile water
Microscope slides
Yeast extract glucose broth tubes at pH 3.0, 5.0, 7.0 and 9.0
Thioglycollate tubes

PROCEDURE:

1. Choose two areas of the skin that differ in terms of moisture and degree of exposure to the outside environment.
2. Swab these areas and isolate microorganisms from each site by streaking onto nutrient agar plates. **Note:** The swabs can be moistened in sterile water.
3. Design a protocol to characterize one isolate in terms of cellular morphology and growth in a number of environmental conditions. (Hint: See Exercise 8 for a discussion of various environmental conditions in which microbes grow. Also,

exercise 6 will give you ideas on how to characterize your microbes morphologically.)
4. Have the protocol approved by your instructor and proceed with the experiment using the materials supplied.
5. Record your results in the RESULTS section in any format you choose.

REFERENCES

Brock, T.D., et al. *Biology of Microorganisms,* 7th ed., Englewood Cliffs, NJ: Prentice-Hall, 1994.

Murray, P., et al. *Manual of Clinical Microbiology,* 6th ed., Washington, DC: American Society for Microbiology Press, 1995.

Schaechter, M., et al. *Mechanisms of Microbial Disease,* 2nd ed., Baltimore: Williams and Wilkins Publishers, 1993.

Youmans, G.P. *The Biological and Clinical Basis of Infectious Diseases,* Philadelphia, PA: W.B. Saunders Co. 1986.

RESULTS

Experimental procedure:

Results of experiment:

REFLECTIONS

1. Did you observe any differences in the microbiota of the two different areas of the skin you examined? What were they?

2. Can you make any correlations between the ranges of pH, salt concentrations, and temperature at which your isolate grew and the characteristics of the area you sampled? If yes, what are they?

3. Describe your isolate in terms of its energy requirements (chemolithotroph or chemoorganotroph) and carbon requirements (autotroph or heterotroph).

4. The mouth has a complex community structure that illustrates a number of interactions between microbes. Describe the interactions that result in the formation of dental plaque.

SECTION VI

MEDICAL MICROBIOLOGY

You have just completed a section in which you learned that microbes live in many different types of habitats, including on our bodies. In Exercise 31, the focus was on those symbiotic microbes that do us no harm. Now you will study the microbes that cause disease. You may have already experienced the effects of some of the disease-producing microbes you will study. You will also see how pathogens are tested for their sensitivity to antibiotics and learn how epidemiologists study diseases. This section then leads us to a study of how our bodies protect us from the pathogens.

EXERCISE 32

SPUTUM, PUS, AND OTHER SLIMY STUFF

Pathogenic Gram-Positive Cocci of the Respiratory Tract, Wounds, and Abscesses

This exercise begins the study of some important procaryotic microorganisms that cause disease (pathogens). The Gram-positive cocci are significant pathogens and are the subject of numerous chapters in medical textbooks. Their medical importance and virulence properties will be briefly explained and you will have the opportunity to identify some of the significant species. This, however, is only a cursory look at these important pathogens and the interested student should take a medical microbiology course to gain a greater appreciation of this group of pathogens.

It was Monday and Alice was anxious about preparing the food for a large family reunion she was catering on Saturday. She was testing a new recipe when she accidentally sliced her finger. She put adhesive tape on the cut and continued her work. On Thursday, she began preparing the large amount of potato salad that would be served at the reunion. She had noticed increased swelling, redness, and warmth at the site of her cut, but continued preparing the salad. On Saturday, her entire hand was inflamed and after catering the reunion, Alice decided to visit the emergency room. An aspirate of some pus from her finger revealed Gram-positive cocci in clusters and a physical exam showed she had an elevated temperature and white blood count. The culture of the aspirate grew Staphylococcus aureus and Alice was treated successfully over the course of the next week with oxacillin, because the bacterium was resistant to penicillin.

Two days after the picnic, the local health department was notified that ten people who were at the reunion on Saturday had developed severe vomiting and diarrhea. The health department contacted Alice and obtained samples of the leftover food. They isolated S. aureus and detected a staphylococcal toxin in the potato salad. The bacteria from the contaminated food were of the same strain, detected by phage typing, as the ones isolated from Alice's abscess and were, therefore, likely to have been introduced into the food by Alice. That week Alice learned a tough lesson about food handling—one she and the rest of her crew will never forget!

BACKGROUND INFORMATION

The story above is about one of the most important human pathogens, S. aureus. It causes a tremendous variety of human diseases, more so than any other pathogen. Staphylococci, along with streptococci that are also Gram-positive cocci, are the most frequent causes of skin and soft-tissue infections as well as respiratory infections. Therefore, both organisms are studied here in the context of these two highly different body sites—the respiratory tract, and skin and tissue.

TABLE 32.1 Some Virulence Factors Common to Respiratory Tract Pathogens

Virulence Factor	Effect	Microorganism
Lipoteichoic acids in cell wall	Adherence to surfaces	*Staphylococcus aureus* *Streptococcus pyogenes*
Fimbriae (finger-like surface structures)	Adherence to surfaces	*Escherichia coli* *Haemophilus* sp.
Capsules	Protection from phagocytosis Adherence to surfaces	*Streptococcus pneumoniae* *Neisseria meningitidis*
Intracellular multiplication	Evasion of host immune defenses	*Chlamydia* sp. *Mycobacterium tuberculosis*
Toxin production	Damage to host tissue	*Corynebacterium diphtherium* *Bordetella pertussis* *Staphylococcus aureus*

A. The Respiratory Tract and Its Infections

The respiratory tract begins with the oral and nasal passages and extends into the lungs. It is one of the major connections between the outside environment and the interior of the body. If it were not for the numerous defense mechanisms of the respiratory tract, including nasal hairs, mucous membranes, and coughing reflexes, we would be constantly plagued with infections caused by microorganisms in our environment. When respiratory infections do occur, it is because microorganisms have evaded our defense mechanisms by several means. The most common virulence factor is the ability of the bacterium or virus to adhere to the mucosal surface of the respiratory tract despite the presence of normal bacterial flora. **Table 32.1** lists other virulence factors common to pathogens of the respiratory tract.

Table 32.2 lists the microorganisms that cause respiratory tract infections. These include microbes that infect the upper respiratory tract, as in the nose or pharynx, and those that cause lower respiratory tract infections, such as pneumonia. This is not a complete list and in some cases, the microbe can be a member of our normal flora but become pathogenic under certain circumstances.

B. Infections Associated with Wounds, Abscesses, and Soft Tissue Lesions

When the skin or mucosal surface is interrupted (broken), a wound or abscess can occur. This interruption can be the result of surgery, trauma, or disease. What microbe infects the skin depends on the location of the wound such as the skin, bowel, or ulcers, or the

TABLE 32.2 Respiratory Tract Pathogens

Common Pathogens (May Be Normal Flora in Some Individuals)	Definite Pathogens (Never Found as Normal Flora)
Streptococcus pyogenes *Streptococcus pneumoniae* *Staphylococcus aureus* *Neisseria meningitidis* *Moraxella catarrhalis* *Enterobacteriaceae* *Haemophilus influenzae* *Candida albicans*	*Corynebacterium* *diphtheriae* *Mycobacterium tuberculosis* *Mycoplasma pneumoniae* *Chlamydia pneumoniae* *Bordetella pertussis* *Histoplasma capsulatum* Viruses

predisposing condition or event such as diabetes, immunosuppression, burns, or bites. Infections of abrasions and burns, as well as boils and ulcers, are often caused by microorganisms that inhabit the skin or mucosal surfaces. These infections are also often caused by nosocomial (hospital-acquired) microorganisms such as *Pseudomonas aeruginosa, S. aureus* and *Klebsiella*. Infections of bites can be caused by oral flora such as streptococci or oral anaerobes. Surgical wounds, especially of the bowel, are the result of enteric pathogens and anaerobes. **Table 32.3** lists some of the bacteria generally encountered in abscesses or wound infections.

Upon close examination of each list of pathogens, you should have noticed that staphylococci and streptococci appear in both lists. Both are Gram-positive cocci that are described in more detail below.

TABLE 32.3 Wound and Abscess Infections

Staphylococcus aureus
Streptococcus pyogenes
Microaerobic streptococci
Enterococci
Enterobacteriaceae, including *E. coli, Proteus, Morganella,*
  and *Providencia*
Pseudomonas sp.
Candida sp.
Clostridium sp.
Bacteriodes sp.
Fusobacterium sp. and other anaerobic bacteria

C. The Staphylococci

The staphylococci appear microscopically as Gram-positive cocci in grape-like clusters (**Figure 32.1**). The formation of clusters is due to the tendency of the bacterium to divide in multiple planes. Staphylococci thrive very well on most conventional media because they have few nutritional requirements. Their colonies are convex, opaque, smooth, and circular, growing 1 to 2 mm in diameter after 18 to 24 hours of incubation. They can produce white, grey-white, or yellow colonies depending on the species. Some staphylococcal species also produce hemolysins when grown on blood agar media.

There are about thirty recognized species of staphylococci and thirteen are found as part of the normal flora of humans. *S. aureus* is the major pathogen in the group, although several other species such as *Staphylococcus epidermidis* and *Staphylococcus saprophyticus* have documented clinical importance. *S. aureus* is carried in the noses of 10% to 40% of the

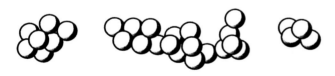

Figure 32.1 Staphylococci—cocci in grape-like clusters.

human population, including those working in health-care settings. *S. aureus* may be isolated from abscesses, boils or carbuncles, and from patients with pneumonia, bacteremia, and endocarditis (inflammation of the lining of the heart). *S. aureus* also produces toxins that cause food poisoning (something Alice found out), scalded skin disease, and toxic shock syndrome. Healthy individuals who get a staphylococcal infection will not normally have a serious infection. Typically, only those people whose defenses are compromised by injury, have prior viral infections, have deficiencies in their immune system, or have their normal flora altered by antibiotics or immunosuppressive agents acquire serious staphylococcal infections. The second clinically significant staphylococcus is *S. epidermidis*. It grows abundantly on numerous areas of the skin and is a recognized part of our normal flora. Most of the time it is acknowledged as a contaminant of specimens collected from infected individuals, but on occasion, especially in immunocompromised patients, it can be a pathogen. Some strains of the bacterium can produce a slime layer that promotes adherence to the surfaces of catheters and other plastic biomedical devices. *S. saprophyticus* has been found to cause urinary tract infections in young females. The other species of staphylococci are uncommon pathogens for humans. Another related member of staphylococci is *Micrococcus luteus*. It is a saprophyte of humans and is found on skin, in water, and in soil. It is included here as an example of normal flora that only rarely causes infection.

The staphylococci can be differentiated from each other and from other Gram-positive cocci by several biochemical tests. Staphylococci are **catalase positive** (unlike the streptococci), are always non-motile, ferment glucose, are resistant to bacitracin, and are oxidase negative. *S. aureus* produces the enzyme **coagulase** (one of its virulence properties), which differentiates it from the other usually non-pathogenic species. **Table 32.4** lists the species and characteristics used to differentiate some of the staphylococci we will investigate.

TABLE 32.4 Differentiation of Some Clinically Significant Staphylococci

Test	*S. aureus*	*S. epidermidis*	*S. saprophyticus*	*M. luteus*
Catalase	+	+	+	+
Coagulase	+	−	−	−
Oxidase	−	−	−	+
Bacitracin	Resistant	Resistant	Resistant	Sensitive
Novobiocin	NA	Sensitive	Resistant	NA

NA = Not applicable.

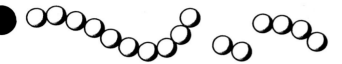

Figure 32.2 Streptococci in pairs and chains.

D. The Streptococci

The streptococci are **catalase negative** Gram-positive cocci that usually appear microscopically in chains or pairs (**Figure 32.2**). Most species belong to the genus *Streptococcus*, but some have been put in a related genus called *Enterococcus*. Some strains prefer a reduced oxygen tension and 5% to 10% CO_2 for adequate growth. Streptococcal colonies are about 1 mm in diameter, grey-white, raised, and translucent. They grow well on supportive media such as sheep blood agar. **Supportive media** are media that allow most nonfastidious microorganisms to grow at normal rates without any particular microorganism having a growth advantage. On sheep blood agar, the streptococci may demonstrate **beta (β), alpha (α),** and **gamma (γ) hemolysis** (**Table 32.4**). Beta hemolysis is complete lysis of the red blood cells evidenced as clearing around the colony, while alpha hemolysis is an incomplete or partial lysis of the red cells resulting in a green color around each colony. The term gamma hemolysis is really a misnomer because it means no hemolysis. Hemolytic reactions are differential characteristics that are useful in classifying the streptococci. Other classification systems use groupings of A, B, C, etc., which are based upon an extractable carbohydrate found in streptococcal cell walls, and at least eighteen have been described.

The pathogenic streptococci of major clinical significance include *S. pyogenes, Streptococcus agalactiae, S. pneumoniae,* and *Enterococcus faecalis. S. pyogenes* causes infections of the upper respiratory tract such as strep throat, and skin, such as impetigo. Respiratory infections caused by *S. pyogenes,* if left untreated, can lead to rheumatic fever and kidney disease, such as acute glomerulonephritis, especially in children. *S. agalactiae* causes neonatal sepsis (pathogens or toxins in the blood) with a mortality rate as high as 75% in newborns. The enterococci are infectious agents of the urinary tract, wounds, endocarditis, and septicemia. The last species of clinical significance is *S. pneumoniae.* It is the leading cause of community-acquired bacterial pneumonia in the United States, especially in infants and children. *S. pneumoniae* possesses a capsule that protects it from our immune system.

There are many tests used to differentiate the species of streptococci. **Table 32.5** contains some of the tests that identify several of the most important streptococci. These tests will be used to identify your unknown streptococcus.

PURPOSE

- To learn about important pathogens of the respiratory tract, wounds, and abscesses
- To learn how the important pathogenic Gram-positive cocci (staphylococci and streptococci) are identified

THE EXERCISE

MATERIALS:

Sheep blood agar plates (BA)
Bacitracin disks
Optochin disks
Novobiocin disks
0.5 McFarland barium sulfate standard
Two unknown broth cultures in brain heart infusion (BHI) broth
3% H_2O_2
Coagulase plasma
PYR reagent and color detector
Mueller-Hinton agar plates (MH)
Oxidase reagent
Candle jar or CO_2 incubator

TABLE 32.5 Differential Characteristics of Some Clinically Significant Streptococci

	S. pyogenes (Group A)	*S. agalactiae* (Group B)	*S. pneumoniae* (No group)	*E. faecalis* (Group D)
Hemolysis	β	β	α	β, α, or γ
Bacitracin	Sensitive	Resistant	NA	Resistant
CAMP Test	−	+	NA	−
PYR Test	+	−	−	+
Optochin	NA	NA	+	−

NA = Not applicable; PYR = Pyrrolidonyl arylamidase.

PROCEDURE:

1. Obtain two unknown broth cultures. These unknowns are possible causes of infection in the two case studies (A and B) listed below.
2. Design a protocol to identify the bacterium in each culture. The organisms can be any of the Gram-positive cocci discussed above.
3. Show your protocol to your instructor and then proceed with the isolation and identification of your pathogens. All suspected streptococci should be incubated under increased CO_2. Following the case studies are the procedures for performing the differential tests needed to identify these bacteria.
4. As you begin to identify each unknown from case A and B, record your findings and report your results as if you were a medical microbiologist. This means you will make daily observations, indicate the tests you performed, record the results of each test, and make your diagnosis. Use the RESULTS sheets provided to record your information. **Note:** You may have used a similar format to record and report your results in Exercise 18.

Case A

A 43-year-old male, unemployed postal worker was in good health until 3 days before he was admitted to the hospital. At admission he had a productive cough with yellow sputum and chest pain on the left side. He denied having fevers, chills, or night sweats. However, he did admit to being an intravenous (IV) drug user (although not for the past year). HIV testing 2 years ago was negative. An x-ray film showed fluid in his lungs. He was started on IV antibiotics after the laboratory cultured a bacterial pathogen from his sputum. Despite receiving antibiotics, he remained very sick for two days before showing improvement. What did the lab culture show?

Case B

A 23-year-old homeless woman was brought to the hospital after the police found her incoherent and wandering in a local park. Her temperature was 103°F. There were some small lumps on her fingers and some pustules on her skin. She had a heart murmur. The laboratory cultured the material aspirated from her skin and also drew blood for culturing. The same bacterium was isolated from both the abscess and the blood. What was that bacterium?

TESTING PROCEDURES

Bacitracin Sensitivity Test

This test is used to presumptively differentiate Group A streptococci from other β-hemolytic streptococci. It is important to test only β-hemolytic colonies because some α-hemolytic streptococci, such as *S. pneumoniae*, are sometimes inhibited by bacitracin. Bacitracin sensitivity serves as an adequate presumptive test for Group A streptococci. In reality, approximately 5% to 10% of β-hemolytic streptococci sensitive to bacitracin are not Group A. Therefore, further confirmatory tests are needed for a final identification. However, even in clinical practice, only a presumptive identification is given because both group A and non-Group A infections are treated with the same antibiotics. Bacitracin can also be used to differentiate staphylococci from micrococci. The former are resistant and the latter are sensitive.

MATERIALS:

Sheep blood agar plate (BA)
0.04 unit bacitracin disk

PROCEDURE:

1. Inoculate a BA plate with a colony and streak for a heavy confluent growth. Make several stabs into the agar with a needle to enhance the hemolytic reaction.
2. Place a bacitracin disk in the center of an area of expected confluent growth.
3. Incubate at 35°C for 18 to 24 hours.

INTERPRETATION:

Bacitracin sensitive: Any zone of inhibition surrounding the bacitracin disk
Bacitracin resistant: The organism grows to the edge of the disk (no zone of inhibition)

Coagulase Test

The test for the production of coagulase is the single most accurate criterion for the differentiation of pathogenic from nonpathogenic staphylococci. One pathogenic species, *S. aureus*, produces coagulase. Coagulase promotes thrombin production which in turn binds fibrinogen of rabbit plasma. This results in the formation of a fibrin clot and agglutination of the bacteria. Other species of staphylococci, called the coagulase-negative staphylococci (CNS), do not possess the enzyme and, therefore, do not form a clot. A probable reaction scheme is shown below:

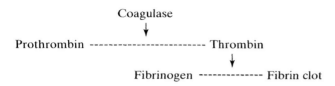

MATERIALS:

Lyophilized rabbit plasma that is reconstituted and used in 0.5 ml aliquots

PROCEDURE:

1. Inoculate a tube containing 0.5 ml of rabbit plasma with a visible inoculum from an isolated colony.
2. Incubate the tube at 35°C for 1 to 4 hours.
3. Examine the tubes for the formation of a clot that cannot be resuspended by gentle shaking. Most strains of *S. aureus* produce clots within 3 hours and frequently within 30 minutes. If the test is not positive within 4 hours, incubate overnight and reexamine the next day.

INTERPRETATION:

Positive: Formation of a clot within 4 to 24 hours
Negative: No clot formation within 24 hours

Novobiocin Sensitivity Test

Susceptibility to novobiocin will presumptively distinguish between two common CNS, *S. saprophyticus* and *S. epidermidis*. The former species is resistant to novobiocin, while the latter is susceptible. Several other species of CNS are also resistant to novobiocin. However, if a CNS is isolated from a urinary culture and it is novobiocin resistant, it is most likely *S. saprophyticus*.

MATERIALS:

Mueller-Hinton agar plates
Saline or broth
0.5 McFarland barium sulfate standard
5 μg novobiocin disks

PROCEDURE:

1. Suspend several colonies in broth or saline to a density matching that of a 0.5 McFarland barium sulfate standard.
2. Spread the suspension with a swab over the entire Mueller-Hinton agar plate to obtain confluent growth.

3. Place the novobiocin disk on the plate.
4. Incubate the plate at 35°C for 18 hours.

INTERPRETATION:

Resistant: Diameter of the zone of inhibition is <16 mm
Susceptible: Diameter of the zone of inhibition is >16 mm

CAMP Test

The presumptive identification of Group B streptococci can be made by performing the CAMP test. The CAMP factor is an extracellular, protein-like substance produced by Group B streptococci. It enhances the hemolytic activity of some staphylococcal strains to produce an even more potent hemolysis. Therefore, whenever Group B member *S. agalactiae* and *S. aureus* come into close proximity on a sheep blood agar plate, an increase in the β-hemolytic activity will be noted. This can be seen in the form of an arrowhead or flame-shaped clearing at their juncture (**Figure 32.3**). The CAMP phenomenon was first described in 1944 by Christie, Atkins, and Munch-Peterson, hence the name "CAMP."

MATERIALS:

Sheep blood agar plates (BA)
β-lysin producing *S. aureus*

PROCEDURE:

1. Inoculate the BA plate with *S. aureus* along a line down the center of the plate.
2. Make another single streak with a portion of the streptococcal colony to be identified, perpendicular to the *S. aureus* streak (**Figure 32.3**). The two streak lines *must not touch* each other.

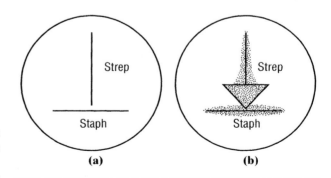

Figure 32.3 The CAMP test: (a) the method of inoculation, and (b) the arrowhead lysis after growth.

3. Several unknown streptococcal colonies can be placed perpendicular to the same streak line of *S. aureus* as long as the lines do not overlap and are labeled properly.
4. Incubate the plate at 35°C for 18 to 24 hours.

INTERPRETATION:

Positive: A zone of increased lysis which assumes the shape of an arrowhead at the junction of the two streak lines (**Figure 32.3b**)
Negative: No enhanced hemolysis

Optochin Sensitivity Test

Optochin inhibition is a useful test that will distinguish *S. pneumoniae* from other α-hemolytic streptococci. *S. pneumoniae* is susceptible to low concentrations (≤5μg) of ethyl hydrocuprein hydrochloride (optochin). To perform this test, a paper disk impregnated with optochin is applied to the streaked area of a BA plate containing the suspected streptococci. The inhibitory zones obtained by *S. pneumoniae* significantly exceed those obtained by other α-hemolytic streptococci.

MATERIALS:

Sheep blood agar plates (BA)
Optochin sensitivity disks

PROCEDURE:

1. Heavily inoculate a section of a BA plate with the isolate to be tested. More than one organism can be inoculated on each plate.
2. Apply an optochin disk to the center of the streaked area using aseptic technique. Tap the disk to ensure adequate contact with the agar surface.
3. Invert the plate and incubate aerobically (not CO_2) for 18 to 24 hours at 35°C. Although some *S. pneumoniae* require CO_2 for initial isolation, it has been found that the zones of inhibition are decreased when the test is done in increased CO_2.
4. Measure the size of the zone of inhibition.

INTERPRETATION:

Sensitive: ≥15 mm zone of inhibition
Resistant: <15 mm zone of inhibition

PYR Test

Some bacteria such as *E. faecalis* and *S. pyogenes* possess the enzyme pyroglutamyl aminopeptidase.

This enzyme hydrolyzes an amide substrate and forms β-naphthylamine. β-naphthylamine can be detected by the formation of a bright red end product when it is combined with a cinnamaldehyde reagent.

MATERIALS:

PYR filter paper
Cinnamaldehyde reagent

PROCEDURE:

1. Obtain a small amount of the colony to be tested and rub it on the surface of PYR impregnated filter paper.
2. Add a drop of freshly reconstituted cinnamaldehyde reagent and look for the formation of a red color within 5 minutes.

INTERPRETATION:

Positive: Bright red color within 5 minutes
Negative: Orange color or no color change

Catalase Test

Refer to Exercise 18.

Oxidase Test

Refer to Exercise 15.

REFERENCES

Baron, E.J., et al. *Bailey and Scott's Diagnostic Microbiology*, 9th ed., St. Louis: Mosby–Year Book, 1994.

Blazevic, D.J. and Ederer, G.M. *Biochemical Tests in Diagnostic Microbiology*. New York, NY: Wiley and Sons, 1975.

Christie, R., et al. A Note on a Lytic Phenomenon Shown by Group B Streptococci. *Australian Journal of Biological Medical Science*, 23(1944): 197-200.

Howard, B.J., et al. *Clinical and Pathogenic Microbiology*. St. Louis: Mosby–Year Book, 1987.

Isenberg, H.D., et al. *Clinical Microbiology Procedures Handbook*. Washington, DC: American Society for Microbiology Press, 1992.

Murray, P.R., et al. *Manual of Clinical Microbiology*, 6th ed., Washington, DC: American Society for Microbiology Press, 1995.

Case A:
Day 1:

Day 2:

Day 3:

Unknown number _____   Identification _____

Reported by:_____

Case B:
Day 1:

Day 2:

Day 3:

Unknown number _____   Identification _____

Reported by:_____

EXERCISE 33

PATHOGENS OF THE URINARY AND GASTROINTESTINAL TRACT

The *Enterobacteriaceae*

This exercise continues your study of some important pathogenic bacteria. These bacteria are Gram-negative rods which belong to the family *Enterobacteriaceae.* Their medical importance will be briefly explained and you will have an opportunity to identify some of the significant species. Just as in the previous exercise, it should be kept in mind that this is only a cursory examination of these pathogens and the interested student should take a medical bacteriology course to gain a greater appreciation of these important microorganisms.

Julie is a 23-year-old accountant who had been married for 6 months. She suddenly developed lower back pain, dysuria (pain upon urination), and urinary frequency. She called her doctor, who asked her to visit the office and supply the laboratory with a clean-catch urine sample. Although Julie felt miserable, she did not have a fever. The laboratory reported that she had some hematuria (blood in the urine) along with Gram-negative rods. Julie's doctor prescribed antibiotic treatment before the laboratory reported isolating Escherichia coli that was sensitive to a variety of antibiotics.

In the next 6 months Julie had three more urinary tract infections (UTIs). Each was diagnosed with clinical symptoms (pain on urination and increased frequency of urination) and laboratory findings (colony counts of 10^5 of a single bacterium). Each responded

to treatment with antibiotics for 1 week. It was decided after her fourth recurrent infection that she would be put on long-term antimicrobial therapy. The treatment worked well and her UTIs did not return.

BACKGROUND INFORMATION

Julie's UTI is common in young women. The infections are usually caused by members of the *Enterobacteriaceae,* such as *E. coli.* Members of this family cause gastrointestinal (GI) discomfort or diarrhea, as well. Therefore, these organisms are studied in this exercise as pathogens in both the urinary and GI tracts.

A. The Urinary Tract and Its Infections

The urinary tract is a system that starts at the kidneys and includes the ureters, bladder, and urethra. The majority of the system (the kidneys, ureters, and bladder) is relatively sterile because of the downward flow of urine and the sloughing of epithelial cells to which bacteria may be attached. The resident flora of the system are those microorganisms that live in close proximity to the urethra. Sometimes these microorganisms, especially the fecal bacteria, ascend the urinary tract and cause infection. Because of the ready access of bacteria to the urinary tract, it is not surprising that they are second in incidence only to infections of the respiratory tract.

A UTI is primarily one of two types; a **cystitis** (infection of the bladder) or a **pyelonephritis** (infection of the kidneys). More than 90% of UTIs are caused by normal intestinal tract bacteria. These infections are more common in women than men due at least partially to the short female urethra. However, men over age 60 with prostatic hypertrophy (enlargement of the prostate) and people with tumors or neurological disorders also have an increased incidence of UTIs. In addition, anything introduced into the bladder, such as a catheter, carries a risk of infection. Therefore, it is not surprising to learn that UTIs are the leading cause of nosocomial infections in the United States, and are also a common source of bacteremia (bacteria in the blood).

UTIs are usually caused by one predominant bacterium. It will colonize the urinary tract and dominate all other potential pathogens. Most urinary tract infections are caused by members of the family *Enterobacteriaceae*. Of this family, *E. coli* is the predominate pathogen in both uncomplicated and complicated infections (such as patients with structural or neurological abnormalities). **Table 33.1** lists, in order of frequency, the most common bacterial causes of UTIs. One factor which allows the *Enterobacteriaceae* to cause infection is their ability to adhere to the mucosal surface (epithelial cells) of the urinary tract. This prevents them from being washed out by the flow of urine. The adherence factor in some strains of *E. coli* is in the form of pili (sometimes called fimbriae) which allow them to stick to the surface of epithelial cells. Once UTI pathogens colonize the bladder, they can spread to the kidneys (pyelonephritis) and into the bloodstream (sepsis) if not treated.

B. The Gastrointestinal Tract and Associated Infections

The Gastrointestinal Tract consists of the stomach and intestines. The bacterial flora of the GI tract is established within the first several weeks after birth and remains essentially the same for the rest of our lives. The stomach is relatively bacteria-free because of its high acid content. On the other hand, the intestines of the normal adult contain from 10^{11} to 10^{12} viable bacteria per gram of feces. The predominant bacteria

TABLE 33.1 Agents of Uncomplicated Urinary Tract Infection

Escherichia coli
Proteus mirabilis
Klebsiella pneumoniae
Enterobacter sp.
Enterococcus sp.
Staphylococcus saprophyticus
Other *Enterobacteriaceae*

are non–endospore-forming anaerobes, but many members of the family *Enterobacteriaceae*, especially *E. coli*, are normal intestinal residents, too. Infectious diarrhea may be caused by bacteria, viruses, and protozoa.

The most common bacterial agents of **gastroenteritis** (intestinal disease) are species of *Salmonella*, *Shigella*, and *Campylobacter*. They cause enteric fevers, food poisoning, and bacillary dysentery. Other bacteria of significance are *Yersinia enterocolitica*, *Clostridium difficile*, *Vibrio*, *Aeromonas*, and certain serotypes of *E. coli*. The clinical picture in acute diarrheal illness (loss of abnormally large volumes of liquid stool) is usually the same for all etiological agents.

Bacteria that cause diarrheal illness do so predominately by two mechanisms: invasion of the intestinal mucosa and production of enterotoxins. Bacteria that invade the epithelial lining of the intestine (*Shigella*) cause inflammation and infection (dysentery). Bacteria that produce toxins (*Vibrio cholerae*) cause the bowel to lose its ability to absorb water, which results in watery stools and dehydration.

Table 33.2 contains a list of the most common bacterial agents of diarrheal illness and sources of these bacteria. Keep in mind, however, that other microorganisms such as viruses and protozoa also cause GI discomfort. In fact, in the United States, the leading cause of diarrhea is rotavirus.

C. The Enterobacteriaceae

Members of the family *Enterobacteriaceae* are by far the most frequently encountered bacteria isolated in the clinical laboratory (50% of all clinically significant isolates). Besides being normal inhabitants of our GI tract, they are also found in water, soil, and plants. They are associated with abscesses, pneumonia,

TABLE 33.2 Some Bacterial Agents of Gastrointestinal Infections

Organism	Source
Salmonella sp.	Contaminated food, especially poultry
Shigella sp.	Fecal-oral contact
Escherichia coli	Human feces and contaminated food
Campylobacter sp.	Farm animals and contaminated food
Yersinia enterocolitica	Animal products
Vibrio sp.	Contaminated water and shellfish
Bacillus cereus	Contaminated foods

meningitis, and septicemia as well as infections of the urinary and intestinal tract. The *Enterobacteriaceae* are Gram-negative rods that vary in size and grow readily on supportive media such as sheep blood agar. Their colonies are large and dull gray on these media. Depending on their metabolic capabilities, they also grow on many types of **selective** and **differential** media. Selective media contain inhibitors such as dyes and salts which inhibit certain groups of bacteria. For instance, MacConkey agar inhibits growth of Gram-positive cocci while allowing Gram-negative rods to grow. Differential media allow organisms to be partially or completely identified based on biochemical reactions of the medium (e.g., MacConkey agar). The three important metabolic characteristics of the *Enterobacteriaceae* are: they reduce nitrates to nitrites; they ferment glucose; and they are oxidase negative.

In the last several decades, the identification schemes of the *Enterobacteriaceae* have undergone many changes. DNA hybridization, antibiotic susceptibility patterns, and computerized identification programs have supplemented the traditional biochemical and serological means of identification. The standard by which all organisms are identified is a series of biochemical reactions in test tube media. Today, many laboratories are using miniaturized or automated biochemical identification systems because of time and cost constraints. We will use one of these systems called API 20E (bioMérieux Vitek, Inc., Hazelwood, Mo.) to identify one isolate in this exercise. A second isolate will be identified with a few traditional biochemical media. **Table 33.3** contains a list of the common pathogenic *Enterobacteriaceae* you will be identifying in this exercise. This table also gives the biochemical results from traditional tubed media that you will use to identify your unknown. When the rapid API system is used, a computer-generated key

will be supplied by your instructor to identify your unknown. An explanation of the differential media and API system are included in the procedure.

PURPOSE

- To learn about important pathogens of the urinary tract and gastrointestinal tract
- To learn how the important pathogenic *Enterobacteriaceae* are identified

THE EXERCISE

MATERIALS:

MacConkey agar plates (MAC)
Motiliy-indole-ornithine tubes (MIO)
Urea agar slants
API 20E strips (bioMérieux Vitek, Inc.)
Voges-Proskauer reagents
Demonstration tubes of all media and bacteria listed in **Table 33.3**
Triple sugar iron (TSI) agar slants
Citrate agar slants
API 20E Codebook (bioMérieux Vitek, Inc.)
Kovacs reagent
10% ferric chloride
0.85% sterile saline (5 ml)
Pasteur pipets
Sterile mineral oil

PROCEDURE:

1. You will be given two unknown bacteria on MacConkey agar plates. The unknowns are associated with the two case studies that follow. **Note:** Normally an oxidase test would be performed to verify the Gram-negative rod is an *Enterobacteriaceae*. However, both of your unknowns are from this family of

TABLE 33.3　Selected Biochemical Reactions of Some Enterobacteriaceae

Organism	Lactose Fermentation	Sucrose Fermentation	H₂S	Motility	Indole	Ornithine	Citrate	Urea
Escherichia coli	+	+	−	+	+	+	−	−
Klebsiella pneumoniae	+	+	−	−	−	−	+	+
Enterobacter aerogenes	+	+	−	+	−	+	+	−
Proteus mirabilis	−	−	+	+	−	+	+/−	+
Salmonella, most serotypes	−	−	+	+	−	+	+	−
Yersinia enterocolitica	−	+	−	−	+/−	+	−	−
Shigella serogroups A, B & C	−	−	−	−	+/−	−	−	−

ᵃTable adapted from Farmer, J.J. III, in Manual of Clinical Microbiology. Washington, D.C.: American Society for Microbiology Press, 1995.

bacteria and an oxidase test cannot be performed with a colony from the MacConkey plate because interfering substances (i.e., crystal violet) may cause false positive reactions. For these reasons, you will not perform an oxidase test on either of your unknowns. The nitrate reduction reaction is also unnecessary and will not be performed.

2. Proceed with the identification of each of these pathogens using the traditional tubed media (TSI, MIO, Citrate and Urea) for case A and the API 20E strip for case B.

3. Following the case studies is a description of each medium including the MacConkey agar plate. Also included is the procedure for inoculating the API strip and analyzing the results.

4. Observe the demonstration tubes of all the bacteria set up by your instructor. **Note:** Observing these media will give you a better idea of positive and negative reactions for each test.

5. Use the sheets in the RESULTS section to record your daily observations as you did in Exercise 32.

Case A

A 20-year-old male was rendered quadraplegic from an automobile accident 6 months ago. He is a resident of an extended care rehabilitation unit at a city medical center. Routine urine cultures are done on all residents once a week. On this occasion, he was found to have a microorganism in significant numbers ($>10^5$) in his urine. What is his pathogen?

Case B

Two days after eating in a Mexican restaurant on a trip to San Diego, a 25-year-old graduate student experienced a sudden onset of abdominal pain, fever, and watery diarrhea. A day later, she still felt ill and the diarrhea was worse with her stools now containing mucus and blood. She decided to visit the health service after returning to campus and the laboratory cultured a sample of her stool. The laboratory isolated this bacterium. What is it? Is it a fecal pathogen? If not, what caused her diarrhea?

MEDIA AND TESTING

MacConkey Agar (MAC)

MAC is a highly selective and differential medium. The selectivity of the medium comes from the addition of certain inhibitors, such as crystal violet, which inhibits the growth of Gram-positive organisms and yeasts. MAC also allows for

the differentiation of lactose-fermenting bacteria (LF) from non–lactose–fermenting bacteria (NLF). LF colonies are red, surrounded by an opaque zone of precipitated red bile. This is because the acids produced as a result of lactose fermentation turn the neutral red bile salt indicator red (acid pH). NLF colonies do not produce acids and precipitate bile and are, therefore, colorless and transparent. MAC is often used in clinical microbiology laboratories to isolate Gram-negative rods from feces, urine, and other clinical specimens.

BACTERIAL IDENTIFICATION USING TRADITIONAL TUBE MEDIA

Triple-Sugar-Iron (TSI)

The fermentation of three sugars in triple-sugar-iron agar is one of the preliminary methods of identifying Gram-negative rods. The three sugars are lactose, sucrose, and glucose (in one-tenth the concentration of the other two). The iron in TSI is supplied from ferrous sulfate. It, along with sodium thiosulfate, allows for the detection of hydrogen sulfide gas (H_2S) producers. This is indicated by a blackening of the medium. TSI contains no inhibitory substances and four protein compounds (beef extract, yeast extract, peptone, and proteose) which makes it nutritionally very rich and able to grow many fastidious species. It contains a phenol red indicator which is red at pH 7.4 and yellow at pH 6.8. When the medium is made, it is allowed to solidify in a slanted position. This essentially creates two reaction chambers within the same tube. The slant portion is exposed to oxygen and its surface is aerobic while the lower portion or "butt" is relatively anaerobic, allowing fermentation to take place (**Figure 33.1**).

For the *Enterobacteriaceae*, glucose is the preferred energy source and is fermented first. As a result, the entire tube becomes acidic (yellow) in 8 to 12 hours. After the recommended 18 to 24 hour incubation period, the butt will remain acidic due to the formation of acids during fermentation, but the slant will revert to alkaline (red). This is due to the oxidation of the fermentation products under aerobic conditions and because the peptones are oxidized to alkaline amines. If, however, the bacterium can also ferment lactose and/or sucrose, the large amount of fermentation acids produced will more than neutralize the alkaline amines and leave the slant acidic (yellow). The CO_2 and H_2 produced during fermentation are indicated by the presence of bubbles or

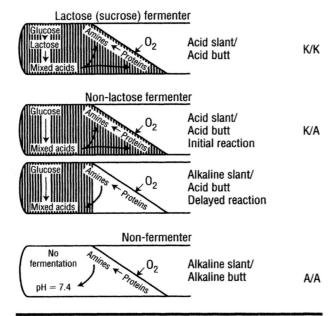

Figure 33.1 Three general types of reactions produced by bacteria growing on TSI agar.

cracks in the agar and the H_2S is manifested by a blackening of the medium.

MATERIALS:

TSI agar slants
An isolated colony on agar

PROCEDURE:

1. Using a straight wire needle, touch the top of a well-isolated colony.
2. Stab the TSI agar through the center of the medium to the bottom of the tube and then streak the surface of the slant.
3. Leave the cap on loosely and incubate the tube at 35°C for 18 to 24 hours. *Do not* incubate the tube longer than 24 hours because aerobic oxidation of lactose and/or sucrose will eventually take place and the slant will revert to an alkaline state.

INTERPRETATION:

Nonfermenter: Alkaline slant/alkaline butt (K/K)
Glucose fermenter only: Alkaline slant/acid butt (K/A)
Glucose, lactose and/or sucrose fermenter: Acid slant/acid butt (A/A)
Note: K/A and A/A patterns can be accompanied by gas production and/or a black precipitate of ferrous sulfide

Motility-Indole-Ornithine Test

Motility-indole-ornithine (MIO) is a semisolid tubed media used to identify members of the family *Enterobacteriaceae*. Three characteristics (indole production, motility, and ornithine decarboxylase activity) are all determined in one tube, saving time and money. Each reaction will be discussed individually below.

A. Motility

A microorganism's ability to move by means of flagella can be determined by performing a motility test in a medium such as MIO. Motile bacteria will move in semisolid agar. This can be determined by stabbing the agar with an inoculum and observing whether the bacteria move away from the original stab line. Motile bacteria move and grow throughout the entire tube while nonmotile bacteria, such as *Klebsiella*, grow only along the stab line (**Figure 33.2**). It is important to stab the tube only once and pull the inoculating needle straight out along the stab line.

B. Indole Production

The principle and testing procedure of the indole test is explained in Exercise 15.

C. Ornithine Decarboxylase

Certain organisms have the ability to decarboxylate ornithine to putrescine. This proceeds under anaerobic conditions according to the following equation:

$$\text{Ornithine} \xrightarrow[\text{Pyrodoxal phosphate}]{\text{Ornithine decarboxylase}} \text{Putrescine} + CO_2$$

The medium, which also contains glucose, initially changes from purple to yellow because of acid produced from glucose fermentation. When the glucose

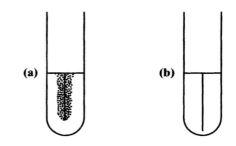

Figure 33.2 The appearance of bacteria growing in semisolid agar: (a) motile and (b) nonmotile.

is used up, the bacterium decarboxylates ornithine, and the alkalinity caused by the amine, putrescine, causes the yellow color to revert back to purple. To ensure that fermentation rather than oxidation occurs, an oil overlay must be used when using a broth medium. However, since MIO is a semisolid medium, no oil overlay is required unless the medium is incubated for more than 24 hours.

MATERIALS:

MIO semisolid tubed medium
An isolated colony on agar

PROCEDURE:

1. With a straight inoculating needle, obtain an isolated colony and inoculate the medium by inserting it *once* through the center of the medium to the bottom of the tube.
2. Incubate the tube at 35°C for 18 to 24 hours.
3. Note the motility and ornithine decarboxylase reactions.
4. Add 1 to 2 drops of Kovac's reagent and determine indole production.

INTERPRETATION:

Motility: Bacterial growth extending out from stab line. Sometimes the growth is diffuse throughout the medium.

No motility: Bacterial growth is confined along the stab line. The rest of the medium is clear.

Indole positive: Red color in the upper aqueous layer.

Indole negative: Light yellow color in the upper aqueous layer.

Ornithine decarboxylation: Purple color throughout the medium.

No ornithine decarboxylation: The medium is yellow except for a small rim of purple at the agar surface.

Citrate

The citrate utilization test is another means of differentiating bacteria. This test is used to determine if a microorganism has the ability to utilize citrate as its sole source of carbon and inorganic ammonium salt as its sole source of nitrogen. The original citrate broth was modified by Simmons with the addition of agar and an indicator, brom thymol blue. This indicator is green at pH 6.8 and blue at pH 7.6 or greater. The exact nature of the alkaline reaction produced by some microorganisms is not clear. It is probably not due to the release of ammonia from ammonium salts, but is more likely to occur because excess CO_2 is gen-

erated. CO_2 is generated when citrate is cleaved to oxaloacetate, which in turn is decarboxylated to pyruvate and CO_2. The excess CO_2 may combine with sodium and water to form sodium carbonate which is alkaline enough to change the indicator from green to deep blue. It is important to minimize the carry-over of any nutrients from other culture media and to use a light inoculum when performing this test. Growth on citrate without the pH change to alkalinity usually indicates the microorganism does not belong to the family *Enterobacteriaceae*.

MATERIALS:

Simmon's citrate agar slants
An isolated colony on agar

PROCEDURE:

1. Streak a portion of an isolated colony on the agar slant. Remember to use a small amount of inoculum to prevent false positive results.
2. Incubate the tube, cap loosened, at 35°C for 18 to 24 hours.

INTERPRETATION:

Positive: Growth with a deep blue color
Negative: Absence of growth and no color change after 4 days

Urease Test

The principle for the urease test was explained in Exercise 15. Refer to that exercise for inoculation of the media and interpretation of the test.

BACTERIAL IDENTIFICATION USING THE API SYSTEM

The identification of your unknown from case B will be done using an API 20E system (**Figure 33.3**). The API strip is a standardized miniaturized version of conventional procedures for identifying Gram-negative

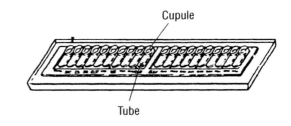

Cupule

Tube

Figure 33.3 The API 20E identification system.

bacilli. The system has twenty miniature capsule reaction chambers that perform twenty-three standard biochemical tests. Once the biochemical reactions have taken place (in 18 to 24 hours), the test results are converted to a seven-digit profile. Identification can then be made with the aid of conventional differential charts or by using the Analytical Profile Index (API Codebook). This system is one of many systems used by clinical laboratories on a daily basis. The advantage of such systems over tubed media will be evident to you after you have performed the testing.

To set up the API strip on your fecal isolate follow these instructions:

a. Aseptically obtain a well isolated colony from your MAC plate and suspend the bacteria in 5 ml of sterile saline.

b. The API strip is incubated in a plastic tray with a lid. Place 5 ml of tap water in the incubation tray to provide a humid atmosphere, and place the strip in the tray.

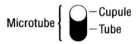

c. Using a sterile Pasteur pipet, transfer the bacterial suspension to each microtube in the API strip. To do this, tilt the strip and fill the tube section of the microtube by placing the pipet against the side of the cupule. Slowly fill the tube so as not to entrap air bubbles in the bottom. Fill the tube portion only to the bottom lip of the opening.

d. Fill both the tube and cupule section of the CIT, VP, and GEL tubes. **Note:** The test names, abbreviations, and reaction results are listed below.

e. Overlay the ADH, LDH, ODC, H$_2$S, and URE cupules with mineral oil.

f. Put the lid on the chamber, label the strip with your name and unknown number, and incubate the strip at 35°C to 37°C for 18 to 24 hours.

g. If the GLU is negative, reincubate another 24 hours. **Note:** You will only be working with organisms from the family *Enterobacteriaceae* and by definition these organisms all ferment glucose.

h. After incubation, add 1 drop of ferric chloride to the TDA cupule.

i. Add 1 drop of Kovac's reagent to the IND cupule.

j. Add 1 drop of a-naphthol and 1 drop of KOH (VP reagents) to the VP cupule.

k. Read all the reactions, and derive the seven-digit code number by scoring each set of three reactions on the API strip which accompanies the strip or on the RESULTS page. A negative reaction counts as zero.

l. Refer to the API 20E Codebook for identification.

A. Tests on the API strip

O-nitrophenyl-β-D-galactoside (ONPG)
Arginine dihydrolase (ADH)
Lysine decarboxylase (LDC)
Ornithine decarboxylase (ODC)
Citrate (CIT)
H$_2$S
Mannitol (MAN)
Sorbitol (SOR)
Sucrose (SUC)
Amygdalin (AMY)
Urea (URE)
Tryptophan deaminase (TDA)
Indole (IND)
Voges-Proskauer (VP)
Gelatin (GEL)
Glucose (GLU)
Inositol (INO)
Rhamnose (RHA)
Melibiose (MEL)
Arabinose (ARA)

B. Results of API 20E tests

Tube	Reaction	
	Positive	**Negative**
ONPG	Yellow	Colorless
ADH	Red or orange, red (36-48 hr)	Yellow, yellow or orange (36-48 hr)
LDC	Red or orange, red (36-48 hr)	Yellow, yellow or orange (36-48 hr)
ODC	Red or orange, red (36-48 hr)	Yellow, yellow or orange (36-48 hr)
CIT	Turquoise or dark blue	Light green or yellow
H_2S	Black deposit	No black deposit
URE	Red or orange, red (36-48 hr)	Yellow, yellow or orange (36-48 hr)
TDA	Brown-red	Yellow
IND	Red ring	Yellow
VP	Red	Colorless
GEL	Diffusion of black pigment	No diffusion of black pigment
GLU	Yellow or gray	Blue or blue-green
MAN	Yellow	Blue or blue-green
INO	Yellow	Blue or blue-green
SOR	Yellow	Blue or blue-green
RHA	Yellow	Blue or blue-green
SAC	Yellow	Blue or blue-green
MEL	Yellow	Blue or blue-green
AMY	Yellow	Blue or blue-green
ARA	Yellow	Blue or blue-green
Nitrate reduction	Red; bubbles are yellow after addition of reagents and zinc	Yellow; orange after reagents and zinc
NO_2	Red; bubbles are yellow after addition of reagents and zinc	Yellow; orange after reagents and zinc
N_2 gas	Red; bubbles are yellow after addition of reagents and zinc	Yellow; orange after reagents and zinc

REFERENCES

Baron, E.J., et al. *Bailey and Scott's Diagnostic Microbiology*, 9th ed., St. Louis: Mosby–Year Book, 1994.

Blazevic, D.J. and Ederer, G.M. *Biochemical Tests in Diagnostic Microbiology*. New York: Wiley and Sons, 1975.

Howard, B.J., et al. *Clinical and Pathogenic Microbiology*. St. Louis: Mosby–Year Book, 1987.

Isenberg, H.D., et al. *Clinical Microbiology Procedures Handbook*. Washington, D.C.: American Society for Microbiology Press, 1992.

Murray, P.R., et al. *Manual of Clinical Microbiology*, 6th ed. Washington, D.C.: American Society for Microbiology Press, 1995.

RESULTS

Case A:

Day 1: Observation of MAC plate and inoculation of tubed media

Day 2: Observation of results

TSI:

MIO:

Citrate:

Urea:

Unknown number _____   Identification _____

Reported by:_____

Case B:
Day 1: Observation of the MAC plate and inoculation of API strip

Day 2: Reading the results

Unknown number _____   Identification _____

Is this a fecal pathogen?_____ If not, what do you think caused her diarrhea?

Reported by:_____

EXERCISE 34

SLEUTHING FOR A PARASITE

> The previous two exercises allowed you to become familiar with procaryotic pathogens, especially those of humans. This exercise will focus on another human pathogen, *Giardia,* an intestinal parasite found worldwide.

You and a friend decide to go backpacking for several days in a wilderness area. As you pack your supplies, you realize that water may be a problem. You know you could carry enough for 2 days, but 3 may be stretching it. You decide that if worse comes to worst, drinking stream water will have to do. However, you have heard of parasites that you should be concerned about. After all, diarrhea a week after your trip would not leave you with pleasant memories. Upon investigating your alternatives, you learn that filtering water removes the most common parasite, Giardia lamblia. *Your task now is to find filters that could be used to supply you with safe mountain water. You soon realize that many different size filters exist and you need to determine what pore size will filter out this diarrheal parasite. What size filter did you end up taking on your hiking trip?*

BACKGROUND INFORMATION

Protozoa from the genus *Giardia* have been studied by microscopists for more than 300 years. In fact, it is believed that van Leeuwenhoek reported through his writings to the Royal Society of London on the actively moving form of the parasite (trophozoites) from his own diarrhoeic specimens. Since this was before the time of Koch who proved the germ theory of disease, it is not known whether van Leeuwenhoek actually associated these "animalcules a-moving very

prettily" with his diarrhea. It is known, however, that he suffered from chronic diarrhea for many years.

G. lamblia is a flagellated protozoan that inhabits the small intestine of the host. Humans, domestic dogs, and wild animals such as beavers and muskrats can serve as hosts to the microorganism. **Giardiasis,** the infection with *G. lamblia,* is acquired by ingestion of water and food contaminated with feces or direct person-to-person fecal-oral contact. The infective form of the parasite is the cyst form. It can survive for long periods of time in a suitable environment outside the host. Because it can survive in fresh water, it is one of the most common causes of waterborne diarrheal disease. Outbreaks of giardiasis are frequent in day-care centers, residential institutions, and among campers. Transmission also occurs during sexual activity, particularly oral-anal contact. In giardiasis the most common symptom is a protracted, or prolonged, diarrhea. If left untreated, the diarrhea, which can be mild or acute, may last for weeks or months with periodic episodes of remission and exacerbation. Malabsorption of nutrients is usually the result of prolonged infection and the classic signs of weight loss and chronic fatigue are usually the result. Diagnosis comes from examination and identification of the organism in fecal specimens. In addition, enzyme immunoassay (Exercise 41) and fluorescent-antibody antigen detection systems (Exercises 7 and 42) are available when stool samples, duodenal (intestinal) aspirates, or a biopsy of the small intestine are repeatedly negative for the organism.

Giardia has a simple asexual life cycle existing as either of two different stages, the **cyst** or the **trophozoite (Figure 34.1)**. Flagellated trophozoites attach to the intestinal mucosa and are responsible for the pathogenesis of the disease. Cysts, which are passed from the body in the fecal mass and are reingested by a new host, represent the resting and infective stage

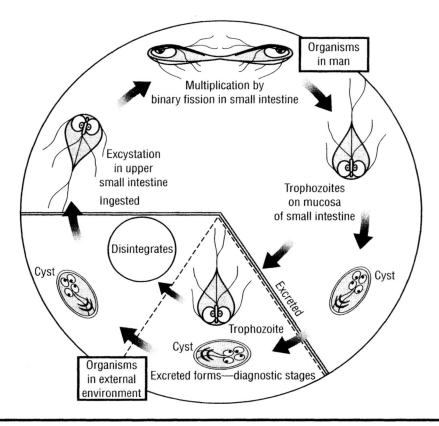

Figure 34.1   Life cycle of *G. lamblia.*

of the organism. Cysts are oval and have four nuclei, although only two may be visible in light microscopy. (**Figure 34.2a**). They are excreted by individuals with formed stools and are passed on to other people by fecal contamination of water or food. After cysts are ingested, trophozoites are formed. Trophozoites are pear-shaped and motile (**Figure 34.2b**). They possess eight flagella and two nuclei. They also have two rigid structures called axonemes which occupy the entire length of the organism. Underneath the trophozoite is a disk-like depression that is used to attach to the surface of an epithelial cell. Once attached to the epithelial surface of the small intestine, the trophozoite multiplies by binary fission and soon millions of trophozoites cover the surface of the small intestine. Then, by a still unknown process, they are stimulated to form cysts in the lumen of the small intestine, are excreted in the stool, and the cycle starts again.

In this exercise, you will observe the stages of the parasite and calculate their average size. With this information, you should be able to determine the filter size necessary to filter this pathogen from drinking water.

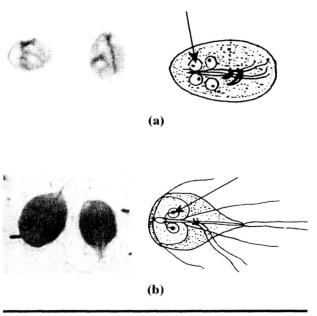

Figure 34.2   The two stages of *G. lamblia:* (a) cyst, and (b) trophozoite. Note the nuclei (arrow).

PURPOSE

- To observe, measure, and calculate the average size of the parasite, *G. lamblia*
- To learn about the life cycle and pathogenic potential of *G. lamblia*
- To determine what filter pore size would be best to take camping

THE EXERCISE

MATERIALS:

Culture of *G. lamblia* and/or prepared stained slides of the cyst or trophozoite stages
Lugol's iodine
Coverslips
Microscope with a reticle eyepiece that allows measurement in micrometers
Microscope slides

PROCEDURE:

1. Obtain a prepared slide or make an iodine preparation of a culture of *G. lamblia*. The iodine prep is made by placing a drop of Lugol's iodine on a slide and with a pipet, adding 1 to 2 drops of the culture and mixing well. A coverslip is placed on the suspension.
   CAUTION: In culture, only trophozoites (non-infectious stage) predominate and cysts are extremely rare. However, the sample should still be handled according to the biohazard precautions stipulated in this manual and by your instructor. All materials (slides, coverslips, pipets, etc.) should be properly disposed of in biohazard containers. Avoid ingesting any of the culture.
2. Place the slide on the microscope and begin searching for the parasite. Start your observations using the low (10×) and high (40×) objectives, and then add oil and move to oil immersion (100×) once a possible trophozoite or cyst is located. A calibrated eyepiece or reticle should be in place. It may have markings that have the following divisions:

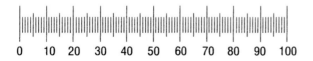

Note: Some reticles are marked in 50 units instead of 100, so determine the type of reticle in your microscope before beginning. Using the 10× objective, 1 unit equals 10 micrometers (0.01 mm) and 10 units of the scale equal 100 micrometers. Using the 40× objective, 1 unit on the scale equals 2.5 micrometers (0.0025 mm) and 10 units equal 25 micrometers. If you used the 100× objective, what would each unit be equal to?

3. Find either the cyst or trophozoite stage of *G. lamblia* and center it under the markings. Count the number of lines that span both the length and width of a cyst or trophozoite. If possible, find 2 to 5 different organisms and measure both the cyst and trophozoite. So that you are not measuring the same organism twice, read the microscope slide following the pattern below:

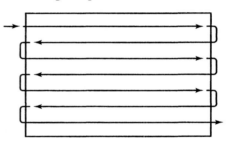

4. Record your results in the RESULTS section and calculate the average size of the parasite. To calculate the size of the microorganism, average the number of lines for the length and width of each stage of the pathogen. Then multiply the number of lines counted by the factor given for the objective lens you used to measure the organism (see above).

REFERENCES

Baker, J., and Muller, R. *Advances in Parasitology*. Vol. 32. San Diego: Academic Press Inc., 1993.

Katz, M., et al. *Parasitic Diseases,* 2nd ed. New York: Springer-Verlag, 1989.

Murray, P., et al. *Manual of Clinical Microbiology*, 6th ed. Washington, D.C.: American Society for Microbiology Press, 1995.

Thompson, R., et al. *Giardia: From Molecules to Disease*. Cambridge: CAB International, 1994.

RESULTS

Measurements of each of the stages you were able to observe:

	Cysts			Trophozoites		
	Length	Width	Objective used	Length	Width	Objective used
1.	_____	_____	_____	_____	_____	_____
2.	_____	_____	_____	_____	_____	_____
3.	_____	_____	_____	_____	_____	_____
4.	_____	_____	_____	_____	_____	_____
5.	_____	_____	_____	_____	_____	_____

Average number of units for each of the stages:

Cyst: Length _____ units   Trophozoites: Length _____ units

Width _____ units   Width _____ units

Average length and width of the organism in micrometers for each of the stages:

Cyst: _____

Trophozoite _____

REFLECTIONS:

1. Which camping filters will filter out the *Giardia* cysts and trophozoites?

    a. Filter pore size: 15.0 μm _____

    b. Filter pore size: 10.0 μm _____

    c. Filter pore size: 5.0 μm _____

    d. Filter pore size: 1.0 μm _____

2. Why is it necessary for several stool cultures to be analyzed before *Giardia* cysts or trophozoites are found?

3. Are antibiotics such as penicillin or ampicillin effective against this pathogen? Why or why not?

4. Is *G. lamblia* a eucaryotic or procaryotic microorganism? What feature that you may have observed led you to this conclusion?

EXERCISE 35

PASSING THE GERM

You just learned about procaryotic and eucaryotic pathogens in the last three exercises. This exercise will focus on how some pathogens are transmitted to new hosts. The transmission routes studied in this laboratory are through human contact and by eating contaminated food.

Cindy and her husband were working parents with two small children. Cindy, a certified nutritionist, worked part-time at a local hospital. On the days she went to work, Cindy took Mike (age four) and Michelle (almost two) to the ABC Day Care facility. They enjoyed playing with friends. One day Mike was fussy but seemed to sleep fine that night, so Cindy took both of them to the day care the next day. That afternoon when Cindy picked up Mike and Michelle, she noticed some raised vesicles on Mike's neck. Cindy lifted his shirt and he was covered with vesicles on his chest and back. One of the day-care providers walked over and commented,"Oh yes, I forgot to tell you. Two of his friends were diagnosed with chicken pox 3 days ago!" Cindy could only imagine what the next 2 weeks would be like.

BACKGROUND INFORMATION

With the recent approval of a chicken pox vaccine, Mike and Michelle would now be protected against chicken pox. However, until widespread use of the vaccine occurs, chicken pox is a good example of how quickly diseases can be transmitted. Young children, especially those in day care facilities, transmit "germs" by such mechanisms as coughing, runny noses, and dirty hands. In fact, children can be

thought of as little infectious disease factories, passing pathogens on to siblings and of course, Mom and Dad. Day care centers not only harbor viruses (respiratory and intestinal) but also bacterial pathogens such as strep throat (*Streptococcus pyogenes*), protozoan parasites (*Giardia lamblia*), and worms (pinworms). The same can be said of other institutional settings such as military barracks, extended care facilities, and college dormitories. This is because humans are one of the primary reservoirs and vectors of infectious disease.

The most common means of disease transmission is through aerosols, such as coughs and sneezes. However, this exercise focuses on three other means of disease transmission. You will explore how organisms can be passed from person to person by touch; observe organisms that are transmitted sexually; and discover how food can harbor microorganisms.

As mentioned above, a common means of disease transmission is through human contact. Human contact is often through hands (with a touch, handshake, etc.). Most bacteria present on hands are transient. They are transferred to the hands by constant contact with the environment, including water. It follows, therefore, that hands are one of the ways bacteria can be transferred from one person to another, through hand-to-hand contact. This exercise will use a bacterium (*Micrococcus luteus*) to demonstrate the transfer of bacteria from one person to another by touching fingertips. *M. luteus* produces yellow colonies so it can be readily recognized and distinguished from other bacteria that reside on skin. After the bacterium is transferred, each person will wash his or her hands to determine whether hand washing removes *Micrococcus* and any normal flora from the skin. The transfer of the bacterium is done with the help of "sticky" caramel candy. The number of microorganisms transmitted will be detected by touching nutrient agar plates with your fingertips. The transferred microbes will be deposited on this supportive medium and give rise to colonies which can be distinguished from other normal skin microbes.

A second means of disease transmission is through sexual contact. There are numerous sexually transmitted infectious agents which cause disease, ranging from mild inflammation of the urethra (e.g., urethritis due to chlamydia) to fatal suppression of the immune system (e.g., HIV). These microorganisms can be bacteria such as those that cause chlamydia, gonorrhea and syphilis; viruses such as HIV (AIDS), herpes virus, hepatitis B virus and papillomaviruses (genital warts); and protozoa such as *Trichomonas*. Since bacteria are the easiest to study in the laboratory, this exercise will focus on two bacteria that are the most common sexually transmitted diseases (STDs) of sexually active men and women, *Chlamydia trachomatis* and *Neisseria gonorrhoeae*.

Chlamydia were once thought to be viruses because they are obligate intracellular parasites. However, they are Gram-negative bacteria, which depend upon host cells for the manufacture of ATP. Because of this dependency, they cannot be propagated on agar media, but instead must be grown in cell culture media. Chlamydia replicate in the cytoplasm of host cells such as McCoy cells, a cell line obtained from mice.

Chlamydia undergo an interesting developmental cycle (**Figure 35.1**). The infectious particles are small rigid structures called **elementary bodies** (EB) which attach to the surface of a susceptible host cell. Somehow the host cells are induced to engulf the EB. As a result, the EB become enclosed in a cytoplasmic vesicle without being destroyed by enzymes within the host. The EB then reorganize to more metabolically active forms called **reticulate bodies** (RB). The RB multiply for 18 to 24 hours at which time they reorganize or condense again into EB particles. It is at this point, when the EB and RB are still enclosed within a vesicle, that they can be stained with iodine and observed microscopically. This is because the EB and RB are rather compact and primarily contain glycogen. Glycogen, like starch, stains brown with iodine. Therefore, the EB and RB appear as dark-brown round bodies at 400× magnification. After 35 to 40 hours, multiplication ceases and the host cell ruptures to release a large number of infectious EB, which attach to other host cells and start the cycle again.

C. trachomatis is the most common bacterial STD. It is four to five times more common than *N. gonorrhoeae* and is one of the most prevalent pathogens in the world. In developing countries, *C. trachomatis*

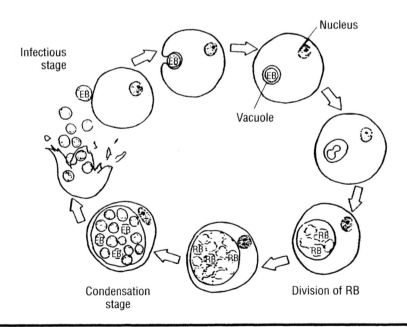

Figure 35.1 The life cycle of chlamydia.

primarily causes blinding trachoma (scarring of the cornea), while in the United States it causes genital infections in an estimated four million people each year. In many individuals with genital infection due to chlamydia, the symptoms can be mild or non-specific or there may be no symptoms at all; these individuals are called asymptomatic carriers. In both men and women, untreated infections can persist for months and lead to serious complications such as infertility and sterility. Fortunately, laboratory techniques can be used to identify the organism, and antibiotics are available to treat chlamydia infection.

In this laboratory you will observe the EB and RB of *C. trachomatis* in a slide culture cell preparation. The slides have been stained with concentrated iodine so that the dark brown particles can be observed. In clinical laboratories, fluorescent antibodies are used to identify chlamydia from cell culture and sometimes from the original clinical sample because the antibodies are more specific and sensitive for a smaller number of organisms. In addition, other rapid diagnostic techniques are being developed that will aid in the tracking and prevention of this STD.

Gonococci (*N. gonorrhoeae*) are Gram-negative cocci which usually occur in pairs with flattened adjacent sides, similar in appearance to a coffee bean. Although they will grow intracellularly within leukocytes (**Figure 35.2**), gonococci do not require host cells to survive and reproduce. Instead, they grow on several specialized agar media. One such medium is called chocolate agar, an enriched medium that supports the growth of many microorganisms. It contains sheep red blood cells that supply free hemoglobin, and NADH. Both are important for the growth of *N. gonorrhoeae*.

In order for these nutrients to be released, the red blood cells are added to the medium while it is still very hot. This lyses the cells and gives the medium the appearance of chocolate; thus, the name chocolate agar. Gonococci also require a moist environment with increased CO_2 and they only grow within narrow temperature (35°C to 37°C) and pH ranges (7.2 to 7.6). This makes them harder, but not impossible, to grow and isolate from clinical specimens.

Once gonococci are introduced into the vagina or urethra, they attach to epithelial cells lining these surfaces and begin to multiply. Gonococci possess pili and proteins which allow them to attach to receptors on the surface of host cells and prevent the pathogen from being washed away by vaginal discharges or the strong flow of urine. Once attached, the gonococci multiply rapidly and spread upward in the urethra in the male and through the cervix in the female. There they eventually invade host cells and thus are sheltered from antibodies and phagocytes. At that point, they can cause inflammation and scarring of tissues. In advanced cases, the gonococci invade the bloodstream and cause infections at distant sites such as joints and skin (skin lesions).

Gonorrhea is the second leading STD. However, because chlamydia is not a reportable infectious disease in all states, gonorrhea is the most frequently reported STD in the United States. Humans are the only host and reservoir for gonococci, and both men and women can carry gonococci as asymptomatic carriers. This is a major reason gonorrhea is hard to control. The incidence of gonorrhea has dropped in the last decade because of more reliable diagnostic tests and antibiotics. However, the incidence of

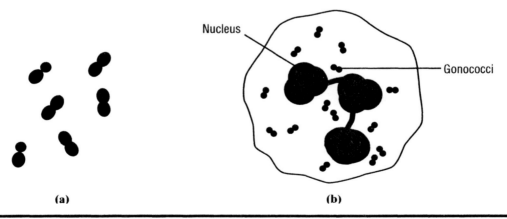

(a)   **(b)**

Figure 35.2 A drawing showing (a) the bean-shaped diplococci of N. gonorrhoeae, and (b) intracellular diplococci within a polymorphonuclear white blood cell.

drug-resistant (penicillin-resistant) strains has increased. Therefore, scientists are focusing their efforts on development of a vaccine. This has proven to be difficult because of strain variability. Controlling this STD will require even more sensitive diagnostic tests and a vaccine that will produce an immune response to all possible strains of *N. gonorrhoeae*, a tall but not insurmountable task. In this exercise, you will observe gonococci growing on chocolate agar and observe the small bean-shaped diplococci in Gram-stained preparations.

Another important method of disease transmission is the eating of contaminated food. Most foods, especially foods without preservatives, are perfect culture media for microorganisms. These organisms not only spoil food, causing a foul taste, but they also cause disease by producing infection or producing toxins resulting in food poisoning. This spoilage is especially evident in meat. Meat is very moist and full of nutrients. It spoils quickly if not consumed soon after purchase. Meat that comes from the muscle of animals is initially sterile, but can be quickly contaminated during processing and handling, like grinding and packaging. Most meat is preserved for a short period of time by refrigeration. The decreased temperatures from refrigeration *slow* the reproduction of most pathogens. However, in order to completely prevent food poisoning, food must be thoroughly heated to kill pathogenic bacteria and the toxins they produce. Food poisoning can cause severe diarrhea, and when bacteria produce toxins, the poisoning can be life-threatening, as in cases of botulism or hemolytic uremic syndrome.

During this part of the exercise, you will work in groups to evaluate the quantity of bacteria present in hamburger left unrefrigerated. This number is compared to the quantity of bacteria from hamburger that has been refrigerated and hamburger that has been cooked. To determine the bacterial count per gram of hamburger, the hamburger is diluted, colonies are counted, and the number of microorganisms per gram of hamburger is calculated. Each group will report their results and a comparison of the refrigerated and unrefrigerated hamburger samples will be made.

PURPOSE

- To learn three ways diseases are transmitted: hand-to-hand contact, sexual contact, and ingestion of contaminated food
- To perform testing that illustrates hand-to-hand transfer of organisms

- To observe organisms responsible for sexually transmitted diseases
- To examine pathogens carried by food and methods of preserving food

THE EXERCISE

Part A: Hand-to-Hand Transmission

MATERIALS:

Nutrient agar plates
Caramel candy (several inoculated with yellow-pigmented *M. luteus*)

PROCEDURE: Work in groups of five or six

Day 1

1. Arrange yourselves in rows.
2. Obtain a nutrient agar plate and divide the bottom of the plate in half with a marker. Label one side "before" and the other "after." Be sure to label your plate with your name and your place in your row (e.g., 1st, 2nd, 3rd).
3. The first person in each row should unwrap the inoculated caramel and roll it in the fingers of one hand several times.
4. At the same time, all the others in the row should unwrap their uninoculated caramels and roll them in their fingers.
5. The *first* person (the one with the inoculated candy) then touches fingertips with the *second* person in the row. Remember, the sticky fingers touch each other.
6. Then the first person inoculates the "before" side of the agar plates by gently but firmly touching their sticky fingertips to the surface of the medium.
7. The second person in the row rubs fingers with the third person and inoculates the "before" side of the medium as the first person did.
8. Moving down the row, each person rubs fingers with the next person before inoculating their agar plate.
9. After inoculating the "before" side of the plate, each person washes their hands thoroughly with soap and water. Allow the hands to air dry without touching anything, and no towel drying.
10. Finally, touch the same fingers used in the hand-to-hand transfer to the "after" side of the agar plate.
11. Each plate is incubated at 30°C until the next laboratory period.

Day 2

1. Arrange each plate from your row in a sequence.
2. Examine the "before" and "after" sides of each plate and estimate the number of yellow-pigmented colonies.
3. Record the results for your group in the RESULTS section. **Note:** The first people in your row may have numerous red-pigmented colonies in a confluent growth pattern. This can be recorded as too numerous to count (TNTC).

Part B: Observing Chlamydia and Gonococci

MATERIALS:

Prepared slides of iodine-stained *C. trachomatis*
Gram-stained slides of *N. gonorrhoeae*
Cultures of *N. gonorrhoeae* growing on chocolate agar

PROCEDURE:

1. Observe the prepared slides of *C. trachomatis* using low (10×) and high (40×) dry objectives (oil immersion is unnecessary). **Note:** These slides are prepared from shell vials which contain a monolayer of cells on a coverslip. The vials were inoculated with chlamydia and incubated for 48 hours. The cells and bacteria were then stained with iodine. The coverslip was removed and placed on a drop of mounting fluid on a slide. Your instructor will explain the procedure more thoroughly.

2. Observe the slides and look for *C. trachomatis*, which appear as dark brown bodies within the host cells.
3. Record your observations in the RESULTS section.
4. Observe *N. gonorrhoeae* growing on chocolate agar plates and describe its characteristic growth in the RESULTS Section.
5. Prepare a smear of *N. gonorrhoeae* and Gram stain it according to the procedure described in Exercise 6.
6. Describe or draw the Gram reaction and cellular morphology of *N. gonorrhoeae* in the RESULTS section.

Part C: Bacteria in Hamburger

MATERIALS:

10 grams of unrefrigerated hamburger
10 grams of refrigerated hamburger
10 grams of cooked hamburger
90 ml of sterile water
Sterile homogenizer
Glass rod culture spreader
Bunsen burner
TSA plates
9 ml dilution blank tubes (water)
Sterile pipets
Alcohol in a beaker

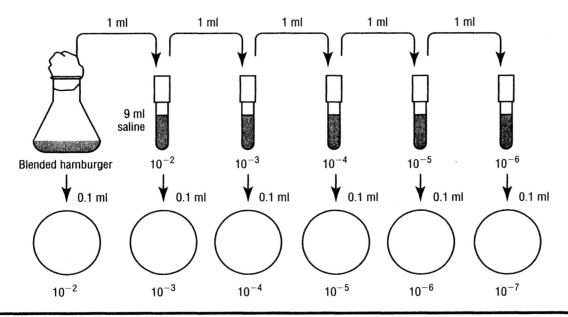

Figure 35.3 Serial dilutions and plating procedure for inoculating the plates.

PROCEDURE: Work in groups of five or six

The same procedure will be performed for the refrigerated hamburger, unrefrigerated hamburger, and cooked hamburger.

Day 1

1. Add hamburger to a blender containing 90 ml of sterile water and thoroughly blend. This gives a 1:10 dilution.
2. Transfer 1 ml of the blended hamburger to a 9 ml dilution tube. Proceed to transfer 1 ml from each dilution to a new sterile dilution blank to achieve dilutions of a least $1:10^6$ of the hamburger (**Figure 35.3**). Refer to Exercise 17 to review the procedure for making serial dilutions.
3. Transfer 0.1 ml from each dilution (including the first dilution in the blender) to a sterile TSA plate (**Figure 35.3**). Spread the inoculum evenly over the plate using a glass culture spreader (see Exercise 20). Label each plate with the dilution. **Note:** Remember that because 0.1 ml was put on each plate, the dilution is actually 10 times more than the dilution blank being used.
4. Incubate the plates at 37°C until the next laboratory period.

Day 2

1. Count the number of colonies that have developed on each plate. Some plates may contain too many colonies to enumerate. Other plates may contain too few colonies to obtain an accurate estimate of the number of microbes present in the hamburger. Therefore, count each plate that contains between 30 and 300 colonies.
2. Record your results in the RESULTS section, along with the results from the other group(s).
3. Calculate the number of microorganisms present per gram of hamburger.

REFERENCES

Baron, E.J., et al. *Bailey and Scott's Diagnostic Microbiology*, 9th ed. St. Louis: Mosby–Year Book, 1994.

Brock, Thomas D., et al. *Biology of Microorganisms*, 7th ed. Englewood Cliffs, NJ: Prentice-Hall, 1994.

Murray, P.R., et al. *Manual of Clinical Microbiology*, 6th ed. Washington, DC: American Society for Microbiology Press, 1995.

RESULTS

HAND-TO-HAND TRANSFER

Record the number of colonies on each plate.

	Number of Colonies of *M. luteus*		Other Colonies	
	Before Washing	**After Washing**	**Before Washing**	**After Washing**
1st person	_____	_____	_____	_____
2nd person	_____	_____	_____	_____
3rd person	_____	_____	_____	_____
4th person	_____	_____	_____	_____
5th person	_____	_____	_____	_____
6th person	_____	_____	_____	_____

SEXUALLY TRANSMITTED ORGANISMS

Chlamydia trachomatis

Slide observations

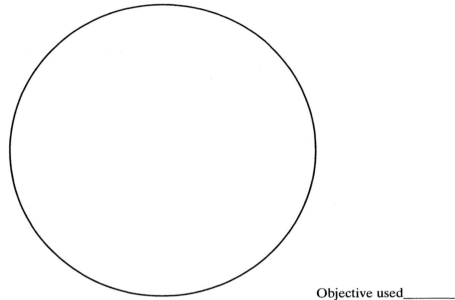

Objective used_____

Neisseria gonorrhoeae

a. Plate morphology

b. Slide observations

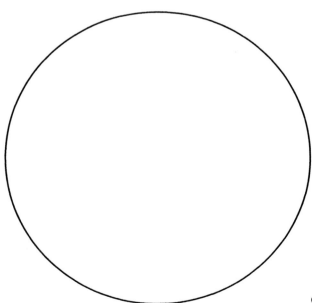

Objective used_____

● Record plate counts of:

BACTERIA IN HAMBURGER

	Number of Colonies		
Final Dilution	Refrigerated Hamburger	Unrefrigerated Hamburger	Cooked Hamburger
10^{-2}	————————	————————	————————
10^{-3}	————————	————————	————————
10^{-4}	————————	————————	————————
10^{-5}	————————	————————	————————
10^{-6}	————————	————————	————————
10^{-7}	————————	————————	————————
Number of organisms/ gram of hamburger	————————	————————	————————

● **REFLECTIONS**

1. How far was *M. luteus* transferred? Was there a dilution effect?

2. Did washing your hands remove all the *M. luteus* from your plate? Explain.

3. Write a scenario in which contact (other than aerosol contact) with another human caused disease transmission.

●

4. The unusual developmental cycle of chlamydia organisms makes it similar to what other types of microorganisms?

5. Why will *N. gonorrhoeae* grow on some mucosal surfaces of our bodies and not on our outer skin, stomach, or intestines? What does this tell you about survival on a toilet seat?

6. Compare the number of bacteria in the three types of meat. Did refrigeration make a difference? Did cooking the hamburger make a difference?

7. You probably determined that bacteria were growing in one of the meat cultures. Name three bacteria that would be pathogenic to humans and cause food poisoning, and describe how you would identify one of the pathogens. Hint: See Exercise 33 and the *Enterobacteriaceae.*

8. What bacterium has a strain that caused severe food poisoning and death (resulting from the ingestion of undercooked hamburger and a specific brand of apple juice)?

WHO (OR WHAT) IS TO BLAME?

It is difficult for us to imagine a time when the role of microbes as agents of disease was not accepted. But in fact, it was only a little more than 100 years ago that the germ theory of disease was proven by the work of Robert Koch. The experimental approach used by Koch still serves as a guideline for relating a particular disease to a particular microbe. But other types of evidence can be used to establish such a relationship—epidemiological evidence. In this exercise, you will explore both approaches.

Diane, a gastroenterologist, was thinking about one of her patients as she walked to the gate for her flight home. She had just attended a gastroenterology meeting where she learned of studies linking a bacterium, Helicobacter pylori, to ulcers. The session regarding the bacterium's role in causing ulcers was a heated one. For years, medical students had been taught that ulcers result from overproduction of acid caused by stress and other factors. Many physicians in the audience were not willing to abandon this long-held belief, and argued strongly against the possible role of H. pylori.

The next day Diane asked her nurse to call Frank, the patient she had been thinking about on her flight home. Frank was a 50-year-old executive with a long history of gastric ulcers. Despite treatment with the best drugs available for blocking excessive acid production, Frank's ulcers always recurred. When Frank arrived in the office later that day, Diane performed an endoscopic examination and obtained a biopsy to test for H. pylori. The results were positive. After talking to Frank, he agreed to try a different therapy. Diane put Frank on a 2-week regimen of tetracycline, metronidazole, and bismuth subsalicylate (Pepto-Bismol). After

2 weeks, Frank's symptoms had decreased. About 2 months later, Diane performed another endoscopic examination which revealed Frank's stomach inflammation and ulcer were gone. Diane saw Frank on a yearly basis for the next several years and was glad to learn that he never had a recurrence of ulcers.

BACKGROUND INFORMATION

The story behind the cure of Frank's ulcers began in 1979 in Australia. While examining stomach biopsies, Dr. J. Robert Warren noticed the presence of numerous spiral bacteria below the stomach's mucous layer. Interestingly, the bacteria were only evident in specimens where there was clear evidence of inflammation. This initial observation led to studies, many done with Barry Marshall (one of Warren's students), which developed methods for culturing the bacterium. These studies linked the bacterium to both gastric and duodenal ulcers.

Initially Warren and Marshall's work was not widely accepted by physicians. The prevailing belief (supported by many studies) was that ulcers result from increased acid production caused by a variety of environmental factors, including stress and diet. The therapy for ulcers was to eat bland foods and treat with drugs that neutralized stomach acid and prevented acid production. However, ulcers were difficult to cure, and once diagnosed, an individual was likely to have relapses throughout life.

How could Warren and Marshall clearly establish the link between the bacterium, now called *Helicobacter pylori*, and ulcers? The best method is to carry out a set of procedures called **Koch's postulates** (**Figure 36.1**). According to Koch's postulates, the microbe must be found in a diseased organism (**Figure 36.1a**); it must be isolated in pure culture from diseased organisms (**Figure 36.1b**); the disease must be experimentally reproduced in another susceptible organism (**Figure 36.1c**), and then the microbe reisolated in pure culture from that organism (**Figure 36.1d**).

Though logical and apparently easy to execute, in reality, Koch's postulates can be difficult to fulfill, especially for human diseases. For instance, when

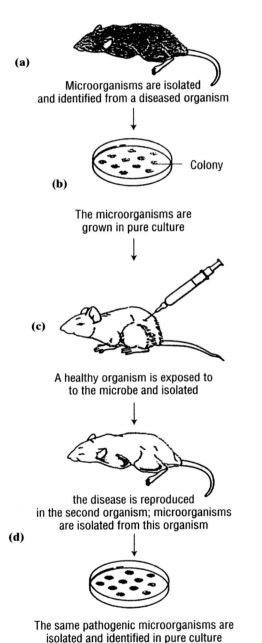

(a)

Microorganisms are isolated and identified from a diseased organism

↓

Colony

(b)

The microorganisms are grown in pure culture

↓

(c)

A healthy organism is exposed to to the microbe and isolated

↓

the disease is reproduced in the second organism; microorganisms are isolated from this organism

(d)

↓

The same pathogenic microorganisms are isolated and identified in pure culture

Figure 36.1 Demonstration that a bacterial disease satisfies Koch's postulates.

Warren first observed *H. pylori* in stomach biopsies, he wondered if others had noted it. Indeed, he found that similar observations had been made almost 100 years earlier, but because the bacterium *could not be cultured*, no further studies were conducted and the observation was forgotten. There are numerous human pathogens which have not been cultured, or are very difficult to culture. Furthermore, think about applying Koch's postulates to AIDS. Who would volunteer to be the experimental organism in a study to prove HIV is responsible for causing AIDS? The application of Koch's postulates to AIDS raises another problem. How can Koch's postulates be fulfilled if the disease develops after many years?

Fortunately, other types of evidence besides fulfillment of Koch's postulates can be used to relate a specific microbe to a specific disease. Such evidence comes from epidemiological studies. **Epidemiology** is a discipline that studies disease in populations. From the data collected, epidemiologists attempt to learn why certain members of the population become ill while others do not. The risk factors may include exposure to a particular microbe in a particular time or place, and in a particular manner. Furthermore, epidemiological studies can help identify societal, environmental, and personal characteristics that put a person at risk for developing disease.

Epidemiological studies are either **descriptive** or **analytical.** Descriptive studies characterize the distribution of disease in a population. The parameters include geography, age, and time of year. Such studies are useful for providing the first hint that a certain factor might be involved in causing disease, but they can not establish causality. Analytical studies are the most powerful epidemiological studies because they establish the role of a risk factor in causing disease. There are two designs for analytical studies, **cohort** and **case-control.** Descriptive studies and the two types of analytical studies are described in more detail below.

In descriptive epidemiological studies, a variety of measures are used. Two of the more common measures are **prevalence** and **incidence.** Prevalence is a measure of the number of existing cases in a population at any point in time (see box). Incidence, however, measures the number of new cases diagnosed over time (see box). The prevalence and incidence of disease in populations of different age, geographical location, socioeconomic group, or with a particular medical history, often provide the first clues as to causes of disease.

Establishing the cause(s) of a disease is done in analytical studies using either the cohort or case-control design. In a cohort study, the medical histories of

Prevalence indicates the number of existing cases in a population at any point in time, calculated using the following formula:

$$P = \frac{C}{N}$$ or expressed as a percent $$P = \frac{C}{N} \times 100\%$$

where
P = Prevalence
C = Number of existing cases
N = Size of population being studied

Incidence is a measure of the occurrence of new cases over a period of time, calculated using the following formula:

$$I = \frac{C}{PT}$$

where
C = Number of new cases
PT = Person-time (the time individuals are at risk for developing the disease); a subject at risk of disease and observed for 1 year contributes 1 person-year of observation.

a population of individuals (the cohort) are obtained at the beginning of the study (their initial status). Then the individuals are monitored over time, focusing on a disease of interest (e.g., lung cancer). In its simplest form, the individuals in the cohort are divided into two groups. One group has been exposed to a risk factor (e.g., smoking cigarettes) and the other has not. At the end of the study, the number of people contracting the disease in each group is compared (**Figure 36.2a**). It is important to note that in a cohort study, exposure to a risk factor is not intentionally done. This would be unethical. Rather, an existing population showing differences in exposure status serves as the study group. It should also be noted that the cohort study just described looks forward in time. That is, it is a **prospective study.** Cohort studies can also be **retrospective** and look back in time. In such studies, medical records that detail exposure and disease status might be used. (**Figure 36.2b**).

Case-control studies can be prospective or retrospective, as well, but are more often retrospective (**Figure 36.3**). In a case-control study, a clearly defined

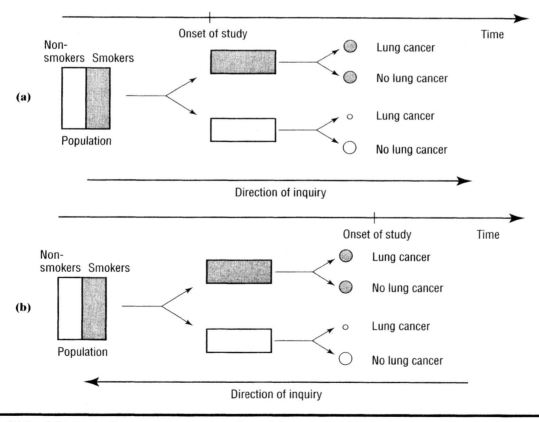

Figure 36.2 Schematic diagram of cohort studies of the relationship between smoking and lung cancer: (a) a prospective study, and (b) a retrospective study.

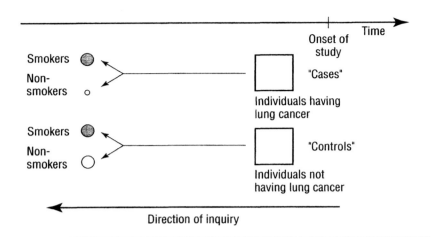

Figure 36.3 Schematic diagram of a retrospective case-control study of the relationship between smoking and lung cancer.

population is used as the source population for identifying individuals with the disease (**cases**) and individuals without the disease (**controls**). In the best designed case-control studies, case individuals are matched to control individuals on a number of variables (e.g., age, gender, smoking habits, diet, and overall health), except exposure to the suspected risk factor. As a result, each case-control pair will fall into one of four combinations of exposure status (**Table 36.1**). Two types of case-control pairs are important in showing a relationship between disease and a risk factor. One type of pair is the one in which the case individuals have been exposed, but the control individuals have not (case/control = +/−). The other type of pair is the one in which the case individuals have not been exposed, but the control individuals have (case/control = −/+). If exposure to a factor (e.g., smoking) does indeed put an individual at higher risk for disease (e.g., lung cancer), then the number of "+/−" pairs (smoker/non-smoker) should be greater than the number of "−/+" pairs (non-smoker/smoker). In other

words, the ratio, called the **odds ratio,** of "+/−" pairs to "−/+" pairs will be greater than one. However, if the factor does not put those exposed to it at higher risk, then the number of "+/−" pairs is approximately equal to the "−/+" pairs, and the odds ratio is 1. The odds ratio when there is no difference in frequency of the two pairs is also called the **null value.**

Let's consider a hypothetical case-control study where the odds ratio is calculated to be 3.6. How does the epidemiologist decide if 3.6 truly reflects a higher risk of disease for individuals exposed to the factor? This is a problem common to all studies of populations. If all humans on Earth were part of the study, then we would know that 3.6 was at least a weak factor in causing the disease being studied. But studies do not examine all humans on the planet. Rather, they study small subsets. This introduces the problem of sampling error. To solve the problem as it applies to the odds ratio, the 95% confidence interval around the odds ratio is calculated. The 95% confidence interval is a range of values one might expect to observe for

TABLE 36.1 The Matched Pairs of a Hypothetical Case-Control Study of the Relationship Between Smoking and Lung Cancer

	Number of Control Individuals Who Smoked		Number of Control Individuals Who Did Not Smoke	
Number of case individuals who smoked	+/+	413[a]	+/−	327[b]
Number of case individuals who did not smoke	−/+	13[c]	−/−	7[d]

[a]This is the number of matched pairs where both case and control individuals smoked (+/+).
[b]This is the number of matched pairs where the case individuals smoked, but the control individuals did not (+/−).
[c]This is the number of matched pairs where the case individuals did not smoke, but the control individuals did (−/+).
[d]This is the number of matched pairs where neither the case individuals nor the control individuals smoked (−/−).

similar study groups. Theoretically, if the odds ratio was calculated for 100 similar study groups, 95 times out of 100, the odds ratio would fall within the 95% confidence interval. Only 5 out of 100 times would it fall outside the interval due to chance. The question being asked is whether or not the null value lies within the confidence interval. If the null value falls within the confidence interval, then that says the null value and odds ratio are not significantly different. The difference between the two is due to chance factors alone. In other words, exposure to the risk factor does not put one at higher risk for disease. However, if the null value falls outside the 95% confidence interval, then only five times out of 100 would a difference this great be due to chance factors alone. Therefore, the difference between the odds ratio and the null value is said to be significant, and the factor clearly shown to put those exposed to it at higher risk for developing disease. The formulas used by epidemiologists to calculate the odds ratio and to determine the 95% confidence interval around it are shown in the boxes below.

In this exercise, you will gain experience in using both Koch's postulates and epidemiological evidence to show that a particular microbe causes a specific disease. In Part A, you will design an experiment that applies Koch's postulates to show that the Gram-negative rod, *Erwinia carotovora*, causes a disease of carrots called soft rot (**Figure 36.5**). Soft rot is so named because the carrot has an affected area that becomes soft and mushy as the disease progresses. The affected area may also become discolored and slimy due to an exudate that oozes through cracks in the infected area. The bacterium is frequently spread to carrots by insects. The insects feed on the carrot, causing wounds that provide access for the bacterium to underlying tissues of the carrot. In Part B, you will be given data based on several epidemiological studies that examined the role of *H. pylori* in causing gastric and duodenal ulcers. You will analyze these data and come to your own decision about the role of this bacterium in causing ulcers.

PURPOSE

- To use Koch's postulates to demonstrate the role of a bacterium in causing a plant disease, soft rot of carrot
- To learn and use some of the standard measures employed by epidemiologists to relate a microorganism or other factors to a disease

---

Calculation of the Odds Ratio Using the Data Presented in Table 36.1

$$\text{Odds Ratio} = \frac{\text{Number of } +/- \text{ matched pairs}}{\text{Number of } -/+ \text{ matched pairs}}$$

$$= \frac{327}{13} = 25.2$$

Determination of the 95% Confidence Interval Around the Odds Ratio Calculated in the Previous Box

$$95\% \text{ CI} = (\text{OR}) \, e^{\left[\pm\sqrt{\frac{1}{+/-} + \frac{1}{-/+}}\right]}$$

$$= (25.2) \, e^{\left[\pm\sqrt{\frac{1}{327} + \frac{1}{13}}\right]} = (25.2) \, e^{[\pm\sqrt{0.08}]} = (25.2) \, e^{[\pm 0.28]}$$

Lower boundary = 19.0   Upper boundary = 33.3

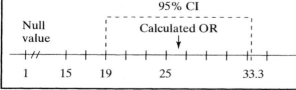

| 1 | 15 | 19 | 25 | 33.3 |

CI = confidence interval; OR = odds ratio.

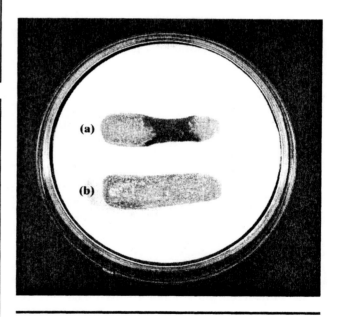

Figure 36.5   A carrot (a) infected with *E. carotovora*, and (b) an uninfected carrot.

THE EXERCISE

Part A: Koch's Postulates

MATERIALS:

Carrot with soft rot
Nutrient agar plates
Razor blades or scalpels
Bunsen burner
Gram-stain reagents
Healthy carrot
Inoculating loop
Alcohol in a beaker
Microscope slides
Microscopes

PROCEDURES: Work in groups of two or three

1. Compare the appearance of a carrot with soft rot to the healthy carrot.
2. Design an experimental protocol, using Koch's postulates as guidelines (**Figure 36.1**), that will allow you to identify the bacterium responsible for causing soft rot. **Note:** Remember that the bacterium normally infects carrots through breaks in the carrot's surface. Also remember to set up a control. A single carrot can be cut into smaller pieces, some of which can be exposed to the microbe (**Figure 36.1**) and the other pieces can be controls.
3. After consulting with your instructor about your protocol, carry out the experiments you have outlined.
4. Record the procedures you used and the results you obtained in the RESULTS section.

Part B: Epidemiological Analysis

1. Examine the summaries of epidemiological studies presented below. Each is based on actual studies done to investigate the role of *H. pylori* in causing ulcers and other diseases.
2. Do the analysis requested for each data set and record your answers in the RESULTS section.

Study 1

In 1985, advertisements were placed in local newspapers to recruit subjects for a study on the prevalence of *H. pylori* in individuals with a history of recurring gastric ulcers or duodenal ulcers. The data are presented in the table at the top of the next column. Calculate the prevalence of *H. pylori* infection in individuals with gastric ulcers. Do the same for individuals with duodenal ulcers. Finally, calculate prevalence for all ulcer patients in this study.

Individuals With Ulcers	Number of Individuals Infected with *H. pylori*	Number of Individuals Not Infected
Gastric ulcers	62	31
Duodenal ulcers	94	13

Study 2

In 1987, advertisements were placed in local newspapers to recruit subjects for a study on the prevalence of *H. pylori* in a population of healthy adults. All respondents were questioned thoroughly. Any respondents reporting gastrointestinal symptoms, a history of ulcers or other gastrointestinal disorders, or a history of using antacids or other gastrointestinal medicines were excluded from the study. A total of 113 individuals participated in the study. All were tested for infection by *H. pylori*, and all were given an endoscopic examination to look for any evidence of inflammation in their stomachs. The data are presented in the table below. Calculate the prevalence of *H. pylori* infection in each age group. Calculate the prevalence of infection in the entire study group. Calculate the prevalence of infection in those with clear evidence of gastritis (by endoscopic examination), and those with normal stomachs.

Study 3

In 1965, a group of Japanese-American men living in Hawaii served as a study group for the Honolulu Heart Program. These men also served as a source of subjects for a subsequent case-control

Age	Number Infected with *H. pylori*	Number Not Infected
18 - 29	2	18
30 - 39	7	15
40 - 49	7	13
50 - 59	8	13
60 - 69	7	8
70 - 91	5	10

Endoscopic Results	Number Infected with *H. pylori*	Number Not Infected
Gastritis	36	6
Healthy stomach tissues	0	71

Type of Ulcer in Case Individuals		Number of Matched Pairs	
		Controls Infected	**Controls Not Infected**
Gastric ulcer (n = 150)	Cases infected	107	32
	Cases not infected	10	1
Duodenal ulcer (n = 65)	Cases infected	48	12
	Cases not infected	3	2

study. Between 1967 and 1968, blood was drawn from the participants in the heart study and stored for the next twenty years. Over that time, individuals diagnosed with either gastric ulcers or duodenal ulcers were identified. At the end of the 20 years, a total of 215 men had been identified as having ulcers (150 had gastric ulcers; 65 had duodenal ulcers). They served as the cases in the case-control study. They were matched with 215 men from the same population that were never diagnosed with ulcers. These ulcer-free individuals served as the controls in the case-control study. The sera of both case individuals and control individuals were tested for antibodies to *H. pylori*, and four different matched pairs designated for each type of ulcer. The results are shown in the table above. Calculate the prevalence of *H. pylori* infection for both the cases and the controls. Calculate the odds ratio and the 95% confidence interval around the odds ratio.

REFERENCES

Agrios, G.N. *Plant Pathology*, 3rd ed. San Diego: Harcourt, Brace-Jovanovich, 1988.

Blaser, M.J. 1996. The Bacteria Behind Ulcers, *Scientific American* 274(1996):104-107.

Blaser, M.J. 1992. Hypotheses on the Pathogenesis and Natural History of *Helicobacter pylori*–induced Inflammation, *Gastroenterology* 102(1992):720-727.

Dooley, C.P., et al. Prevalence of *Helicobacter pylori* Infection and Histologic Gastritis in Asymptomatic Persons, *New England Journal of Medicine* 321(1989):1562-1566.

Greenberg, R.S. *Medical Epidemiology*. Norwalk, CT: Appleton and Lange, 1993.

Nomura, A., et al. *Helicobacter pylori* Infection and Risk for Duodenal and Gastric Ulceration, *Annals of Internal Medicine* 120(1994):977-981.

Peterson, W.L. *Helicobacter pylori* and Peptic Ulcer Disease, *New England Journal of Medicine* 324(1991):1043-1048.

RESULTS

Record the procedures and results of the experiment you designed to show that *E. carotovora* causes soft rot.

PROCEDURES:

RESULTS:

Record your analysis of the epidemiological studies below.

Study 1:
Prevalence of infection in gastric ulcer patients:

Prevalence of infection in duodenal ulcer patients:

Prevalence of infection in all ulcer patients:

Study 2:
Prevalence of infection in healthy adults by age group:

Prevalence of infection in entire study group:

Prevalence of infection in those with and without gastritis:

Study 3:
Prevalence of infection in those having and not having ulcers:

Odds ratio and 95% confidence interval around odds ratio:

REFLECTIONS

1. Did you isolate one bacterium from the infected carrot? Explain.

2. If you isolated more than one bacterium from the infected carrot, which was responsible for causing soft rot? Explain.

3. Did you have any evidence that this bacterium was *E. carotovora*? Explain.

4. Was there any evidence in the ulcer studies for age being a factor in infection by *H. pylori*? Explain.

5. Based on the three ulcer studies, do you think being infected with *H. pylori* increases the risk of developing ulcers? Explain.

6. Is there any evidence in the three ulcer studies that infection by *H. pylori* puts one at risk for any other gastrointestinal disorders? Explain.

7. Design a prospective cohort study using students on your campus to test the association between infection by *H. pylori* and ulcers.

EXERCISE 37

TOO MUCH RESISTANCE

After identifying important pathogens and studying how they are transmitted, the next step is to learn how these microorganisms are tested for their sensitivity to antibiotics. This is one of the most important functions clinical laboratories provide for physicians and their patients. There are several methods for testing a microorganism's sensitivity to an antibiotic. You will perform one of the common methods used in many medical laboratories.

It was 2:00 A.M. when Sharon was called by the hospital to draw blood for blood cultures on a 32-year-old woman. Sharon, a clinical laboratory scientist, obtained the blood from Elizabeth, who had just started spiking intermittent fevers. A day earlier Elizabeth had delivered her sixth child, a boy, after a traumatic delivery which eventually ended up in an emergency cesarean section. Sharon obtained enough blood for microbiological culturing and a white blood cell (WBC) count. After placing the blood cultures in the incubator, Sharon performed a WBC count on Elizabeth's blood. The WBC was elevated to 25,000/mm^3 (normal = 5,000-10,000/mm^3), one of the signs of sepsis (blood infection). The next day a Gram-negative rod similar to E. coli was observed in the blood cultures and Elizabeth was started on intravenous antibiotics. While identifying the organism, Sharon also performed susceptibility testing so she could advise the physician on the antibiotic to use. Elizabeth was still feverish 2 days later and was switched to a new antibiotic. Sharon identified the organism as E. coli and determined that it was sensitive to several antibiotics including tetracycline, ampicillin, cephalothin, and gentamicin. For the next week, a pat-

tern kept repeating itself. Elizabeth would spike fevers every 2 days and then be switched to a new antibiotic. As the laboratory staff continued to isolate E. coli from Elizabeth's blood, Sharon began to notice a disturbing pattern. Each time the organism was isolated and antibiotic testing performed, it was sensitive to fewer and fewer antibiotics. Finally, the E. coli was sensitive to only one antibiotic (gentamicin). Elizabeth remained in the hospital and after 8 days, another doctor on call (a surgeon) reevaluated her case and noticed a swollen and tender abdomen. He decided to take her to surgery and reopen the incision. When he did, he found a small piece of gauze left from the cesarean section and a large abscess. He removed both and placed a drainage tube through her incision. She continued to spike fevers and 4 days later was sent to a larger metropolitan hospital. Unfortunately, a week later, Elizabeth died from kidney and liver complications caused by a drug-resistant E. coli.

BACKGROUND INFORMATION

This story about Elizabeth happened 25 years ago, when drug resistance was not as prevalent. Today, because of widespread antibiotic use, pathogenic microorganisms have become more and more drug resistant. We now have multiple-drug–resistant microorganisms that are not sensitive to any antibiotics. Combinations of drugs that are **synergistic** (that is, the combination of two is more effective than the total additive effect of the agents if given separately) are now often used for life-threatening infections. It was once thought that antibiotics would always be available to treat infections, but we have now entered an era of increased antibiotic resistance that has been compared to the pre-antibiotic era. Pharmaceutical companies are retooling their research and development programs so that new antimicrobial agents can be developed. Hopefully, we can stay one step ahead of the pathogens as they mutate to resistance—an ever vicious cycle.

The term **antibiotic** was coined from the word antibiosis, meaning against life. Antibiotics are substances produced by microorganisms that inhibit the growth of other microorganisms. The first antibiotics were chemicals secreted by microorganisms such as fungi, for example, penicillin from *Penicillium* sp. Now many **antimicrobial agents**—any chemical substances inhibiting the growth of microorganisms—are synthetic molecules. Antibiotics should not be confused with **antiseptics** or **disinfectants.** Antiseptics kill most organisms and can be applied to the skin or mucous membranes. They are, however, rarely safe enough to be taken internally like antibiotics. Disinfectants are agents that also kill microorganisms, but are restricted to use on inanimate objects such as tables, dishes, or floors. They are not safe for ingestion or application to living tissue.

After resistant microorganisms were first observed, it became evident that methods for testing a bacterium's susceptibility to antibiotics were needed to guide the therapy of a patient. Several *in vitro* (in glass or culture) methods were developed to determine a bacterium's susceptibility to different antimicrobial agents. One commonly used method will be used in this exercise. It is called the **agar diffusion method.** Two types of agar diffusion methods will be used. The first is called the disk diffusion method. It involves placing commercially prepared antibiotic-impregnated disks of known concentration on a fresh inoculum of bacteria. The bacteria are plated on a standard agar

medium called Mueller-Hinton (MH) agar. MH agar is a specially designed agar with specific nutrients, a pH of 7.4, and cation concentrations that allow for diffusion of a wide variety of antibiotics. It is particularly important to use MH when testing the antibiotics sulfonamide and trimethoprim, which are antagonized by increased levels of para-aminobenzoic acid (PABA) and thymidine found in non-MH media. The plates with the disks are incubated and then observed. The antimicrobial agent will diffuse away from the disk in decreasing concentrations (**Figure 37.1**) until at some point it is insufficient to prevent bacterial growth. A clear area of no growth around the disk is called the **zone of inhibition.** The zone is measured and according to predetermined standards, the bacterium is said to be either sensitive, have intermediate sensitivity, or be resistant to the antibiotic in question.

During this exercise you will test the susceptibility of two bacteria to four antibiotics. You will be able to observe whether each antibiotic inhibits the growth of a Gram-positive bacterium (*Staphylococcus epidermidis*) and a Gram-negative bacterium (*Escherichia coli*).

The second agar diffusion method is called the **Etest.** The Etest (developed by AB Biodisk, Solona, Sweden) is a relatively new method for performing antimicrobial susceptibility testing. It is done by placing a strip with a defined antimicrobial gradient on an inoculated agar plate and incubating the plate as in the disk diffusion method (**Figure 37.2**). The strip has fifteen two-fold dilutions over a continuous gradient and the results generated are a measure of the

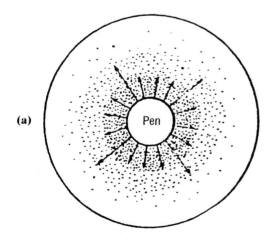

(a)

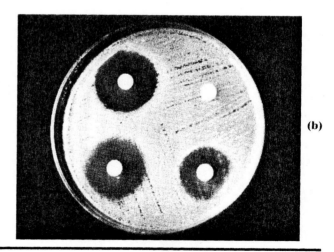

(b)

Figure 37.1 (a) Diffusion of an antibiotic through the agar, and (b) MH plate with antimicrobic disks. Note the zone of inhibition around three of the disks. (Pen = Penicillin.)

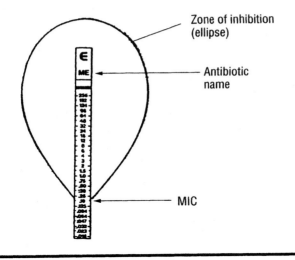

Figure 37.2 The Etest strip.

antimicrobial agent's **minimum inhibitory concentration (MIC)**. The MIC is a quantitative result rather than a category result (resistant, intermediate, or susceptible). MIC is the lowest concentration of an antibiotic expressed in µg/ml that prevents the growth of the bacteria being tested. MIC results provide the physician with guidelines for determining if a given dosage of antibiotic will be sufficient. However, there is no clear evidence that MIC results are more useful to physicians than category results. Nevertheless, because easier semi-automated and automated methods are available, many clinical laboratories now report MIC results. The MIC for the Etest is read where growth intersects the strip and an elliptical zone of inhibition forms (**Figure 37.2**). Several of these strips can be placed on one large plate, or a single small agar plate can be used to test one antimicrobic. These strips are costly and many laboratories only use them to test single specific antibiotics against a particularly resistant or fastidious organism. An example of this is the testing of *Streptococcus pneumoniae* with penicillin (**Figure 37.3**). It has been found that 30% of *S. pneumoniae* strains are now resistant to penicillin. In this lab you will test one of your organisms with one Etest strip on a MH agar plate.

PURPOSE

- To learn procedures for testing bacterial susceptibility to antimicrobial agents
- To compare the susceptibility of a Gram-positive organism and a Gram-negative organism to several antibacterial agents

THE EXERCISE

MATERIALS:

Three MH agar plates (100 mm)
An Etest strip (AB Biodisk North America, Piscataway, N.J.) of one of the antibiotics listed in **Table 37.3**
Two 4.5 ml tubes of TSB broth
Pipet pump
Forceps
A variety of antibiotic disks listed in **Table 37.1** and **Table 37.2**
Sterile swabs
Overnight broth cultures of *E. coli* and *S. epidermidis*
Two sterile 1 ml pipets
Alcohol

PROCEDURE: Work in pairs

Part A

1. Use a 1 ml pipet to transfer 0.5 ml of the overnight broth of *E. coli* to 4.5 ml of TSB. **Note:** This will provide a 1:100 dilution of the broth culture, or approximately 10^8 cells/ml.
2. Repeat step 1 with *S. epidermidis* and a second TSB tube.

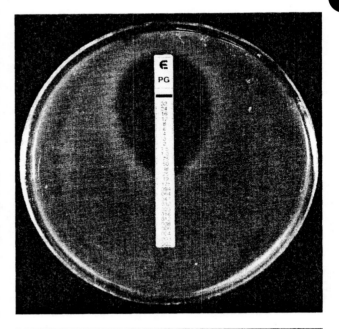

Figure 37.3 Testing the susceptibility of *S. pneumoniae* to penicillin using the Etest. The MIC is 0.25 µg/ml or intermediate sensitivity.

TABLE 37.1 Zone Size Interpretive Standards for Selected Antibiotics and Staphylococci[a]

Antimicrobial Agent	Disk Content (µg)	Zone Diameter (mm)		
		Resistant	Intermediate	Susceptible
Amoxicillin-clavulanic acid	20/10	≤19		≥20
Ampicillin	10	≤28		≥29
Ampicillin-sulbactam	10/10	≤11	12-14	≥15
Cefazolin	30	≤14	15-17	≥18
Cefotaxime	30	≤14	15-22	≥23
Ceftriaxone	30	≤13	14-20	≥21
Cephalothin	30	≤14	15-17	≥18
Chloramphenicol	30	≤12	13-17	≥18
Ciprofloxacin	5	≤15	16-20	≥21
Gentamicin	10	≤12	13-14	≥15
Imipenem	10	≤13	14-15	≥16
Tetracycline	30	≤14	15-18	≥19
Trimethoprim-sulfamethoxazole	1.25/23.75	≤10	11-15	≥16
Nitrofurantoin	300	≤14	15-16	≥17
Norfloxacin	10	≤12	13-16	≥17
Sulfisoxazole	250 or 300	≤12	13-16	≥17
Trimethoprim	5	≤10	11-15	≥16

[a]NCCLS. 1993. *Methods for Dilution Antimicrobial Susceptibility Tests for Bacteria That Grow Aerobically,* 3rd ed. Approved standard M7-A3. NCCLS, Villanova, PA.

TABLE 37.2 Zone Size Interpretive Standards for Members of the Family *Enterobacteriaceae*[a]

Antimicrobial Agent	Disk Content (µg)	Zone Diameter (mm)		
		Resistant	Intermediate	Susceptible
Amoxicillin-clavulanic acid	20/10	≤13	14-17	≥18
Ampicillin	10	≤13	14-16	≥17
Ampicillin-sulbactam	10/10	≤11	12-14	≥15
Cefazolin	30	≤14	15-17	≥18
Cefotaxime	30	≤14	15-22	≥23
Ceftriaxone	30	≤13	14-20	≥21
Cephalothin	30	≤14	15-17	≥18
Chloramphenicol	30	≤12	13-17	≥18
Ciprofloxacin	5	≤15	16-20	≥21
Gentamicin	10	≤12	13-14	≥15
Imipenem	10	≤13	14-15	≥16
Tetracycline	30	≤14	15-18	≥19
Trimethoprim-sulfamethoxazole	1.25/23.75	≤10	11-15	≥16
Nitrofurantoin	300	≤14	15-16	≥17
Norfloxacin	10	≤12	13-16	≥17
Sulfisoxazole	250 or 300	≤12	13-16	≥17
Trimethoprim	5	≤10	11-15	≥16

[a]NCCLS. 1993. *Methods for Dilution Antimicrobial Susceptibility Tests for Bacteria That Grow Aerobically,* 3rd ed. Approved standard M7-A3. NCCLS, Villanova, PA.

3. Immerse and saturate a sterile cotton swab in the 1:100 dilution of the broth culture of *E. coli*. Remove excess liquid by rotating the swab against the tube wall above the liquid surface.

4. Apply an even inoculum over the entire surface of the MH plate in the following manner: Use the swab to divide the plate into four quadrants (**Figure 37.4a**). Move the swab back and forth over half of the plate (**Figure 37.4b**). Turn the plate 90° and swab another half of the plate (**Figure 37.4c**). Turn another 90° and do the same (**Figure 37.4d**). Finally, turn the last 90° and reswab the remaining two quadrants (**Figure 37.4e**). Each quadrant should be swabbed in two directions. Before discarding the swab, circle the entire rim of the agar several times. The instructor will demonstrate this procedure. **Note:** This manner of inoculating a plate ensures confluent growth of bacteria over the entire plate.

5. Using a marker, label the plate *E. coli* and divide the bottom of the plate into four sectors.

6. Inoculate and label the second MH plate with *S. epidermidis* in the same manner as in steps 1 through 4.

7. Select four antibiotic disks for testing. Use the same four antimicrobial agents for each bacterium. If possible, use the same antibiotic that will be used in the Etest procedure. **Note:** The antibiotic disks have a code written on each disk. Record the abbreviated code when you apply the disk to the plate.

8. To place the disks on each plate, use forceps and sterilize them by dipping them in alcohol and flaming them. Obtain an antibiotic disk from the cartridge, place it in the center of the sector you have labeled, and gently press on the center of the disk. Repeat this procedure with the other plate and organism. **Note:** Do not touch the agar surface with the forceps or lay them on the bench, or they will have to be resterilized. Also, do not move the disk once it has been placed on the plate; the antibiotic is immediately absorbed into the agar.

9. Invert each plate (disks will not come off) and incubate the plates at 35°C for 24 hours.

10. Observe and record your results in the RESULTS section.

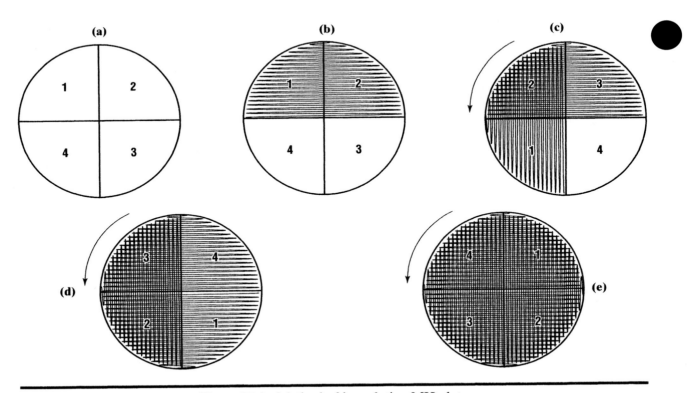

Figure 37.4 Method of inoculating MH plate.

Part B

1. Obtain another MH agar plate. **Note:** Because these strips are expensive, this test may be done in pairs, larger groups, or as a demonstration in class.
2. Repeat the inoculation procedure in Part A, steps 3 and 4, with *E. coli*.
3. Using sterile forceps, obtain one Etest strip and hold the end of the strip labeled E. Make certain the MIC scale faces upward (the antimicrobial agent is on the reverse side).
4. Gently place the strip on the agar plate such that the highest concentration of antibiotic is near the edge of the plate. **Note:** Begin by allowing the end opposite the E to contact the agar first. Also, remove any air bubbles by gently pressing on the strip.
5. Once the strip has been placed on the agar surface, *do not move it*. The antibiotic is immediately released into the agar once it touches the surface. If the strip is accidentally placed upside down,

carefully pick up the strip with sterile forceps and turn it over.

6. Invert the plate and incubate it for 18 to 24 hours at 35°C.
7. Observe the plate and record the MIC results in the RESULTS section. Compare the results to the interpretative standards for the antibiotics listed in **Table 37.3** and determine whether the organism is resistant, intermediate, or susceptible to the antibiotic tested.

REFERENCES

Baron, E.J., et. al., *Bailey and Scott's Diagnostic Microbiology*, 9th ed. St. Louis: Mosby–Year Book, 1994.

Isenberg, H.D., et. al., 1992. *Clinical Microbiology Procedures Handbook*. Washington, D.C.: American Society for Microbiology Press, 1992.

Murray, P.R., et al., *Manual of Clinical Microbiology*, 6th ed., Washington, D.C.: American Society for Microbiology Press, 1995.

TABLE 37.3   MIC Interpretative Standards for Members of the Family *Enterobacteriaceae*[a]

Antimicrobial Agent	MIC (µg/ml)		
	Resistant	Intermediate	Susceptible
Amoxicillin-clavulanic acid	≤8/4	16/8	≥32/16
Ampicillin	≤8	16	≥32
Ampicillin-sulbactam	≤8/4	16/8	≥32/16
Cefazolin	≤8	16	≥32
Cefotaxime	≤8	16-32	≥64
Ceftriaxone	≤8	16-32	≥64
Cephalothin	≤8	16	≥32
Chloramphenicol	≤8	16	≥32
Ciprofloxacin	≤1	2	≥4
Gentamicin	≤4	8	≥16
Imipenem	≤4	8	≥16
Tetracycline	≤4	8	≥16
Trimethoprim-sulfamethoxazole	≤2/38		≥4/76
Nitrofurantoin	≤32	64	≥128
Norfloxacin	≤4	8	≥16
Sulfisoxazole	≤256		≥512
Trimethoprim	≤8		≥16

[a]NCCLS. 1993. *Methods for Dilution Antimicrobial Susceptibility Tests for Bacteria That Grow Aerobically*, 3rd ed. Approved standard M7-A3. NCCLS, Villanova, PA.

RESULTS

Part A

Record your results and those from others in the class in the table below. Write S, I, or R (sensitive, intermediate, or resistant) after measuring the zone size and consulting **Table 37.1** and **Table 37.2**.

Antimicrobial Agent	*S. epidermidis*	*E. coli*

Part B

Record the MIC for your antibiotic and determine if your *E. coli* is susceptible, intermediate, or resistant to the antibiotic you tested using **Table 37.3**.

Antibiotic name _____

MIC value _____

Interpretation _____

Draw the zone of inhibition you obtained around the strip.

REFLECTIONS

1. Did the results of the disk diffusion method agree with the result you obtained from the Etest diffusion method? Were they both sensitive, intermediate or resistant? If not, try to explain why you had discrepancies.

2. Why is it important to run control strains of bacteria when testing a bacterium's susceptibility or resistance to an antibiotic?

3. Did you notice any differences between the Gram-positive *S. aureus* and the Gram-negative *E. coli* in their resistance to any antibiotics? If so, what were they?

4. Are the antibiotics you tested effective against fungi, protozoa, or viruses? Explain.

EXERCISE 38

NAME THAT PATHOGEN

This exercise will allow you to integrate previously learned information about pathogens into a presentation and written paper on a specific disease. This is an interactive presentation and you will work in groups of three. Several weeks will be necessary to complete the assignment; your instructor will set a deadline. You will be graded on both the presentation and paper, and will also have the opportunity to obtain bonus points for correctly diagnosing the pathogen introduced in other presentations. In addition to reviewing your infection and pathogen, this exercise will provide an excellent opportunity for you to review information about other pathogens and the infections they cause.

Once your group has been selected, you will randomly draw the name of an infection and associated pathogen. Based on the information given, you will have the following two-part group assignment:

PART A: WRITING ABOUT THE INFECTION AND PATHOGEN

Your paper should be quite extensive and include up-to-date information about the pathogen and associated infection. Sources of information include textbooks, articles, and possibly the Internet. Do not copy or paraphrase information from textbooks. The following aspects of the disease must be covered in the paper:
  a. Historical information, such as when your pathogen was isolated, and by whom
  b. Symptoms of the infection
  c. Virulence mechanisms of your pathogen which contribute to the infectious process
  d. How your pathogen is isolated from clinical specimens
  e. Some tests used to identify your pathogen
  f. Current treatment of the disease

  g. Prognosis for recovery
  h. Current research that may lead to a vaccine or possible eradication of your pathogen

The writing assignment may be divided up in any reasonable, feasible, and equitable way, and all members should be involved in the writing. Your instructor will give you instructions on the length of the paper and the format in which it should be submitted. It must include appropriate references. The paper is due on the day of your presentation (see Part B).

PART B: PRESENTATION ABOUT THE INFECTION AND PATHOGEN

As a group, you will prepare a presentation for the entire laboratory class. The presentation should be made in a "quiz show" format. This means it is a brief presentation and the rest of the class will only have a short time to "diagnose" the pathogen from the disease you are describing. Each person in the group must play a role in the presentation.

Person 1

Person 1 presents a 3 to 5 minute case history written by your group. The case history must supply all pertinent information necessary to diagnose the pathogen associated with the infection *but not* give it away. Your instructor may have examples of case histories that you can examine, and many medical microbiology textbooks contain case histories that may give you ideas on how to present a case study. *Do not copy them*, but use other references, your class notes, and knowledge to compose your case. Remember, this is a group effort and each person within the group is responsible for the information presented by the others.

PERSON 2:

This person will present, in 1 to 2 minutes, visual materials that point out certain aspects of the disease process or pathogen. These could include pictures of patients with the infection, a Gram-stained slide, cultures showing colony morphology, or biochemical tests and their results. This visual presentation should illustrate certain important features of the infection and pathogen but should not give away the answer. Take care to use descriptive terminology that is neither too informative nor too vague.

After persons 1 and 2 have presented their information, the "audience" will have an opportunity to diagnose the cause of the infection. This will be an open-book and group-oriented effort, but only 1 to 2 minutes will be allowed for quiet discussion and decision making within your group. During the first minute, audience members are allowed to ask questions of the presenters to clarify points (except, of course, what the pathogen is). Each group writes down their diagnosis and gives it to the instructor after the discussion.

PERSON 3

This person will provide the class with the correct "diagnosis" or pathogen associated with the infection. They will quickly summarize why the material presented is diagnostic of the pathogen. Focus should be given to key information that was presented by persons 1 and 2. They should also give any follow-up information on their fictitious patient (i.e., the patient's mortality, therapy, or other information relevant to the case). In addition, presenting group members should be available to answer questions from the instructor or any audience member regarding aspects of the case.

Grading

Your instructor will assign points to the paper your group submitted based on the criteria listed above. In addition, your group will also be graded on the presentation and, depending upon your instructor, points may possibly be awarded for clarity, ingenuity, brevity, quality, accuracy, collaboration, and knowledge of the subject. Bonus points will be given for each correct diagnosis. The group at the end with the most bonus points will receive additional points.

Please make sure that you do not inadvertently reveal your group's pathogen to other class members; after all, you want those extra points. The presentations will be fun and you will find this is a good review of pathogens associated with different infections. Good luck!

SECTION VII

HOST DEFENSES

In the previous section on medical microbiology, you learned about some microorganisms that cause disease, how they are identified, and how bacteria are tested for their susceptibility to antibiotics. In this section, you will learn how our immune system controls pathogens. Our own defense system contains cells (white blood cells) and molecules (antibodies and complement) which function to destroy and clear from our body unwanted microbes. In this section, you will observe your own white blood cells engulfing yeast (phagocytosis) and study methods for observing and measuring antibody production.

EXERCISE 39

PHAGOCYTOSIS

This is the first exercise in which you will study and observe some of our normal host defenses. You may already have some knowledge of our complex immune system and the role that white blood cells (leukocytes) play in destroying bacterial pathogens. During this exercise, you will be able to observe phagocytic cells (PMNs and monocytes) and the role they play in the immune process. You will be observing your own leukocytes as they engulf, or phagocytize, yeast cells.

Joe, a 6-year-old boy, always seemed to be sick. He would get an infection such as a sore throat, abscess, or diarrhea, and it would take him longer than most other kids to get well. His doctor became concerned after one episode when Joe became so ill with pneumonia that he ended up in the hospital. His white blood cell count (WBC) was elevated (26,000/mm³) and he had an increase in polymorphonuclear neutrophils (PMNs)—a sign of bacterial pneumonia.

Joe showed a consistent pattern with most of his infections. This included a slow recovery after treatment with antibiotics and another infection after a short period of good health. His doctor consulted with other physicians and they decided to run several tests to study Joe's immune system more closely. His blood smears showed no abnormal cells and a bone marrow aspirate also revealed no abnormalities or hyperplasia (increased cell number) of any blood cell type (white blood cells, red blood cells, or platelets). Joe also had normal antibody levels, especially immunoglobulin G (IgG). The tests were conducted to determine whether Joe had normal functioning PMNs. The doctors specifically wondered if Joe's PMNs were phagocytizing bacteria. They also wanted to know if the bacteria, once phagocytized, were being destroyed by enzymes within the phagocytic cells. The results of these tests showed that Joe had a very rare genetic defect. He was deficient

in a component of complement called C3. C3, when activated at the site of infection, is deposited on the infectious agent. Neutrophils and macrophages have receptors which bind to C3. Thus, C3 serves as a target on the pathogen, giving the phagocytes something more readily recognized and engulfed. Phagocytosis can take place without C3 complement, but binding of bacteria to PMNs, monocytes and macrophages is greatly enhanced if complement is present. Since this is a genetic defect, Joe probably will suffer from repeated bacterial infections throughout the rest of his life.

BACKGROUND INFORMATION

Our immune system is complex, and one of the ways our body reacts to an infectious agent or injury is through inflammation. During the inflammatory response, **PMNs** migrate out of capillaries and into the infected tissue. A PMN is a white blood cell with a multilobed nucleus. These cells are attracted to the site of infection through a process known as **chemotaxis.** During chemotaxis, certain molecules such as components of the complement system (C5a in particular) encourage phagocytes to migrate toward the infected site where **phagocytosis** begins. The phagocytic cells are PMNs, **monocytes,** and **macrophages.** Monocytes are white blood cells with one large nucleus. Monocytes circulate in our peripheral blood for only about 1 day. They may eventually move into tissues where they mature into a cell called a macrophage. Macrophages have a life span of several months. PMNs and macrophages are the major phagocytic cells of the immune system.

Phagocytosis is the process by which phagocytes ingest, kill, and digest infectious organisms and unwanted cellular debris, such as old cells or particulate matter. The pathogens susceptible to phagocytosis can be intracellular, such as *Mycobacterium tuberculosis,* or extracellular, such as *Streptococcus pneumoniae.* The intracellular pathogens are ingested by macrophages when they are released from a dying cell. The process begins after the phagocytes are attracted to the site of injury and begin to attach to the microorganism(s). Attachment is accomplished because phagocytes have certain receptors (non-specific) on their cell surface to which the microorganism can be attached (**Figure 39.1**). This attachment is enhanced if IgG (specifically the Fc portion of IgG) and another component of complement (C3) is activated; this is a process called **opsonization**.

Opsonization with C3 and IgG helps bind the microorganism to the membrane of the phagocyte. Once the membrane is activated by the presence of the microbe, pseudopodia extend out around the microorganism and engulf it, forming a **phagosome** within the cell. Once in the cell, specific lysosomes containing hydrolytic enzymes fuse with the phagosome and start to destroy the microorganism (**Figure 39.2**) Sometimes undigested remnants of the microorganism are left and they are released from the cell.

Joe's story shows how complicated the immune system is and how a deficiency in a component of the system can have serious impact. Joe has normal functioning phagocytes, but the enhanced binding of these phagocytes to pathogens was compromised. **Table 39.1**

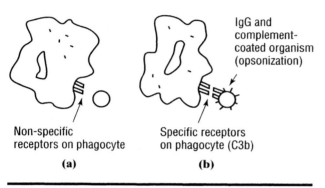

Figure 39.1 Attachment of a microorganism to a phagocyte: (a) non-specific and (b) specific.

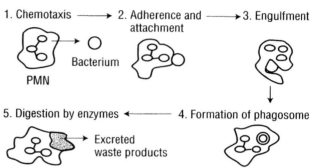

Figure 39.2 Phagocytosis and digestion of a trapped bacterium.

TABLE 39.1 Differences in the Binding of Phagocytes to Bacteria During Phagocytosis

Mechanism of Binding	Illustration of Binding	Amount of Binding
Direct binding of phagocyte to bacterium which is part of our innate immunity. (Joe's body can do this.)	Bacterium	+/−
Antibody (IgG), which acts as an opsonin and bridge to allow bacterium to attach to Fc receptor of phagocyte. (Joe's body can do this.)	Fc receptor / IgG	+
Complement (C3b) activated on the surface of the bacterium, which acts as an opsonin and binds the bacterium to the phagocyte via receptors. (Joe's body cannot do this.)	C3b complement	+ +
Both IgG and C3b acting as opsonins, greatly enhancing phagocytosis. (Joe's body cannot do this.)	IgG / C3b	+ + + +

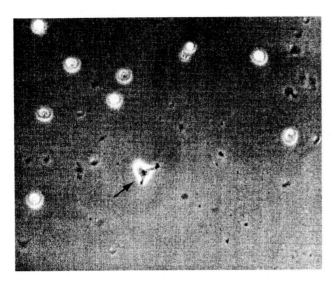

Figure 39.3   A PMN sending out pseudopodia as it begins to migrate toward yeast cells (arrow).

illustrates Joe's deficiency of C3 complement and how this affects Joe's ability to fight off infections.

During this exercise you will see PMNs in your own blood engulf yeast cells. As you watch this process, try to observe the entire sequence of events which includes chemotaxis (movement of PMN to yeast cell), adherence, engulfment, and phagosome formation (**Figures 39.2 and 39.3**). You will also stain your cells after phagocytosis has occurred using a common blood cell stain (Wright's stain) and observe ingested yeast cells within your PMNs.

PURPOSE

- To observe phagocytosis by microscopically examining PMNs and monocytes as they ingest yeast cells
- To understand the mechanism of phagocytosis

THE EXERCISE

MATERIALS:

Lancet
Disposable gloves
Heparinized capillary tubes
Microcapillary centrifuge
Coverslips
RPMI 1640 cell culture medium with 25 mM Hepes
   buffer
Toothpicks
Wright-Giemsa stain

Staining racks
Proper discard containers for the lancet, capillary
   tubes, gauze, slides, etc.
Alcohol swabs
Gauze
Suspension of yeast cells (~10^8 cells/ml)
Clay for sealing capillary tubes
Microscope slides
Humid incubation chamber, as used in Exercise 13
Pasteur pipets with bulb
Phosphate buffer (pH 6.4)
Safety glasses

PROCEDURE:

1. After wiping your finger with an alcohol swab, stick your finger with the lancet (see the Tips on Collecting Blood box). Your instructor will demonstrate this procedure. **The hand not being stuck should be gloved!**

   CAUTION: *Work only with your own blood.* **Discard the lancet in a proper sharps container. Discard all blood contaminated materials (gauze, gloves, capillary tubes, slides, etc.) in autoclave bags or autoclavable containers.**

2. Place the capillary tube in the blood and let the tube fill until at least one-half full.

3. Insert the capillary tube into the sealing clay and remove; this plugs one end of the tube. **Note:** After the bleeding has stopped, this hand can be gloved.

Tips on Collecting Blood

1. Allow your finger to dry after using the alcohol swab and before sticking it.
2. Hold your finger below the level of your heart (don't fight your heart).
3. Shake and squeeze the tip of your finger until it turns red.
4. Use a quick sharp jab of the lancet and stab the side of your fingertip (off center).
5. Do not stick your thumb or first finger; they usually have thicker and tougher skin. Instead, stick the index or fourth finger.
6. After sticking your finger, wipe the first drop away and take the second large drop. The first drop has tissue juices.
7. When collecting blood in capillary tubes, hold the tube parallel to your finger, not perpendicular.

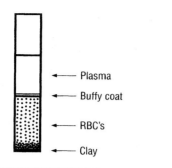

Figure 39.4 Capillary tube with blood.

4. Place the tube in the microcapillary centrifuge and balance it with another capillary tube filled with the same amount of fluid.

5. Spin the tube for 2 minutes. **Note:** If a microcapillary centrifuge is unavailable, leave the capillary tube in the clay in a vertical position and let it stand for at least 1 hour. Eventually gravity will separate the cells from the plasma. The capillary-tube should look like that shown in **Figure 39.4.** The area on top of the red blood cell (RBC) layer is called the **buffy coat**. The buffy coat contains the highest concentration of WBCs and it is this layer that you want to extract and observe.

6. Your next task is to break the capillary tube at the buffy coat.

CAUTION: Wear eye protection when snapping the tube. Be careful not to cut yourself. The tube may break unevenly and produce a sharp edge.

To break the tube, carefully use a glass rod etching device or file to etch the capillary tube. Then grasp the capillary tube between two hands. Position your forefingers and thumbs at the etched point and snap the tube (**Figure 39.5**). Some RBCs may be present in the plasma fraction, but not enough to interfere with observations of phagocytosis. If you do not have a glass etching device, place the tube at the edge of the counter and snap the tube at the interface.

7. Carefully tap the portion with the fluid (plasma) and cells onto a coverslip. The coverslip is placed on a glass slide for easier handling. Also place a drop at the end of another glass slide (**Figure 39.6**). Steps 8 through 11 will be carried out for both the coverslip and slide. Discard the tubes in a biohazard container. **Note:** Sometimes small pieces of glass from the capillary tube end up on the coverslip or slide.

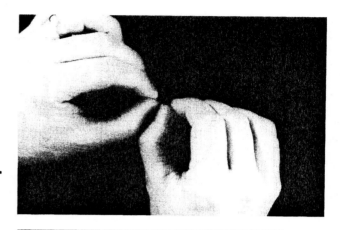

Figure 39.5 Breaking the capillary tube.

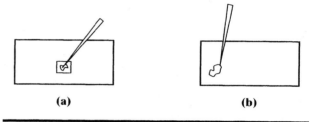

(a)   **(b)**

Figure 39.6 Tapping the buffy coat with plasma onto (a) a coverslip, and (b) slide.

These can be removed with forceps. The forceps should be flamed after use.

8. Dispense 1 drop of RPMI 1640 cell culture medium with Hepes buffer next to the fluid. **Note:** The medium ensures that the PMNs do not die while they are phagocytizing the yeast.

9. Dispense 1 drop of suspended yeast cells (*Saccharomyces cerevisiae*) next to the fluid.

10. Mix the three suspensions together with a toothpick. Discard the toothpick in a biohazard container.

11. Place both the slide with coverslip and the second slide in a humid incubation chamber and incubate for 5 to 10 minutes at 37°C. **Note:** It is important that the mixture on the slide and coverslip does not dry while incubating. Keep the lid closed on the chamber and make sure the paper is thoroughly moistened during incubation.

12. After 5-10 minutes, remove the slide with the coverslip and carefully invert the coverslip onto the slide. Let the fluid on the coverslip settle for 1 minute before observing. **Note:** You have made a wet mount of phagocytes and yeast cells.

13. Continue to incubate the other slide for an additional 45 minutes in the humid chamber.

14. Observe the slide with the coverslip under 40× power. The suspension is best observed using phase microscopy.

15. Watch as the PMNs send out pseudopodia and begin to engulf the yeast cells (**Figure 39.3**). Record your observations in the RESULTS section. If you study different cells long enough you may be able to see the entire process: chemotaxis, adherence, engulfment, and phagosome formation within the PMN. **Note:** The PMNs are larger, irregularly shaped, granular cells, whereas the yeast cells and RBCs are smaller and more round.

16. After the slide has incubated about 1 hour, remove it from the chamber and spread the fluid over the entire slide. This can be done by using another slide or a toothpick. Allow the slide to air dry.

17. Stain the slide according to the following Wright's staining procedure:
    a. Place the slide on a staining rack and cover it with filtered Wright's stain.
    b. Allow the stain to remain on the smear for at least 5 minutes.
    c. Slowly add buffer to the stain until the buffer begins to overflow the stain. Watch for the appearance of a metallic luster. **Note:** Some

stains purchased commercially already have the buffer in them and this step is unnecessary.
    d. After mixing the buffer and stain by gently blowing on the smear, let the slide sit for another 5 minutes. Do not let it dry out.
    e. Gently wash the stain and buffer off the slide with distilled water.
    f. Air-dry the smear or carefully blot the slide between two sheets of bibulous paper.

18. Examine the smear microscopically. Use 40× or oil immersion (100×) to see the ingested yeast. In a properly stained slide, the red blood cells will appear as small pink- to red-colored cells, whereas the white blood cells will appear blue to dark purple with a dark purple nucleus. If the slide is poorly stained, your white blood cells will be faintly stained.

19. Draw your observations in the RESULTS section.

REFERENCES

Beck, W.S. *Hematology*, 5th ed. Cambridge, MA: Massachusetts Institute of Technology Press, 1992.

Lee, R.L., et al. *Wintrobe's Clinical Hematology,* 9th ed. Philadelphia: Lea & Febiger, 1993.

Roitt, I., et al. *Immunology.* New York: Harper and Row, 1989.

Turgeon, M.L. *Immunology and Serology in Laboratory Medicine.* St. Louis: Mosby–Year Book, 1990.

RESULTS

1. Draw and/or describe the events you saw during the microscopic examination of your PMNs engulfing yeast cells.

2. Draw or describe the PMNs you observed with your stained slide.

REFLECTIONS

1. The sample placed on the slide contained plasma, not serum (fluid portion of the blood). What is the difference between serum and plasma?

2. Does plasma contain the IgG and C3 necessary for opsonization?

3. How long did it take your PMNs to engulf the yeast cells?

4. Using your observations, describe phagocytosis in your own words. Think about what happened as you watched a PMN and yeast cell.

EXERCISE 40

ANTIGEN-ANTIBODY REACTIONS

In the last exercise, you observed a critical part of our immune system, phagocytosis. This exercise involves learning and visualizing another important part of the immune system, antibody production. Two tests will be performed that demonstrate the antigen-antibody agglutination reaction. One is the reaction of antibody to the presence of antigen on the surface of streptococcal bacteria, and the other is a hemagglutination reaction of specific antigens on our red cells to antibodies in serum (ABO blood typing).

Sarah just learned that her bisexual brother, Sam, had tested positive for antibodies to the human immunodeficiency virus (HIV). She had many questions to ask including, "Does this antibody test indicate he has an active infection of the virus?" Sam had gone to the doctor 6 weeks prior to this test because he had a week-long fever, swollen lymph glands, and a splotchy rash all over his body. His doctor tested him for HIV because he had admitted to having unprotected sex with a new male partner. The HIV test was negative. However, Sam was counseled to come back for follow-up testing because antibodies to HIV are usually not detectable in the initial phase of infection. It was during the second visit that he learned he was HIV-positive. Both Sarah and Sam learned that a positive HIV antibody test signifies a current infection and that Sam would almost certainly get acquired immunodeficiency syndrome (AIDS). Sam's doctor counseled him about treatment and the progression of HIV infection to AIDS, which can take many years. However, his doctor could only
offer him hope for the possibility of new anti-HIV drugs that would lead to a cure of Sam's infection.

BACKGROUND INFORMATION

AIDS is defined by a set of illnesses and malignancies that results from the immune system being under attack by HIV. This virus will relentlessly and progressively destroy specific cells in Sam's body called **lymphocytes.** There are several types of lymphocytes. One type is called a **T cell,** which originates in the bone marrow and matures in the thymus. One T lymphocyte is the **T helper cell** (T_H). This is the lymphocyte that the HIV virus attacks and destroys. Other types of T cells are called cytotoxic T cells (T_C), delayed-type hypersensitivity cells (T_D) and a distinct class of lymphocytes called natural killer cells (NK). All of the T cells are part of our **cell-mediated immune** (CMI) response (**Figure 40.1**). Refer to your text for a discussion of these types of lymphocytes.

One of the functions of the T_H cell is to stimulate another kind of lymphocyte, the **B lymphocyte.** B cells produce large amounts of **antibody** (immunoglobulins) when presented with the foreign **antigen** of a bacterium or virus. B cells also originate in the bone marrow, but unlike T cells, mature there as well. The production of antibodies is a process called **humoral immunity** or antibody-mediated immunity (**Figure 40.1**).

The stimulation of B cells by T_H is a complex process. When a pathogen enters the body, macrophages are attracted to the microorganism and eventually engulf the foreign invader and digest it (see Exercise 39). During digestion, unique chemical groups of the invading organism are moved to the surface of the macrophage. This creates specific antigenic

278

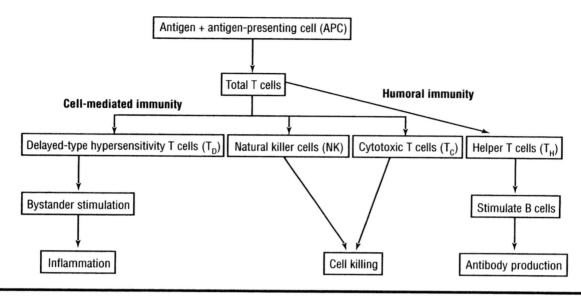

Figure 40.1 The relationship and overview of cell-mediated immunity and humoral immunity.

determinants which are presented to T_H cells. Upon detecting the antigens on the surface of the macrophage, T_H cells stimulate specific B cells to differentiate into plasma cells. Plasma cells secrete antibodies that are specific for the antigen that stimulated its production. The antibody will complex with the antigen (**Figure 40.2**) producing several types of reactions depending upon the location and type of antigen. Some of these reactions include lysis, killing, precipitation, neutralization, and agglutination. The type of reaction you will observe in this exercise is agglutination and hemagglutination, the agglutination of red blood cells.

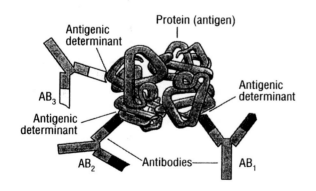

Figure 40.2 Antigen, antigenic determinants, and antibodies. Antigens may contain several different antigenic determinants, each capable of reacting with a specific antibody.

The CMI response plays a major role in fighting HIV. However, infected individuals also mount a large antibody response. Why isn't this enough to check Sam's infection? Unfortunately, much is still unknown about the virus and its impact on the immune system. It is known that T_H cells are killed by HIV, but how that happens is unclear. This decrease in T_H cells is coupled with the fact that HIV is constantly changing its genetic structure and subsequent antigens. Therefore, a new antibody specific for each new antigen has to be produced by the body. Because of the decreased number of T cells, Sam's body will lose the battle and eventually not be able to mount an immune response to the HIV variants or to the numerous opportunistic pathogens that will come his way.

Antibodies are important in our protection against disease. They are also useful in the identification of pathogenic microorganisms. An example is the agglutination test for diagnosing streptococcal infections. In this test, antigen from pathogenic streptococci (Group A *S. pyogenes* and Group B *S. agalactiae*) is agglutinated with antibody contained in commercially prepared antisera. To better observe this barely visible agglutination, the antibodies are attached to latex beads which increases the number of antigen-binding sites (**Figure 40.3**).

In this exercise you will perform a latex bead agglutination test for streptococci. You will also observe hemagglutination of your red blood cells with type-specific antisera. The A and B antigens on

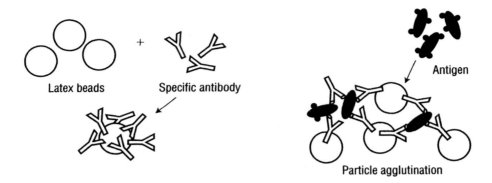

Figure 40.3   Antibody bound to latex beads and agglutination of antigen and antibody.

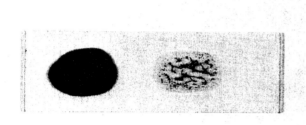

Figure 40.4   A microsope slide showing agglutination when blood is mixed with antisera.

our red blood cells are much stronger antigens and large aggregated clumps will be readily visible when agglutination has occurred. If you have neither A nor B antigen on your red blood cells, you will have no agglutination of either antisera and therefore the cells are blood type O. **Figure 40.4** shows a picture of agglutination when cells clump or aggregate. No agglutination is a smooth suspension of cells and serum.

PURPOSE

- To observe antigen-antibody reactions as demonstrated by agglutination reactions
- To observe the hemagglutination reaction of our red blood cells with type-specific antisera and determine our blood type
- To understand the importance of antibodies and the role they play in our immune system

THE EXERCISE

Part A: Latex Agglutination Testing

MATERIALS:

Group A and B antiserum to *Streptococcus* (PathoDx latex agglutination reagents)

One known and one unknown *Streptococcus* on sheep blood agar plates (BA)

Latex agglutination card

Sterile applicator sticks

PROCEDURE: Work in groups of two or three

1. Obtain a latex agglutination card, one BA plate with an unknown *Streptococcus,* and one BA plate with a known *Streptococcus.*
2. Observe the type of hemolysis that each of your microorganisms exhibits, and from your previous knowledge of streptococci (see Exercise 32), speculate about the type of streptococcus your unknown might be.
3. Carefully pick 4 or 5 β-hemolytic colonies of your **unknown** microorganism with a sterile applicator stick and rub it onto a designated oval on the card. Repeat this step in another oval.
4. In a third oval, rub 4 or 5 colonies of your **known** organism with a sterile applicator stick.
5. Resuspend the latex reagents by gentle inversion. Add 1 drop of Strep A latex to the first oval and 1 drop of Strep B latex to the second oval. Add 1 drop of the specific antisera (A or B) to your known microorganism.
6. Mix the reagent and microorganism with an applicator stick, using a clean end for each oval.
7. Hold the slide under good lighting and gently tilt the slide back and forth. A positive agglutination reaction with one of the latex reagents usually

occurs in 15 to 60 seconds. Do not rock the slide for more than 60 seconds.

8. Record your results in the RESULTS section.

Part B: Blood Typing

MATERIALS:

Anti-A and anti-B blood typing antisera
Sterile lancets
Toothpicks
Proper discard containers for materials contaminated with blood (e.g., gauze, toothpicks, slides, etc.)
Slides
Alcohol swabs
Biohazard disposable sharps container
Gloves

PROCEDURE:

1. Mark two circles on a glass slide with a wax pencil and label them A and B.
2. Have your instructor place a drop of anti-A antisera in the A circle and anti-B antisera in the B circle.
3. Clean the tip of a finger with the alcohol swab and rub the base of the finger toward the cleaned area to increase the blood supply in the fingertip.
4. After wiping your finger with an alcohol swab, stick your finger with the lancet (see the Tips on Collecting Blood box). Your instructor will

---

Tips on Collecting Blood

1. Allow your finger to dry after using the alcohol swab and before sticking it.
2. Hold your finger below the level of your heart.
3. Shake and squeeze the tip of your finger until it turns red.
4. Use a quick sharp jab of the lancet and stab the side of your fingertip.
5. Do not stick your thumb or first finger; they usually have thicker and tougher skin. Instead, stick the index or fourth finger.
6. After sticking your finger, wipe the first drop away and take the second large drop. The first drop has tissue juices.

TABLE 40.1 Expected Results of ABO Blood Typing

Blood Type	Anti-A Antisera (Antibodies)	Anti-B Antisera (Antibodies)
O	−	−
A	+	−
B	−	+
AB	+	+

+ = agglutination; − = no agglutination.

demonstrate this procedure. **The hand not being stuck should be gloved!**

CAUTION: *Work only with your own blood.* **Discard the lancet in a proper sharps container. Discard all blood contaminated materials (gauze, gloves, capillary tubes, slides, etc.) in autoclave bags or autoclavable containers.**

5. Use a toothpick to transfer a drop of blood from your finger to the anti-A sera in circle A. Mix the blood and antiserum to a smooth consistency and discard the toothpick in a proper container. **Note:** You can also squeeze a drop of blood directly onto the slide.
6. Use a second toothpick and obtain a second drop from your finger to add to the anti-B antisera in circle B. Mix the blood and antisera to a smooth even consistency.
7. Slowly tilt the slides back and forth (do not mix the circles) and observe for agglutination. Compare your results with **Table 40.1** listed below and determine your ABO blood type. Record your results in the RESULTS section.

REFERENCES

Brock, T.D., et al. *Biology of Microorganisms*, 7th ed., Engelwood Cliffs, NJ: Prentice-Hall Publishers, 1994.

Salyers, A.A., Whitt, D.D. *Bacterial Pathogenesis, A Molecular Approach*. Washington, DC: American Society for Microbiology Press, 1994.

Schaechter, M., et al. *Mechanisms of Microbial Disease*, 2nd ed. Baltimore: Williams and Wilkins, 1993.

Turgeon, M.L. *Immunology and Serology in Laboratory Medicine*. St. Louis: Mosby–Year Book, 1990.

RESULTS

Part A

Type of hemolysis for known streptococcal species _____

Type of hemolysis for unknown streptococcal species _____

Unknown number _____ Group type _____

Identification of unknown _____

Part B

Agglutination with anti-A antisera (+ or −)_____

Agglutination with anti-B antisera (+ or −)_____

Your ABO blood type_____

REFLECTIONS

1. Streptococci are divided into different groups called serotypes. Consult Exercise 32 or other textbooks and explain what determines the different serotypes (A-O) of streptococci?

2. Why was the known organism given to you to type?

3. What was the source of the antigen for the latex agglutination test you performed?

4. In what fraction of our blood (fluid or cellular) are the immunoglobulins (antibodies) such as IgG or IgM found?

5. Why is it that antigen-antibody complexes are visible in aggregated clumps, and yet red blood cells are microscopic?

6. You may have heard the of the terms "universal donor" and "universal recipient." Refer to **Table 40.1** again and determine which person (Type O, A, B, or AB) is considered a universal donor and which is a universal recipient. Explain your answer.

EXERCISE 41

MEASURING ANTIBODY TITER BY ENZYME-LINKED IMMUNOSORBENT ASSAY (ELISA)

In the previous exercise, you learned about agglutination reactions between antigen and antibody, and how they are important in typing blood and in diagnostic tests. Such reactions can also be used to determine the amount of a specific antibody in the blood (antibody titer), either as a means of diagnosing an illness, monitoring an infection, or showing prior exposure to a pathogen. In this exercise, you will determine antibody titer using a different assay—enzyme-linked immunosorbent assay.

Dr. Landers' first patient of the day was a young man, Jesse, who complained of fever, chills, and malaise. Jesse's symptoms had begun 3 days earlier, and initially he thought he simply had a very bad case of the flu. But he also noticed his lymph glands were swollen and very tender to the touch. When he began to vomit, he decided it was time to contact the doctor. The symptoms Jesse exhibited were characteristic of a number of illnesses including plague and tularemia. Although plague was very rare in Oklahoma, tularemia was relatively common. Unfortunately, the two diseases are easily confused in the initial stages. With that in mind, Dr. Landers began asking Jesse questions about recent events that might help her make the diagnosis. She asked whether Jesse had any recent contact with dead animals such as rabbit or deer, and whether he had been hiking recently. Dr. Landers knew tularemia is spread primarily by two mechanisms—direct contact with carcasses of infected animals, and by tick transmission. When Jesse reported that he had recently been hunting for rabbits and had been very successful, Dr. Landers decided to test him for tularemia. This can be done by testing for antibodies against the bacterium that causes tularemia. Dr. Landers also began treating Jesse with the antibiotic streptomycin. Jesse's initial antibody titer to the bacterium was less than 1:20. Within a few days, Jesse's symptoms eased noticeably; his vomiting stopped, his fever disappeared, and his lymph nodes decreased in size. One week later, when Jesse's antibody titer was tested again, it was found to be ≥1:160; 2 weeks after Jesse's first visit, the titer was ≥1:640. Because of the rise in antibody titer over a 3-week period, Dr. Landers' tentative diagnosis of tularemia was confirmed. Because of the antibiotic therapy, Jesse recovered fully.

BACKGROUND INFORMATION

Tularemia is caused by a Gram-negative, pleomorphic, rod-shaped bacterium called *Francisella tularensis*. It is spread from its mammalian hosts in the wild (usually rabbits, muskrats, and beavers) to humans, either by direct contact, tick bites, ingestion, or inhalation. Although tularemia is relatively uncommon (200 cases of tularemia per year nationwide), in certain regions of the United States (e.g., Oklahoma), the bacterium is endemic in the wild. The severity of the disease varies and is sometimes mistaken for influenza and other illnesses with similar symptoms. In its worst forms, it is rarely fatal, even if patients are untreated. However, tularemia symptoms can resemble plague, and it is important to diagnose the illness as quickly as possible. Unfortunately, *F. tularensis* grows slowly and requires a specialized growth medium. Therefore, it is not always possible to use diagnostic tests that involve culturing the bacterium. Instead, a common test used to diagnose tularemia is to monitor the level of antibodies to *F. tularensis* over time.

Antibody levels to *F. tularensis* can be used to diagnose tularemia because the bacterium, like many pathogens, elicits an **antibody-mediated immune response** (AbMIR). Typically, an AbMIR occurs when certain helper T and B lymphocytes—those having receptors on their surfaces that recognize antigens on the surface of *F. tularensis*—detect *F. tularensis* in host tissues. Once *F. tularensis* is detected, the B lymphocytes proliferate; some progeny become antibody-producing cells (**plasma cells**) and others become **memory cells** that will function to produce antibody in subsequent encounters with the pathogen. If the levels of specific antibodies (antibody titer) are monitored over time, a pattern such as that shown in **Figure 41.1** is often observed. Notice the strong reaction upon second exposure to the antigen. This is due to memory cells which produce antibody and prevent illness from recurring.

In the case of tularemia, antibody to *F. tularensis* is usually undetected in the first week of infection but then begins to appear and continues to rise for several weeks. The increase in titer is often fourfold or greater at 2-week intervals throughout the infection. Thus, fourfold increases in antibody titer over a 1- to 2-week interval is indicative of infection.

Antibody titer can be determined in a number of ways. For tularemia, the best method is the enzyme-linked immunosorbent assay (ELISA). In this method, different dilutions of serum from the infected individual are placed in wells in a microtiter plate (**Figure 41.2**), but only after the wells have first been coated with *F. tularensis* antigen (**Figure 41.3a**). If anti–*F. tularensis* antibodies are present in the patient's serum, they bind the antigen in the well (**Figure 41.3b**). In the next step of the assay, antibody from an animal such as goat is added to the well. This second antibody is specific for the Fc portion of human antibody proteins and will bind to human antibodies in the well. (Remember, the human antibody is bound to the antigen in the well.) The second antibody also has another characteristic of importance—it is covalently linked to an enzyme such as urease or horseradish peroxidase. Such an enzyme-linked antibody is called a conjugated antibody. The enzyme is important because it catalyzes a chemical reaction that is chromogenic; that is, it produces color. Therefore, presence of the conjugated enzyme is easily ascertained. After incubation with the conjugated enzyme, the wells are washed. If no antibody is present in the serum of the patient, the conjugated antibody will be washed away. If antibody is present, the patient's antibody will be bound to the antigen in the well, and the conjugated antibody will bind to the patient's antibodies (**Figure 41.3d**). When the substrate of the enzyme portion of the conjugated antibody is added (**Figure 41.3f**), the reaction occurs and a

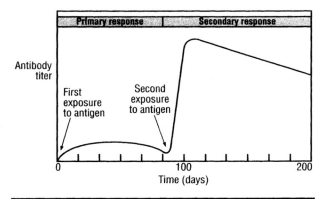

Figure 41.1 Typical antibody titers to a pathogen over time.

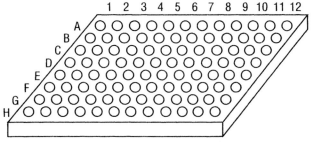

Figure 41.2 A 96-well microtiter plate.

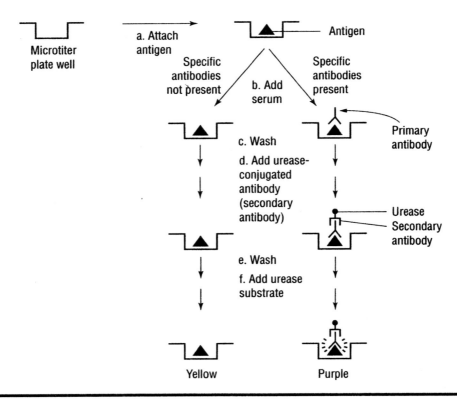

Figure 41.3 An ELISA for detecting and quantifying a specific antibody in serum.

color appears. This color can be observed with the unaided eye or can be quantified with a special spectrophotometer designed to scan microtiter plates. The titer of the antibody is reported as the dilution (or the inverse of the dilution) giving the last positive response. The higher the positive dilution (the more dilute the serum), the higher the titer of antibody in the patient's serum.

In this exercise, you will use the ELISA method to determine the titer of antibodies in rabbit serum to chicken egg albumin. Rabbit serum is used because human serum can be dangerous to work with, since it can contain blood-borne pathogens. The conjugated antibody used in the assay is goat anti-rabbit antibody linked to the enzyme urease. Urease was discussed in Exercise 15. It catalyzes the hydrolysis of urea to ammonia, which increases the pH of the solution. In this assay, bromcresol purple is included as a pH indicator. It is yellow at pH values of 4.2 and below, and purple at pH values of 5.8 and above. Both colors are visible to the unaided eye. Thus, if antibody is present when urea is added, a purple color will be observed; if not, no reaction takes place and yellow is observed. The antibody titer is calculated by determining the last well (dilution), which has a purple color.

PURPOSE

- To perform an enzyme-linked immunosorbent assay (ELISA)
- To calculate antibody titer based on results from an ELISA

THE EXERCISE

MATERIALS:

Chicken egg albumin (10 µg/ml)
Rabbit serum #1 (1/50 dilution)
Dilution buffer (0.01 M phosphate-buffered saline, pH 7.2 containing 0.05% [w/v] Tween-20 and 0.25% [w/v] bovine serum albumin and 0.1% [w/v] sodium azide)
Wash buffer (0.01 M phosphate-buffered saline with 0.05% [w/v] Tween-20)
37°C incubator
0.1 M sodium carbonate buffer, pH 9.6
Rabbit serum #2 (1/50 dilution)
Urea-bromcresol purple reagent, pH 4.8
Microcentrifuge tubes and racks
Micropipetters and sterile tips

Urease-conjugated goat anti-rabbit immunoglobulin (Ig) polyclonal antibodies
96-well microtiter plate with lid (or parafilm)

PROCEDURE: Work in pairs

If desired, a single microtiter plate can be shared by two pairs of students.

Day 1: Attachment of Antigen to Microtiter Plate Wells (Figure 41.3a)

1. Add 200 μl of chicken egg albumin to wells A1 through A10 and to wells C1 through C10 (**Figure 41.2**).
2. Add 200 μl of the sodium carbonate buffer to wells B1 through B10, and to wells D1 through D10. **Note:** The chicken egg albumin is dissolved in the sodium carbonate buffer. Because wells in rows B and D only have sodium carbonate buffer and not chicken egg albumin (antigen), they are control wells.
3. Cover the microtiter plate.
4. Incubate the plate at 4°C either overnight or until the next laboratory period. **Note:** During this period, the chicken egg albumin becomes firmly attached to the wells and cannot be washed out of the wells in subsequent steps.

Day 2

*Part A: Preparation of Dilutions of Rabbit Sera (Primary Antibody) (**Figure 41.4**)*

1. Label 9 microcentrifuge tubes A-2, through A-10 and arrange in order in a microcentrifuge tube rack.
2. Add 0.5 ml dilution buffer to each tube.

3. Label the tube of rabbit serum #1, A-1.
4. Prepare twofold dilutions as show in **Figure 41.4.** **Note:** Below the drawing of each tube is space to indicate the final dilution. Remember the tube of serum you were given is already a 1/50 dilution. Fill in the blank spaces in **Figure 41.4** and then have your figures checked by your instructor. If the values are correct, fill in the appropriate blanks in the RESULTS section.
5. Label the tube of rabbit serum #2, C-1, and make the same set of dilutions as for serum #1, labeling the tubes C-2 through C-10.

*Part B: Binding of the Primary Antibody to Chicken Egg Albumin Attached to Wells (**Figure 41.3b**)*

1. Obtain a microtiter plate with chicken egg albumin attached to wells.
2. Uncover the plate and empty the wells by inverting the plate over a sink. **Note:** This is done with a quick snapping motion over the sink. Any remaining liquid can be removed by briefly inverting the plate onto a paper towel.
3. Fill each well with wash buffer. **Note:** Washing the wells removes any unattached antigen and chemicals that might interfere with subsequent steps of the ELISA.
4. Empty the wells as in step 2.
5. Repeat steps 3 through 4 two more times.
6. Add 200 μl of tube A-1 to wells A1 and B1. Discard the tip.
7. Add 200 μl of tube A-2 to wells A2 and B2. Discard the tip.

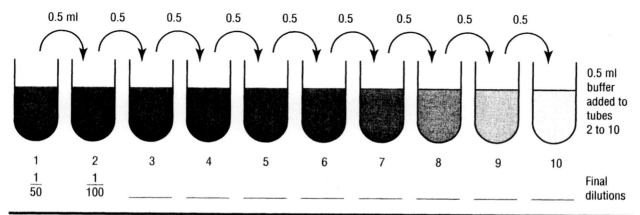

Transfer 0.5 ml from tube 1 to 2, mix, etc.

Figure 41.4 Procedure for doing a two-fold dilution series of rabbit serum. Fill in the space left for recording final dilution before proceeding with the ELISA.

8. Continue down the row by adding 200 μl of tube A-3 to wells A3 and B3, A-4 to wells A4 and B4, etc. Remember to discard the tip after each transfer.
9. Repeat steps 6 through 8 using the dilutions of rabbit serum #2 (tubes C-1 through C-10) and adding 200 μl of each dilution to the corresponding C wells and D wells.
10. Cover the plate and incubate at 37°C for 30 minutes. **Note:** During the incubation period, antibodies in the rabbit sera (primary antibodies) that recognize chicken egg albumin (antigen) will bind the antigen attached to the wells in rows A and C.
11. Empty the wells as in step 2. **Note:** Any primary antibodies not attached to the antigen will be poured out when the wells are emptied.
12. Wash all wells with wash buffer three times, as in steps 3 through 5 (**Figure 41.3c**). **Note:** Any remaining unbound primary antibodies will be washed out of the wells when the wells are washed.

*Part C: Binding of Urease-Conjugated Goat Anti-Rabbit Ig Antibodies (Secondary Antibody) to the Primary Antibodies (**Figure 41.3d**)*

1. Add 200 μl of the urease-conjugated goat anti-rabbit immunoglobulin antibodies (secondary antibody) to each well.
2. Cover the plate and incubate at 37°C for 30 minutes. **Note:** During the incubation period, the secondary antibodies will bind to primary antibodies in the wells.
3. Empty the wells as in steps 3 through 5, Part B. **Note:** Any secondary antibodies not attached to primary antibodies will be poured out when the wells are emptied.
4. Wash all wells at least 2 times with wash buffer, as in steps 3 through 5, Part B (**Figure 41.3e**). **Note:** Any remaining unbound secondary antibodies will be washed out of the wells when the wells are washed.

5. Wash all wells 2 times with distilled water, using the same washing procedure as described in Part B, steps 3 through 5. **Note:** These washes remove all buffer. The buffer must be removed because it interferes with the pH change that will occur as ammonia is produced by the hydrolysis of urea.

*Part D: Detection of Urease-Conjugated Goat Antibodies (Secondary Antibodies) in Wells (**Figure 41.3f**)*

1. Add 200 μl of the urea-bromcresol purple reagent to each well. **Note:** The same tip may be used for each addition if it does not come into contact with the liquid or sides of the wells.
2. Cover the plate and incubate at 37°C for 30 minutes. **Note:** During the incubation period, if secondary antibodies (urease-conjugated antibodies) are in a well, the urease will hydrolyze urea producing ammonia. As ammonia is produced, the pH of the solution increases to greater than 5.8. At pH values >5.8, bromcresol purple is purple. At more acidic pH values, it is yellow.
3. Uncover the plate and examine the wells. Some wells will be purple and others will be yellow. Record the color of each well in the RESULTS section.

REFERENCES

Chandler, H.M., et al. An Investigation of the Use of Urease-antibody Conjugates in Enzyme Immunoassays. *Journal of Immunological Methods* 53(1982):187-194.

Gage, K.L., et al. Nonviral Vector-Borne Zoonoses Associated With Mammals in the United States. *Journal of Mammology* 76(1995)(3):695-715.

Rohrbach, B.W. Tularemia. *Journal of the American Veterinary Medicine Association* 193(1988):428-432.

Turgeon, M.L. *Immunology and Serology in Laboratory Medicine.* St. Louis: C.V. Mosby Co., 1990.

RESULTS

Record the color of the wells in the table below. Use P for purple and Y for yellow. Review the procedures and determine which color, purple or yellow, indicates the presence of antibodies specific for chicken egg albumin in the rabbit serum. After doing so, rescore the results in the table as positive (+) or negative (−).

	Well Number (Rows A, B, C, or D)									
	1	**2**	**3**	**4**	**5**	**6**	**7**	**8**	**9**	**10**
Final dilution of rabbit serum										
Color: A wells (albumin + rabbit serum #1 + conjugated antibody)										
Color: B wells (rabbit serum #1 + conjugated antibody										
Color: C wells (albumin + rabbit serum #2 + conjugated antibody)										
Color: D wells (rabbit serum #2 + conjugated antibody)										

REFLECTIONS

1. What was the titer of rabbit anti-chicken egg albumin antibodies in each rabbit serum? Immunologists and serologists express antibody titer as either the dilution giving the last clear positive result, or as the inverse of the dilution giving the last clear positive result (i.e., 1/640 or 1:640 or 640).

2. Did both rabbit sera contain antibodies to chicken egg albumin? Explain.

3. Consider wells A1, B1, C1, and D1. Draw a cartoon that illustrates the presence and placement of chicken egg albumin, rabbit anti-chicken egg albumin antibodies, and urease-conjugated goat anti-rabbit Ig antibodies in each well when the ELISA is completed.

4. The B and D row wells are controls. What did each set of wells tell you? Suggest another control that would have been appropriate to use.

5. One of the initial tests done when diagnosing AIDS or HIV-infection is an HIV-ELISA. It is used to detect the presence of antibodies specific for HIV antigens in the blood of an individual suspected to be infected with HIV. These antibodies usually appear within the first few months of infection and are detectable throughout most of the infection. When the test results are positive, it means the individual has anti-HIV antibodies in his or her blood, and that he or she is infected by the virus. The HIV-ELISA is very similar to the ELISA you did in this exercise. Using your knowledge of the ELISA performed in this exercise, determine the corresponding components used in the HIV-ELISA and complete the table below.

Components in the ELISA Done in this Laboratory Exercise	Corresponding Components in the HIV-ELISA Test*
Chicken egg albumin (antigen)	
Rabbit serum (primary antibody)	
Urease-conjugated goat anti-rabbit Ig antibodies (secondary antibody)	

* A general description of the component is adequate.

6. Which row of wells done in this exercise would correspond to serum from an individual who is HIV-positive? Which would correspond to serum from an individual who is HIV-negative?

7. Why is it important to get retested for HIV infection if a known exposure has occurred, but the first test is negative?

EXERCISE 42

MONOCLONAL ANTIBODIES

The past two exercises have focused on antigen-antibody reactions and methods for assaying these reactions. This exercise will supply you with information on specific antibodies (monoclonal antibodies) and how they have been used in diagnostic testing. You will use a monoclonal antibody that has been coupled with a fluorescent dye to observe a specific antibody as it binds exclusively to the surface of *Neisseria gonorrhoeae*.

In 1984, two immunologists, Cesar Milstein and Georges J.F. Kohler, shared the Nobel Prize in Medicine. It was just ten years earlier, in 1974, that these two scientists developed a method that continues to have profound medical significance. Kohler was then a postdoctoral fellow in Milstein's laboratory. Milstein, an immunologist at the British Medical Research Council's laboratory in Cambridge, England, had already made important observations about immunoglobulin synthesis at the protein and nucleic acid level. The goal of his new research was to better understand the genetics of antibody diversity. However, when Kohler arrived in Milstein's laboratory, he, like many other researchers, was frustrated because antibodies were difficult to study. This was because plasma cells, which produce antibodies, only lived in cell culture for several days. Therefore, Kohler and Milstein decided to use previously described techniques to immortalize the antibody-forming cell. Their novel idea was to fuse the antibody-forming cell (plasma cell) with a myeloma cell (a cell that can divide indefinitely) and produce a hybrid cell (hybridoma), which would produce an abundance of a specific antibody (monoclonal antibody) indefinitely. They published their results in 1975 (Nature 256:495-497) and were only

slightly aware of the ramifications of the procedure they developed. They had no idea that today monoclonal antibodies would be used extensively in basic and applied research and in diagnostic testing, spawning a multibillion-dollar industry. Many advances in molecular biology have also been possible because of monoclonal antibodies. The experiments performed by Kohler and Milstein demonstrate the importance and unpredicted power of basic science research. These two men pursued their interests for the sake of knowledge and their results had significance far beyond their expectations.

BACKGROUND INFORMATION

The method developed by Kohler and Milstein was quickly adapted to the production of many types of antibodies and today many companies supply researchers and diagnostic laboratories with **monoclonal antibodies.** **Figure 42.1** is an illustration of how **hybridomas** are made to produce monoclonal antibodies. Refer to this figure while reading the following brief description of how monoclonal antibodies are produced.

A desired antigen such as a surface antigen on *N. gonorrhoeae* is injected into a mouse. After several weeks, the mouse produces B cells secreting antibodies to *N. gonorrhoeae* through the normal immune process. The mouse is sacrificed and its spleen, which is rich in B cells, is removed. The B cells are fused with a myeloma cell line, making a hybridoma. A critical element in the Kohler-Milstein experiments was to find a method to recover only the fused cells. Remember that plasma cells die quickly *in vitro* so they weren't a problem. But myeloma cells are immortal and can live forever under the correct conditions. The key that Kohler and Milstein discovered was to use a myeloma cell line that was deficient in the enzyme hypoxanthine-guanine-phosphoribosyltransferase (HGPRT) and grow it in a medium called HAT (hypoxanthine, aminopterin, and thymidine). The

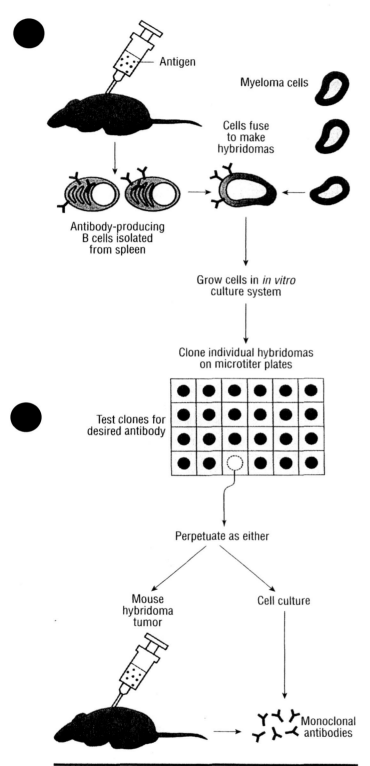

Figure 42.1 The process of producing monoclonal antibodies.

unfused myeloma cells are unable to utilize hypoxanthine and thymidine in HAT for nucleic acid synthesis. They must resort to an alternate pathway, but this pathway is blocked by aminopterin. As a result, unfused myeloma cells cannot synthesize purines for nucleic acid synthesis and they die. The hybridoma cells (fused cells) will grow normally in HAT because HGPRT was provided by the plasma cells during fusion with the myeloma cell.

After the hybridomas have grown, the next step is to pick the clone(s) of interest (e.g., hybridomas which produce antibody to *N. gonorrhoeae*). Usually several distinct clones can be identified and each makes a monoclonal antibody to a different antigenic determinant. All the clones are tested for the desired antibody and each is perpetuated by either growing them in cell culture or injecting them into a mouse. The mouse will produce a large amount of the monoclonal antibody and the antibody can be extracted from its peritoneal cavity. Hybridomas can be frozen and later thawed to be grown again whenever the specific monoclonal antibody is needed. As you can see, this is a cleaner way of producing a specific antibody against a specific antigen, since there are no other antibodies.

Monoclonal antibodies are used in the identification of pathogens such as *N. gonorrhoeae*. Monoclonal antibodies are also used for testing specific drug metabolites and in over-the-counter pregnancy testing kits. The use of monoclonal antibodies in research is also constantly expanding. Besides being used to understand metabolism and our immune system, the use of monoclonal antibodies has spread to genetic engineering, the diagnosis and treatment of cancer, and identification of microbes in the environment.

The monoclonal antibody you will use to identify *N. gonorrhoeae* has a fluorescent dye attached to it. The dye allows us to identify the bacterium using fluorescent microscopy. The binding of the fluorescent compound to the antibody does not interfere with the specificity of the antigen-antibody reaction. In fact, fluorescing cells not only allow us to visually identify certain populations of cells, but to enrich for certain cells, too. Enrichment is accomplished by using an instrument called a fluorescence-activated cell sorter (FACS), which separates fluorescent cells bound to antibody from nonfluorescing cells.

Your task in this exercise is to use a monoclonal antibody specific for *N. gonorrhoeae* and tagged with fluorescein isothiocyanate (FITC) to identify unknown bacteria. The unknowns are Gram-negative cocci that are oxidase positive (*Neisseria*). Refer to Exercise 7 for information on fluorescent anti-body (FA) microscopy and Exercise 31 for information on *N. gonorrhoeae*. The advantages for using this procedure in clinical labs are that testing can be performed from primary culture, only a small inoculum is required, and testing can be performed more quickly than other routine confirmatory procedures.

PURPOSE

- To understand monoclonal antibodies—what they are, how they are produced, and how they are used
- To use a fluorescently labeled monoclonal antibody to identify *N. gonorrhoeae*

THE EXERCISE

MATERIALS:

A chocolate agar plate containing freshly isolated colonies (less than 48 hours old) of two *Neisseria* spp.
Fluorescence-grade microscope slides (two wells)
Humid chamber
Inoculating loop or needle
Pipet tips
Distilled or deionized water
N. gonorrhoeae culture confirmation test kit (Syva Microtrak) with reconstitution diluent and mounting fluid
Micropipetters (5 and 30 μl)
Coverslips
Fluorescence microscope with filter system for FITC (excites at 490 nm and emits at 520 nm)
Note: To save reagent since this can be an expensive procedure, only the instructor will prepare a slide with a positive and negative control.
Optional: To save media, the instructor may choose to supply you with a slide labeled A and B that has been prepared within the last 18 to 24 hours. If *N. gonorrhoeae* is unavailable, a kit for Group A *Streptococcus pyogenes* can be used as a substitute.

PROCEDURE:

1. Obtain a chocolate agar plate that has two unknown *Neisseria* labeled A and B.
2. Obtain a fluorescent-grade glass slide and place 5 ml of distilled or deionized water in each well labeled A and B.
3. With an inoculating loop or needle, very lightly touch five identical colonies from organism A and suspend them in the drop of water in well A. Make a barely visible suspension over the entire well.

Note: A smooth, thin suspension is important because clumps or thick smears may trap stain and cause misinterpretation.

4. Repeat step 3 for organism B.
5. Allow the slide to air dry completely.
6. Gently heat fix the slide by passing it over a flame twice. Be careful not to overheat the slide as overheating will produce uninterpretable results. The slide should be warm but not hot to the touch.
7. Place 30 μl of *N. gonorrhoeae* reagent in each slide well of A and B. Make sure the entire well is covered.
8. Incubate the slides for 15 minutes at 37°C in a well-humidified chamber (see Exercise 13). **Note:** Do not let the reagent dry on the slide because this will cause dense staining around the perimeter of the well.
9. Rinse the slide for 5 to 10 seconds with a gentle stream of distilled water. Hold the slide at an angle and aim the stream of water at the slide surface above the well so that the water flows down over the well. Do not spray the water directly on the well.
10. Shake off the excess water and air dry the slide thoroughly.
11. Add a drop of mounting fluid to each well and place a coverslip over each. Avoid air bubbles.
12. Immediately observe the slides using a suitable fluorescence microscope and a 100× oil immersion objective. Also observe the slide of the positive and negative control prepared by your instructor. **Note:** The cells with monoclonal antibody bound to them will fluoresce an apple-green color. This fluorescence is specific for *N. gonorrhoeae* and indicates a positive result.
13. Record your observations and results in the RESULTS section.

REFERENCES

Brock, T. D., et al. *Biology of Microorganisms*, 7th ed. Engelwood Cliffs, NJ: Prentice-Hall Publishers, 1994.

Kohler, G. and Milstein, C. Continuous Cultures of Fused Cells Secreting Antibody of Predefined Specificity. *Nature* 256(1975):495-497.

Milstein, C. Monoclonal Antibodies. *Scientific American* 243(1980):66-74.

Stevens, C. D. *Clinical Immunology and Serology, a Laboratory Perspective*. Philadelphia: F.A. Davis Co., 1996.

RESULTS

Unknown number_____

Results of fluorescent staining of A:_____

Results of fluorescent staining of B:_____

If you had a positive organism, draw or describe what you saw. Compare your observations to the control organisms (positive and negative control).

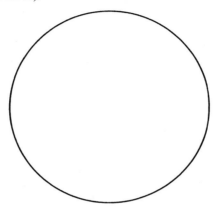

REFLECTIONS

1. Use your text or other sources to learn about one other way monoclonal antibodies are used (other than those already described), and write a short paragraph about it.

2. Before Kohler and Milstein developed their procedure, how were antibodies prepared and studied?

3. There are several methods available for analyzing specific drug metabolites in urine (also called drug testing). Speculate as to why use of monoclonal antibodies is so popular.

4. Name some limiting factors for routine use of fluorescent monoclonal antibodies in identifying organisms.

SECTION VIII

BIOTECHNOLOGY

The diverse metabolic capabilities of microorganisms have made microbes useful for the production of food, beverages, and a variety of other products. Since the metabolism of an organism is dictated by the genetic information contained in its genome, it is now possible to exploit the genetic information of microbes as well. The exploitation of the genetic and metabolic features of microbes has led to the development of an applied science called biotechnology. In this section, you will learn about some of the ways microbes are important to biotechnology.

EXERCISE 43

A DAY OF FEASTING COURTESY OF THE MICROBES

It is easy to focus on the microbes that cause disease, but it is misleading to do so. Most microbes are harmless and many are beneficial. In this exercise, you will learn how humans have exploited microbes for thousands of years, using them to create foodstuffs with a longer shelf life and other desirable characteristics, such as good taste. Bon appetit!

BACKGROUND INFORMATION

The items in bold in the menu are made or grown with the help of microbes. Humans have been exploiting microbes in this way for thousands of years—long before their discovery. For instance, there is evidence that humans have been making wine and other fermented beverages since the very beginning of civilization. Yet the role of microbes in making these beverages was not understood until the mid-1880s. At that time, Pasteur was asked by local vintners to determine why their wines were consistently sour. When Pasteur began his studies, the prevailing belief was that wine fermentation was the result of chemical, not biological, processes. But Pasteur had often observed yeast cells in wine and felt they might be important to alcohol production. His subsequent experiments clearly demonstrated that yeast cells oxidize sugars in grape juice under anaerobic conditions, producing carbon dioxide and ethanol as fermentation products. Furthermore, he showed that other

Suggested Menu

Breakfast
- Bagel with **cream cheese**
- **Coffee**, sugar and cream
- Orange juice

Lunch
- Hot dog smothered with **sauerkraut** and mustard, served on a **whole-wheat hot dog bun**
- **Root beer** and other **soft drinks**
- Potato chips
- **Cottage cheese** with fruit

Supper
- Antipasto: pepperoni slices, hot peppers, assorted **cheeses**
- Salad: lettuce, other greens, **olives** and tomatoes, served with a delightful oil and **vinegar** dressing and topped with a sprinkle of freshly grated **Parmesan cheese**
- Lasagna: layers of pasta, **ricotta cheese**, **mozzarella cheese**, spinach, **mushrooms** and **sausage**, smothered with tomato sauce and topped with a mixture of **Parmesan** and **Romano cheeses**
- **Garlic bread**
- **Fresh garden peas**

Dessert:
- **Frozen yogurt** sundaes with chocolate sauce, whipped cream, and **peanuts**

microbes in the grape juice, bacteria in particular, were responsible for making the wines "sick." This notion of "sick" wines and the role microbes played in causing the "sickness" eventually led to the first clear statement of the germ theory of disease.

Today microbes are used by industry to produce a variety of foods, food additives, pharmaceuticals, and chemicals (**Table 43.1**). In some cases, the desired product is a fermentation product made when microbes are cultivated anaerobically. But there are also a variety of products produced when microbes grow aerobically. Unfortunately for many beginning microbiology students, industry refers to both aerobic and anaerobic industrial processes as fermentations. In this exercise, you have the opportunity to explore the role of microbes in the production of yogurt and sauerkraut.

Yogurt is a fermented dairy product made by the action of two bacteria, *Streptococcus thermophilus* (a Gram-positive coccus) and *Lactobacillus bulgaricus*

(a Gram-positive rod). The inoculum that contains these bacteria is from a starter culture—typically, a previous batch of yogurt. Both bacteria catabolize lactose (milk sugar) and produce the fermentation product, lactic acid. Lactic acid alters the milk protein, casein, and this causes the milk to thicken to a typical yogurt-consistency.

Sauerkraut is also a product of microbial fermentation. The bacteria of importance for sauerkraut production are coliforms (see Exercise 29), *Leuconostoc mesenteroides* (a Gram-positive coccus), and *Lactobacillus plantarum* (a Gram-positive rod). All are found naturally on cabbage (from which sauerkraut is made) and all are lactic acid producers. In addition, *L. mesenteroides* and *L. plantarum* are salt tolerant. Similar bacteria are also important in the production of pickles and vinegar.

In this exercise, you will make yogurt and sauerkraut. You will examine the characteristics of

TABLE 43.1 Products Made by Microorganisms

Product	Microbe
Foods	
Ripened cheeses	*Streptococcus* spp., *Leuconostoc* spp., *Propionibacterium*
Yogurt	*Streptococcus thermophilus, Lactobacillus bulgaricus*
Sausages and hams	*Aspergillus, Penicillium* spp., *Pediococcus cerevisiae*
Coffee beans	*Erwinia dissolvens, Saccharomyces* spp.
Olives	*Leuconostoc mesenteroides, Lactobacillus plantarum*
Sauerkraut	*Leuconostoc mesenteroides, Lactobacillus plantarum*
Soy sauce	*Aspergillus oryzae, Aspergillus soyae, Saccharomyces rouxii*
Tempeh	*Rhizopus oligosporus, Rhizopus oryzae*
Bread	*Saccharomyces cerevisiae*
Sourdough bread	*Saccharomyces exiguus, Lactobacillus sanfrancisco*
Beverages	
Root beer	*Saccharomyces cerevisiae*
Beer	*Saccharomyces carlsbergensis*
Ale	*Saccharomyces cerevisiae*
Wine	*Saccharomyces cerevisiae*
Jamaican rum	Wild yeasts
Antibiotics	
Penicillin	*Penicillium notatum*
Tetracycline	*Streptomyces aureofaciens*
Erythromycin	*Streptomyces erythraeus*
Streptomycin	*Streptomyces griseus*
Enzymes	
β-Amylase (for brewing)	*Bacillus subtilis*
Lactase (digestive aid for individuals with lactose intolerance)	*Escherichia coli*
Streptokinase (breaks down blood clots)	*Streptococcus* spp.
Subtilisins (laundry detergents)	*Bacillus subtilis*

the milk and cabbage during the course of the fermentation. Based on the data you collect, you will draw conclusions about the changes that occur to these foods and the succession of microbes that cause those changes.

PURPOSE

- To prepare some foods that are made in part by the activities of microorganisms
- To learn about the changes made in the starting materials (e.g., cabbage and milk) as the food product is made

THE EXERCISE

Part A: Making Yogurt

MATERIALS:

Powdered milk
Beaker
pH strips
Microscopes
Sterile applicator sticks
Stove or hot plates for heating milk
Whole milk
Plain yogurt containing live culture
Microscope slides
45°C incubator
Six large screw cap tubes or other containers

PROCEDURE: Work in pairs

1. Dissolve 4 g of powdered milk in 100 ml of whole milk in a beaker. **Note:** The powdered milk adds more milk solids and improves the consistency of the yogurt.
2. Heat the solution to boiling.
3. Cool the solution to 45°C.
4. Measure the pH of the milk with a pH strip and record in the RESULTS section. Also note the odor and consistency of the milk.
5. Add 2 ml of plain yogurt to the milk and stir with an applicator stick to mix thoroughly.
6. Prepare a *thin* smear of the milk by mixing a small amount of the milk with a drop of water. Gram stain and examine it (Exercise 6). Note the morphology and Gram reaction of the microbes observed. Determine the percentage of Gram-positive cocci and the percentage of Gram-positive rods in one field or average several fields (percentage Gram-positive cocci in one field = number Gram-positive cocci counted in field/total

number bacteria counted in field × 100). Record your observations in the RESULTS section.
7. Dispense the inoculated milk into 6 screw-cap tubes or other containers. Label the tubes 1 through 6.
8. Incubate the tubes at 45°C for 6 hours.
9. At 1 hour intervals, either you or your instructor should remove a tube and refrigerate it. Remove tube 1 after 1 hour of incubation, remove tube 2 after 2 hours of incubation, and so on until the last tube has been refrigerated. The tubes will remain refrigerated until the next laboratory period.

Day 2

1. Test the pH of the milk in each tube. Record your results in the RESULTS section.
2. Observe the odor and consistency of the milk in each tube. Record your observations in the RESULTS section.
3. Prepare *thin* smears of the milk in each tube by mixing a small amount of the milk with a drop of water. Gram stain and examine the smears.
4. Determine the percentage of Gram-positive cocci and Gram-positive rods in one field of each smear. Record your results in the RESULTS section.
5. Graph the change in pH over time by plotting time on the x-axis and pH on the y-axis.
6. Graph the percentage of Gram-positive cocci and Gram-positive rods over time in a single graph. **Note:** Both graphs can be done on one of the sheets of graph paper provided.

Part B: Making Sauerkraut

MATERIALS:

Cabbage
Knife
pH strips
Gram stain reagents
Wide-mouth canning jar and lid
Salt
Microscope slides
Microscope

PROCEDURE: Work in pairs

1. Remove the outer leaves of the cabbage, as well as any damaged leaves. Wash thoroughly.
2. Cut the cabbage in half, remove the core, then shred the cabbage by cutting each half lengthwise into thin strips.
3. Measure 100 g of shredded cabbage.
4. To the 100 g of shredded cabbage, add 3 g of salt. Mix thoroughly and tightly pack into the

wide-mouth jar. Be careful not to bruise the leaves. **Note:** Due to the difference in salt concentration inside and outside the cabbage leaf cells, water moves out of the cells. This creates the liquid in which the cabbage will ferment.

5. When enough juice is available to sample, remove some and set aside. **Note:** This is the zero-time sample for this experiment.

6. Use a pH strip to measure the pH of the juice collected at zero time. Record the pH in the RESULTS section.

7. Place the lid on the jar and incubate at room temperature for up 21 days or longer.

8. Prepare a Gram stain of the juice removed at zero time. Note the morphology and Gram reaction of the microbes in the juice. Also note their relative abundance. Record your observations in the RESULTS section.

9. At 2, 7, 14, and 21 days, repeat steps 5 through 8 on juice removed from the jar. Record your observations in the RESULTS section.

10. Graph pH change over time.

REFERENCES

Rose, A.H. *Industrial Microbiology.* Washington, DC: Butterworth, Inc., 1961.

Demain, A.L. and Soloman, N.A. *Biology of Industrial Microorganisms.* Menlo Park, CA: Benjamin/Cummings Publishing Company, Inc., 1985.

RESULTS

Record your observations of the milk in the table below.

Time (hours)	pH	Other Observations
0		
1		
2		
3		
4		
5		
6		

Record your observations of the cabbage juice in the table below.

Time (Days)	pH	Observations of Gram Stains
0		
2		
7		
14		
21		

REFLECTIONS

1. At what pH and time did the milk become yogurt?

2. Examine the graphs you generated from making yogurt. Do your graphs support this statement: *L. bulgaricus* grows better at lower pH values than does *S. thermophilus*? Explain.

3. Summarize the changes in microbial population you observed during the cabbage fermentation. Can you correlate the relative abundance of the different microbes with pH changes? Explain.

4. Both sauerkraut and yogurt have a much longer shelf life than fresh milk and cabbage. What characteristics of these fermented foods increase their shelf life?

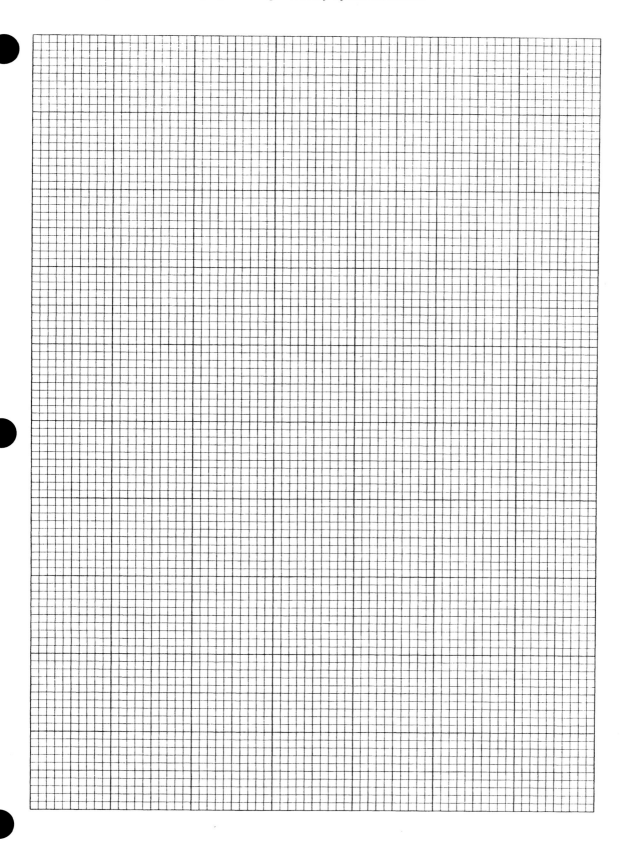

10 X 10 PER INCH

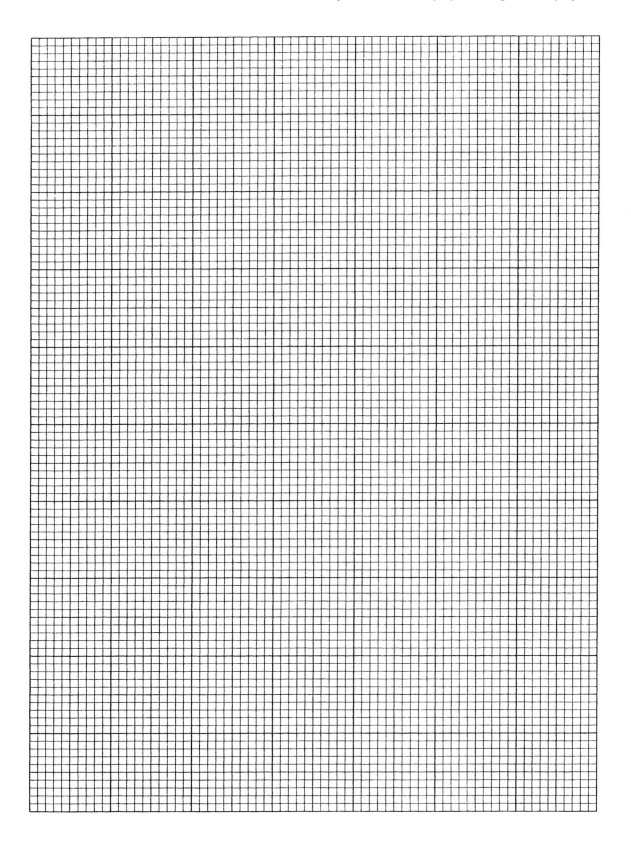

10 X 10 PER INCH

BIOFILMS AND SPACEFLIGHT

Bacteria, through many different mechanisms, can attach and irreversibly adhere to any surface in an aquatic environment. This growth on the surface is called a **biofilm.** Biofilms can spell trouble to space shuttles, industrial water distribution systems, and even huge ships traveling in the ocean. Biofilms are also tremendous problems in medical devices. A film of resistant bacteria can build up in a patient's catheter and be a constant source of infection unless removed. During this exercise, you will observe the resistance of biofilms to disinfectants.

Al is an engineer who works for a large firm that has contracts with the National Aeronautics and Space Administration (NASA). He is responsible for monitoring water quality on the space shuttle before and after each flight. Everything is going well as the technicians begin to fill the 100-gallon water tank on the shuttle 2 months before launch. Al then saturates the water with iodine to kill any microorganisms. About 2 weeks before the flight and just after the shuttle is on the launchpad, Al begins monitoring the water supply for microorganisms. He activates the pumping system and the water goes through a resin cartridge that absorbs most of the concentrated iodine from the water. The cartridge, also called an iodine check valve, releases iodine automatically whenever the level of iodine falls below 2 to 4 mg/L. Al samples the system and sends water samples to a microbiology laboratory for testing. The samples are negative, indicating there are no bacteria isolated. He continues to monitor the water regularly and suddenly, 3 days before the flight, testing indicates 10^6 colony forming units (CFU) of bacteria/ml of water. Normal drinking water

has ~10^5 CFU/ml of heterotrophic bacteria, but NASA's standards for water quality are much more stringent (<1 CFU/ml). The standards are stricter because there is evidence that after humans spend time in microgravity, their immune systems are suppressed. Immunosuppression may lead to increased susceptibility to waterborne organisms that are not normally pathogenic. Al and his associates decide to shock the system by resaturating the water with iodine. After the iodine is removed by the resin cartridge, new samples are taken. It is now 24 hours before launch and test results from the lab indicate the samples still have 10^3 CFU of bacteria/ml of water. Al immediately calls together a group of engineers and consulting microbiologists. He has to make a quick recommendation as to whether NASA should scrub the launch or suspend the water standards. It is too late to start another treatment and test for microorganisms. What will Al do? Will they launch the shuttle?

BACKGROUND INFORMATION

The shuttle will probably be launched because the water standards will be suspended. NASA water standards are very high (<1 CFU/ml) compared to normal drinking water standards (~10^5 CFU/ml). They will launch the shuttle because the risk of infection is small and delaying a spaceflight costs time and money. However, high water standards for the protection of the space crew is not a trivial matter. In addition to the problem of decreased immunity in crews after prolonged spaceflight, there is evidence that bacteria grow faster in microgravity and that they have an increased resistance to antibiotics. Therefore, NASA is constantly studying the problem of maintaining and monitoring pure water systems on their spacecraft. In addition, the international space station will need a system of reclaiming and monitoring contaminated water, or prolonged occupation of the station will not be possible.

One reason for bacteria being present in the water system of the shuttle may have been the formation of a biofilm somewhere in the system. When biofilms are formed, they are extremely resistant to disinfectants or antibiotics. On occasion, there is sloughing of bacteria from the biofilms and this could be the reason bacteria were detected 3 days before the launch. NASA has chosen iodine as the disinfectant for their treatment systems, but scientists have learned that bacteria are becoming more and more resistant to iodine and other disinfectants. In fact, while iodine eliminated bacteria and biofilm formation in simulated space vehicles, it was ineffective in eliminating biofilm formation in a recycled water system. Bacteria such as pseudomonads, which form biofilms, can develop increased resistance to large doses of iodine (1.0 mg/L) over time.

How and why do bacteria form biofilms? Bacteria are remarkably responsive to the environment in which they live. Being responsive is a universal strategy for their survival. It has been found that the cell walls of bacteria growing in nutrient-poor environments differ radically from those bacteria growing in a suspension of nutrients. Cell wall characteristics and enzymatic activity in cells attached to surfaces can be quite different from the characteristics exhibited by planktonic cells, which

are cells in suspension. Furthermore, during the formation of a biofilm, physiological changes may occur. Attached cells change their metabolism to accommodate the new nutrients available for their use.

The formation of a biofilm is illustrated in **Figure 44.1.** Bacterial cells will float along a surface and eventually adhere to it. At first this association is reversible, but eventually it becomes irreversible because the cells form adhesions. These adhesions can be the result of a cell's ability to produce exopolysaccharide (polysaccharides outside the cell), which form a glycocalyx. Within the glycocalyx matrix, the cell divides and forms microcolonies. In addition, bacteria floating nearby the microcolony can be recruited into the matrix and become embedded within it. Eventually an adherent multispecies biofilm is formed.

Sometimes bacteria within biofilms form discrete microcolonies on the surface of metal and the bacteria bind the metal. Their metabolic activity lowers the pH and this results in a pitting or corrosion of the metal. Once pitting of the metal begins, the surface has to be scraped or removed by some other means to prevent further corrosion. Biofouling of industrial pipelines is a source of many kinds of contamination, as well as a source of corrosion. Biofilms can cost an industry millions of dollars when processing systems have to be replaced. They

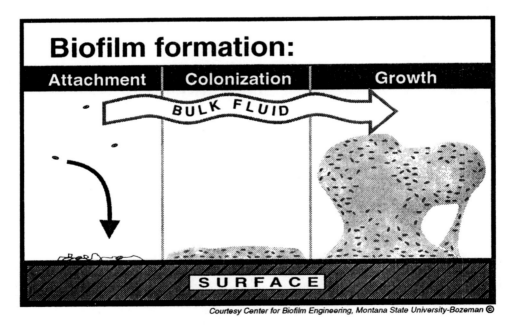

Courtesy Center for Biofilm Engineering, Montana State University-Bozeman ©

Figure 44.1 Biofilm formation due to cell association and adherence (attachment); formation of microcolonies and recruitment of other bacteria (colonization); and biofilm formation (growth).

are also a big concern in the medical community. Bacteria will attach to the inside surface of a patient's catheter or tubing (e.g., intravenous, gastric, or abdominal) and form a biofilm. Because biofilm bacteria are resistant to antibiotics and slough off from the surface occasionally, they are a constant source of infection to a patient. In fact, in most cases when biofilms have formed, the only way to stop the infection is to remove the tubes.

Scientists now believe that controlling biofilms is of major importance in water distribution systems. They have also come to realize that preventing attachment and biofilm formation may require many different methods of physical disruption, disinfection, or filtration. Therefore, the water system in the space shuttle and space station will probable employ combinations of disinfection and filtration methods to stay one step of ahead of bacteria.

During this exercise, you will make biofilms of *Klebsiella pneumoniae* on glass slides. Then you will treat the biofilms and remaining planktonic bacteria with different concentrations of chlorine disinfectant, or bleach. Each group of four people will use a different concentration of bleach and your results will be shared with other groups in the class.

PURPOSE

- To determine resistance of bacteria in a biofilm to the disinfectant chlorine
- To compare the resistance of attached bacteria in a biofilm to bacteria growing in suspension

THE EXERCISE

MATERIALS:

Sterile, wide-mouth 125 ml flask with two microscope slides slanted against each other (**Figure 44.2**)
100 ml of sterile 1/10 strength tryptic soy broth (TSB)
Four nutrient agar plates
Sterile tips
TSB broth
0.5 McFarland standard (barium chloride standard)
Two sterile rubber policemen
Fresh bleach diluted 1:10
10% sodium thiosulfate
Twenty tubes each containing 9 ml of sterile saline
Sterile 1 ml pipets or micropipetters and pipet tips
One beaker with 100 ml of sterile water
One beaker with 100 ml of sterile saline
2- to 4-hour broth culture of *K. pneumoniae*

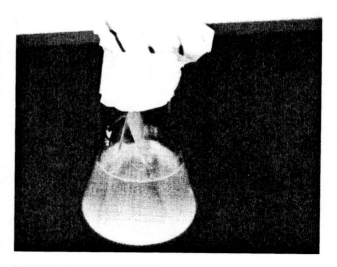

Figure 44.2 Wide-mouth flask with slides after incubation.

PROCEDURE: Work in groups of four

Day 1: Preparation of Biofilm

1. Aseptically pour the 100 ml of sterile 1/10 strength TSB broth into the sterile flask containing two glass slides.

2. Obtain a 2 to 4 hour culture of *K. pneumoniae* and compare the density of the growth in the tube to a 0.5 McFarland standard. Dilute the broth to the equivalent density if necessary. This density is approximately 1×10^8 bacteria/ml.

3. Add 0.01 ml of the diluted culture to the biofilm flask. Diluting 0.01 ml in 100 ml of broth will result in approximately 1×10^4 bacteria/ml in the flask.

4. Incubate the flask on a shaker at room temperature for 18 to 24 hours at 50 to 100 RPM. **Note:** *K. pneumoniae* is nonmotile, so shaking the flask not only speeds up the attachment of cells, but it also provides a flow of nutrients over the surface of the slides, important to biofilm formation.

Day 2: Chlorine Treatment

1. Obtain one nutrient agar plate for each group member.

2. With a marking pen, divide the plate into 6 equal sectors as shown at the top of p. 310. Label the sectors 1 through 6. **Note:** The procedure used for determining the quantity of bacteria in the broth and the biofilm is called a **spot inoculation**

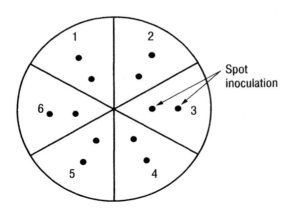

Spot inoculation

procedure. By using this procedure, only one plate is needed instead of six.

3. Each member of the group will perform one part of the study (person A, B, C, or D) and your results will be combined for analysis. Label your plate appropriately (A, B, C, or D). Each person will make the same dilutions and use the same procedure for plating the organism. However, each of you will perform a different part of the experiment prior to diluting and plating.

Person A: Measuring Biofilm Bacteria—No Chlorine Treatment

a. With sterile forceps, carefully remove one of the slides from the flask and place it in a beaker with 100 ml of sterile saline.

b. With a sterile rubber policeman (**Figure 44.3**), scrape the biofilm from both the front and back of the slide into the saline.

c. Thoroughly mix the solution to resuspend any particles in clumps.

d. Remove 1 ml of the solution and add it to the first 9 ml tube of your dilution series. Using a new pipet or pipet tip, mix and transfer 1 ml to the second tube. Use this procedure to dilute the microorganism through five tube dilutions as indicated on top of the following page.

e. Obtain 0.01 ml (10 μl) from tube 1 and spot inoculate one area in the first section of your plate (see drawing of plate above). **Note:** After incubation, you will observe either confluent growth in one spot or isolated colonies (**Figure 44.4**).

f. Repeat this step and inoculate another spot in the· same section of the plate. **Note:** The number of colonies for each replicate of each dilution will be averaged to obtain a more accurate number of the CFU/ml.

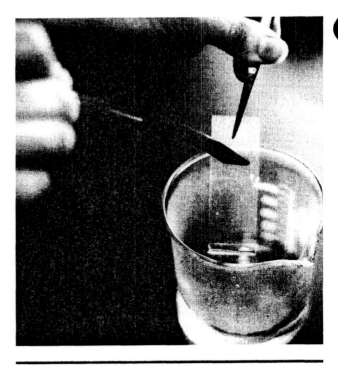

Figure 44.3 A slide with a biofilm of bacteria being scraped with a rubber policeman.

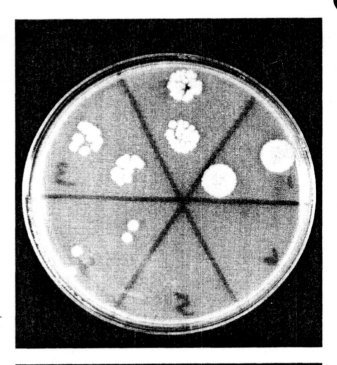

Figure 44.4 A spot inoculation plate.

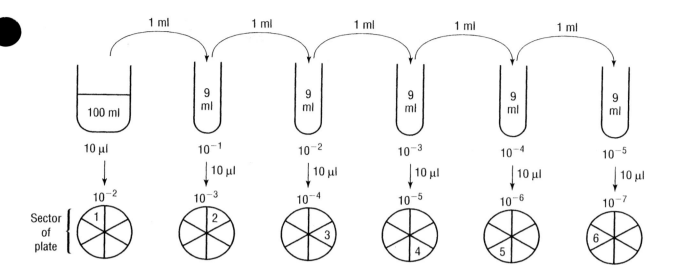

g. Transfer 10 μl from each dilution tube to each corresponding section of the plate (see above). Make a duplicate inoculation with each solution. Use a new pipet tip for each new dilution.

h. Let the plate dry, invert and incubate the plate for 24 hours at 35°C.

Person B: Measuring Biofilm Bacteria—Chlorine Treatment

a. To the beaker containing 100 ml of sterile water, add the appropriate concentration of chlorine bleach. Your instructor will assign your group a concentration to test. **Note:** To obtain 2.5 parts per million (ppm) of chlorine, you would add 0.05 ml of diluted (1:10) bleach to the 100 ml. If you are testing 1.5, 2.0, 3.0 ppm, or other dilutions, make the calculations for determining the amount of chlorine bleach to add.

b. With sterile forceps, carefully remove the other slide from the flask and place it in the beaker of sterile water with bleach.

c. Let the slide stand for 10 minutes.

d. After 10 minutes, add 0.05 ml of 10% sodium thiosulfate to the solution. **Note:** Sodium thiosulfate neutralizes the chlorine to stop the killing effect.

e. With a sterile rubber policeman, scrape the biofilm from the slide (front and back) and try to resuspend any large particles that may not be in suspension. Remove the slide from the solution and follow the same steps for diluting and plating the organisms (steps d through h) as for person A.

Person C: Measuring Planktonic Bacteria—No Chlorine Treatment

a. You will determine the number of bacteria in the suspension. Mix the flask thoroughly to resuspend the organisms that may have settled on the bottom.

b. Follow the same steps for diluting and plating the organisms (steps d through h) as for person A.

Person D: Measuring Planktonic Bacteria—Chlorine Treatment

a. After person C has extracted the quantity needed for their procedure (1.0 ml and 0.01 ml), add bleach to the flask. Use the same concentration of diluted bleach that was used to treat the biofilm.

b. Gently mix the chlorine with the solution of planktonic bacteria and let stand for 10 minutes.

c. After 10 minutes, add 0.05 ml of sodium thiosulfate to stop the reaction.

d. Follow the same steps for diluting and plating the organisms (steps d through h) as for person A.

Day 3: Reading Your Results

1. Each person will determine the CFU/ml on the plate they prepared. To do this, find the dilution that has between 3 and 30 colonies in a spot and count the number of visible colonies (**Figure 44.4**).

2. Average the number from the two replicates and multiple by the dilution factor. For example, if an average of four colonies was observed in sector four of your plate your colony count is 4.0×10^5 CFU/ml.

3. Record your results in the RESULTS section and complete the table with the results from the other people in your group.
4. Share your results with other groups in your class and graph CFU/ml versus chlorine concentration by plotting chlorine concentration on the x-axis and CFU/ml on the y-axis, using either the 2-cycle or 4-cycle graph paper included. Use an × for before and an ○ for after treatment for both biofilm and planktonic organisms.

REFERENCES

Costerton, J.W., et al. Bacterial Biofilms in Nature and Disease. *Annual Reviews in Microbiology* 41(1987):435-464.

McFeters, G.A., et al. Disinfection Susceptibility of Waterborne Pseudomonads and Legionellae Under Simulated Space Vehicle Conditions. (*SAE Technical Paper Series 911402*, 21st International Conference on Environmental Systems, San Francisco, CA, July 15-18, 1991).

Pyle, B.H., et al. Microbiological Concerns and Methodological Approaches Related to Bacterial Water Quality in Spaceflight. (*SAE Technical Paper Series 921232*, 22nd International Conference on Environmental Systems, Seattle, WA, July 13-16, 1992).

Pyle, B.H., et al. Physiological Aspects of Disinfection Resistance in *Pseudomonas cepacia, Journal of Applied Bacteriology* 76(1994):142-148.

Yu, Feipeng P, et al. A Direct Viable Count Method for the Enumeration of Attached Bacteria and Assessment of Biofilm Disinfection. *Journal of Microbiological Methods* 17(1993):167-180.

RESULTS

No Chlorine Treatment Group

Treatment Group	Person A: Biofilm (CFU/ml)	Person C: Planktonic (CFU/ml)
1.5 ppm		
2.0 ppm		
2.5 ppm		
3.0 ppm		
Other: _____		

Chlorine Treatment Group

Concentration of Chlorine	Person B: Biofilm (CFU/ml)	Person D: Planktonic (CFU/ml)
1.5 ppm		
2.0 ppm		
2.5 ppm		
3.0 ppm		
Other: _____		

REFLECTIONS

1. Was there any killing of bacteria in the biofilm and in the planktonic solution with your treatment of chlorine?

2. Using the class information, did increasing the concentration of chlorine affect the number of bacteria in both the biofilm and planktonic culture?

3. Were the biofilms more resistant, the same, or less resistant to disinfection with chlorine bleach?

4. Speculate as to why bacteria associated with biofilms in catheters are much more resistant to antibiotics.

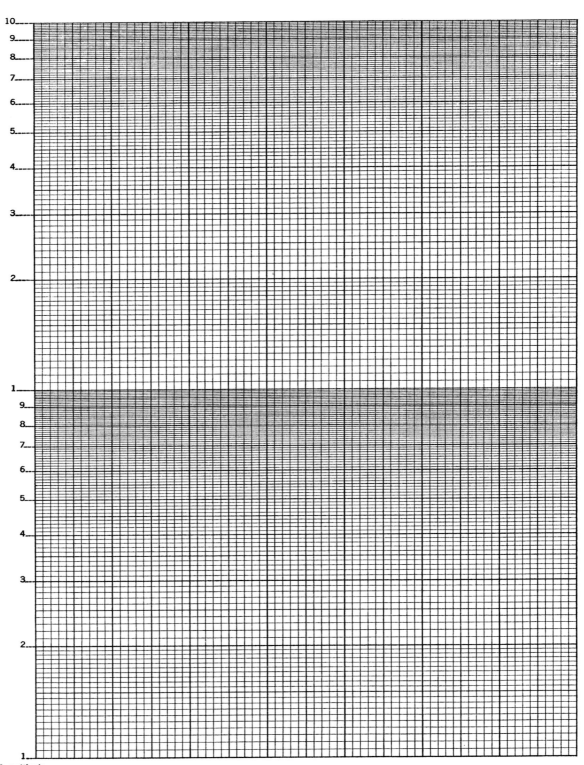

Semi-Logarithmic
2 Cycles x 10 to the inch

SEMI-LOGARITHMIC
4 CYCLES × 10 DIVISIONS PER INCH

EXERCISE 45

THE PROBLEM WITH PACKING MATERIALS

This exercise will allow you to use your knowledge about microbes to solve a problem. Put yourself in this person's place and prove that the product you and your fellow workers have developed is biodegradable. Who knows, you may be solving similar problems someday.

*You have just been hired to work for a large manufacturer who supplies boxes and packing materials to companies all over the world. One of the jobs you are asked to investigate is the development of a biodegradable packing material similar in size and shape to the white packaging peanuts your company already produces (**Figure 45.1**). You and your company are concerned because the current styrofoam peanuts you produce take years to degrade in the environment. After some thinking and work with company engineers and a consulting chemist, you develop a peanut made from cornstarch. It is the same size and shape and will provide the same cushioning effect as the original "peanuts," but it has a darker appearance. You are still faced with the task of convincing your boss that the new cornstarch peanut is biodegradable and should be manufactured. You know that starch is a large molecule that can be broken down to monomers by certain enzymes called amylases, and that many bacteria produce amylases. You also know that starch turns blue in the presence of iodine. You have already designed a medium that contains cornstarch peanuts. Now your task is to design an experiment that will prove to your company managers that these new peanuts will be easily broken down in the environment and that you have produced an environmentally safe product.*

BACKGROUND INFORMATION

Biodegradation of organic materials like the starch peanuts is taking place all the time in our compost piles, landfills, and sewage treatment plants. These processes can be broadly viewed as **bioremediation** because they rely on microorganisms to degrade unwanted wastes. Other bioremediation efforts which have received much more attention are the use of microorganisms (usually bacteria and fungi) to degrade pollutants in soils or waters contaminated with oil, pesticides, or carcinogens. Using microorganisms to degrade substances is attractive because microbes are relatively inexpensive, readily available, and their use avoids costly collection and delivery of materials such as contaminated soils.

There are some problems with bioremediation, though, and it is not a cure for all our environmental contamination problems. Sometimes, microorganisms produce other toxic products during the degradation process. Even if they don't, microbes are only effective at biodegradation if environmental conditions such as temperature and available nutrients, permit their growth, and if they degrade contaminants relatively rapidly. For instance, many microbes degrade some pollutants such as DDT very slowly and fail completely to degrade some synthetic compounds such as plastic polymers.

Your task is to design an experiment that demonstrates biodegradation of packing materials. If you can successfully prove that these new cornstarch peanuts are biodegradable in our environment, these materials will help eliminate one of the major waste materials in our landfills—styrofoam packing materials.

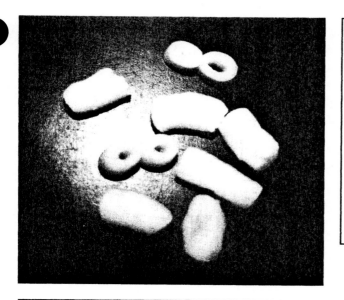

Figure 45.1 Typical packaging "peanuts."

PURPOSE

- To design, conduct, and report on an experiment that tests the biodegradability of cornstarch peanuts

THE EXERCISE

MATERIALS:

Cornstarch "peanut" agar plates
Other supplies or microorganisms as requested
Iodine

PROCEDURE: Work in groups of two to three

1. You will be given agar plates that have been prepared by the procedure above.

Preparation of Peanut Cornstarch Medium

1. Dispense 300 ml of distilled water into an Erlenmeyer flask and warm it in a microwave or on a heating block.
2. Add 6 or 7 cornstarch peanuts and mix until dissolved. This gives approximately a 0.4% solution of starch. The warm water ensures the cornstarch is completely dissolved.
3. Add 6.9 g of nutrient agar to the flask and mix.
4. Autoclave the flask for 15 minutes at 121°C and 15 PSI.
5. Aseptically pour the medium into 8 to 10 Petri plates and allow to solidify for several hours.

Optional: Your instructor may ask that you prepare the plates to give you experience in media preparation.
2. With your group, discuss an experimental approach to test for starch breakdown by bacteria. Remember, both positive and negative controls are an important part of any experimental design.
3. Briefly write down your procedure and have your experiment approved by your instructor before proceeding. Materials are available (within reason), so don't hesitate to be creative in your design.
4. Proceed with your experiment.
5. Record your procedure and results in the RESULTS section.
6. Write a laboratory report explaining the testing procedures and results. Follow the format used in scientific journals (introduction, experimental methods, results, and conclusions) to write your paper. Refer to Appendix B for a discussion of this format.

RESULTS

Record the procedures and results below.

PROCEDURE:

RESULTS:

HOW LENSES, MAGNIFIERS, AND MICROSCOPES WORK

HOW LENSES WORK

The type of lens most familiar to people is the **converging lens.** A converging lens is one that is thicker in the middle than it is at the ends. It is said to be converging because parallel rays of light approaching the lens from one side are bent by the lens in such a way that they all meet, or (converge) at a single point on the other side of the lens (**Figure A.1**). This point is called the **focal point,** and the distance from the focal point to the center of the lens is called the **focal length.**

In **Figure A.1a,** the light rays approach the lens from the left and converge on the right. The figure is drawn like this because the most common convention used in optics is to represent the movement of light rays from left to right. This convention was probably adopted because the scientists developing the theories of optics in the 1600s were European and read from left to right. Had they been Chinese, the convention would probably be that rays move from right to left. We make this point because if **Figure A.1a** was redrawn so that the rays were traveling from right to left, then another focal point would be defined (**Figure A.1b**). In other words, all converging lenses have two focal points, one on either side of the lens, which are the same distance from the center of the lens. The focal point on the left represents the point of convergence of rays coming from the right of the lens; and the focal point on the right represents the point of convergence of rays coming from the left of the lens.

An important question is, why is the light bent by the lens? When light passes through a medium such as air, water, or glass, it travels at a speed slower than

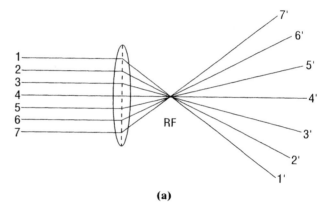

(a)

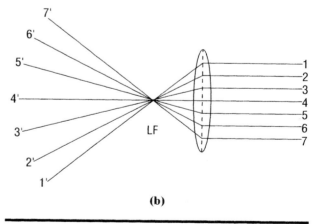

(b)

Figure A.1 Pathway of light through a converging lens: (a) light moving from left to right defines the right focal point (RF); (b) light moving from right to left defines the left focal point (LF).

when it travels through a vacuum. When light passes obliquely from one medium to another, it is bent, or (refracted) at the junction of the two media. We have all had experiences with this phenomenon. Think of what a stick looks like when it is partially submerged in water. It looks as though it is bent; the bend occurs at the junction of the water and the air. If the stick is totally submerged and we are trying to locate it while looking from above the water, its position seems to be slightly shifted in space. Both of these alterations in appearance are the result of the refraction that occurs when light hits the interface of air and water.

It is the ability of a lens to change the path of light that allows it to create an image. What the image looks like, however, is dependent on the location of the object being viewed with respect to the focal point of the lens. **Figures A.2, A.3,** and **A.4** show three possible locations of an object and the image formed in each case. There are features common to each of these figures. The object is an arrow placed to the left of the lens. The top of the object (T for top) is represented by the point of the arrow. From the very tip of the arrow point, light rays are traveling towards the lens at all possible angles. Some of the possible light rays are shown in the inset in **Figure A.2**. Each ray that passes through the lens will be refracted and sent on a new course (except one, but more on that in a moment.) However, trying to see what will happen to all the pos-

sible rays emanating from the tip of the arrow is not practical, and more importantly unnecessary. That's because two particular rays of light are easy to trace, and will serve to define the very tip of the arrow in the image created. The first ray (ray 1) is parallel to the horizontal axis of the lens. This ray is refracted such that it passes through the right focal point (RF) of the lens. The second easily traced ray (ray 2) passes through the center of the lens. The center of the lens is indicated by point C in each figure, and is defined as the junction of the horizontal and vertical axes of the lens. The path of this ray is shown as being unaltered because the bending of the light when it enters the lens is canceled by the bending as it exits. Thus there is no net change in the path of the light.

The two rays described above define the top of the image (T') created by the lens. For each point along the length of the arrow, equivalent rays could be used to define the corresponding point in the image. However, we need only trace those easily traced light rays coming from the bottom of the object. What we see is that for the very bottom tip of the object (B for bottom), only a single ray (ray 3) need be traced. That's because we've simplified matters by placing the bottom of the object on the horizontal axis of the lens. Thus, the ray coming from the bottom point of the object that is parallel to the horizontal axis of the lens is also the ray that passes through the center of the lens. As you can see, that ray

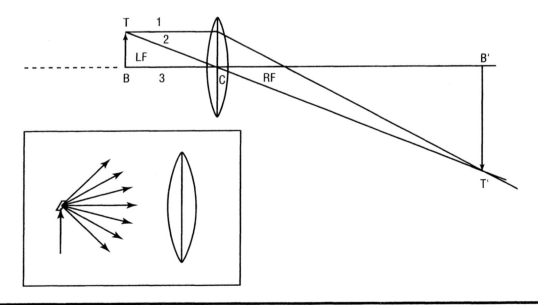

Figure A.2   A real magnified image: **T, B:** top and bottom of the arrow respectively; **T'B':** top and bottom of the image of the arrow; **C:** center of the lens.

passes unaltered through the lens. Now let's examine each figure in closer detail to determine how the placement of the object relative to the left focal point (LF) affects the nature of the image produced.

Figure A.2 shows how a lens can be used to create a **real image** that is larger than the actual object. A real image is one that really exists and can be projected onto a surface such as a wall. When the object is placed between one and two focal lengths from the lens, rays 1 and 2, which come from the top of the object, pass through the lens and meet on the other side at point T'. T', then, is the point of the arrow in the image. Ray 3, which comes from the bottom of the arrow, is used to define the bottom of the arrow in the image. Since the object is a vertical line, by drawing a vertical line from T' to ray 3, B' is located, and we can see the image created by the lens. There are two things to note about this image. First, it is inverted. Second, it is magnified. The object was drawn as 1 cm in length. The image, though inverted, is about 3 cm in length. Thus the image is larger than the object.

Figure A.3 shows the same lens and same object, but this time the object is even farther to the left of the left focal point. In fact, it is slightly farther than twice the focal length of the lens. In this case, rays 1 and 2 meet at a point that is much closer to the right focal point of the lens. As a result, T' and B' are much closer together, and the image of the arrow is real and inverted, but smaller than the actual arrow.

Figure A.4 shows the creation of a very different kind of image—the **virtual image.** A virtual image is created when the object is less than one focal length from the lens. Rays 1 and 2 drawn from the tip of the arrow point pass through the lens, but do not meet on the other side. If you imagine yourself to the right of the lens, then each eye receives one of the light rays. The interpretation the brain makes is that both of these rays are generated from a single point. In essence, the brain extends rays 1 and 2 toward the left (away from the eye) until the two rays meet. That point is defined by the brain as T'. By necessity, ray 3 is also extended to the left. The line drawn from T' to

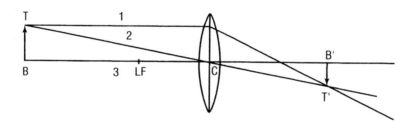

Figure A.3   A real but smaller image. **T, B, T', B',** and **C** are as defined in **Figure A.2.**

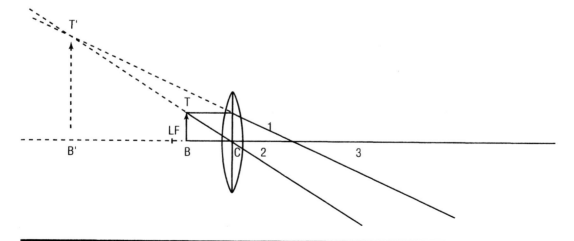

Figure A.4   A virtual image. **T, B, T', B',** and **C** are defined as in **Figure A.2.**

ray 3 defines B', and the line between T' and B' defines the image. This is not a real image, however. It cannot be projected onto a surface like a real image can. In fact, there is no image, only the mind's interpretation that the light rays coming from T and B seem to be coming from T' and B'. Another important difference between a virtual image and a real image is that a virtual image is not inverted. Although the image is not real, it is bigger than the object, so again we see an image that appears to be larger than the object actually is.

A summary is appropriate. If an object is placed more than one focal length but less than two focal lengths from the lens, then the image created will be a real image that is larger than the object. If the object is placed more than two focal lengths from the lens, the image created is real, but smaller than the object. Finally, if the object is placed less then one focal length from the lens, then the image created is a virtual image that is larger than the object. With that understanding of optics, let's look at two common tools for magnifying: the magnifying glass and the compound light microscope.

MAGNIFYING GLASSES AND MICROSCOPES

Magnifying glasses are simple magnifiers that consist of a single lens. If you think back to the times when you have used a magnifying glass, you will probably recall that the object viewed looked larger, but was not inverted. Since the image was upright, this means that the image you saw was a virtual image produced by positioning the object so that it was less than one focal length from the lens of the magnifier.

The compound light microscope uses two lenses sequentially to create a final image. The objective lens has a short focal length and the specimen is positioned between one and two focal lengths away from the lens. Thus, the image produced by the objective lens is a real image. It is inverted and magnified. The ocular lens is positioned such that it creates a virtual image of the real image produced by the objective lens. In other words, the ocular lens is magnifying the image made by the objective lens. The final image, then, is larger and inverted.

Most compound light microscopes look something like the microscope shown in **Figure 4.1** and work in the following way. The specimen being examined is fixed to a microscope slide which is placed on the stage of the microscope. Stage clips are used to hold the slide in place. The light used to view the specimen comes from below the specimen. It may be light from a window or from a separate light source. The light is directed toward the specimen, and the amount of light is controlled by the diaphragm. The beam of light, if directed properly, will strike the specimen on the slide. Three things can happen to the light. It can be scattered by some component of the specimen, it can be absorbed by some component of the specimen, or it can pass through the specimen. The light that passes through the specimen continues up through the objective lens. Many microscopes have two or three different objective lenses of different power located on a revolving nosepiece. A particular objective lens can be used by simply rotating the nosepiece into position above the specimen. The objective lens uses the light passing through it to create a magnified real image in the tube separating the objective and ocular lenses. The focusing knobs located on the arm of the microscope move the stage up or down so that the object is the appropriate distance from the objective and a clear image is created. The image in the tube is then magnified by the ocular lens, as described above, and you see an inverted, backward image. This is important to remember when moving the slide, especially if you are tracking a motile microbe.

Microscopes are one of the major tools used by microbiologists. With the information provided in this appendix, you should have a better understanding of how they function. This knowledge and much practice will make them more useful to you.

WRITING LABORATORY REPORTS

Writing and communicating information is an essential part of the scientific process. When scientists conduct experiments that are unique and lead to new important information, they report the results in scientific journals. This allows others to use the information in their own research projects or teaching. Many exercises in this laboratory manual lend themselves to being communicated in the same way—in the form of a journal article. Writing a laboratory report in this format is a skill that requires a great deal of practice. Below we have provided guidelines for writing a laboratory report, as well as suggestions for more effective writing.

FORMAT OF A LABORATORY REPORT

A laboratory report modeled after a scientific publication should use the following format and contain the following information.

TITLE

The title is brief, but should indicate the important features of the research, for instance: "The Isolation and Characterization of Bacteria From Martian Soil."

INTRODUCTION

In this section, introduce the reader to the research problem. This section often includes a clear statement of any hypotheses being tested. Before stating the hypotheses, describe the observations and experiences that led to their formulation. For instance, if a scientist hypothesizes that Martian microbes are different than Earth microbes, the hypothesis should be accompanied by an explanation or description of earlier observations or other factors that led to its formulation.

EXPERIMENTAL METHODS

In this section, describe how the experiments were done and what tools, media, and reagents were used. Standard microbiological procedures need not be described. Instead, cite the laboratory manual or other sources. For instance, if a Gram stain was done as described in this laboratory manual, cite the manual in the text and include a complete citation for the laboratory manual in the reference section.

RESULTS

Many kinds of data are presented in the results section. Always try to organize data into figures or tables whenever appropriate. It is important to remember, however, that a story is being told—the story of what experiments were done, what data were collected, and how the data were interpreted. Therefore, in the results section, the results are described in general terms in the text and the details are left to tables and figures. The construction of informative figures and tables takes practice. Consult your instructor if you have any questions.

CONCLUSIONS

This is often the hardest section to write, so be prepared to think about, write, and rewrite this section many times. In the conclusions section, the data are interpreted and evaluated. Below is a list of the kinds of information included in the conclusions section:

1. A brief summary of the major results
2. A discussion about whether the results support the hypotheses stated in the introduction
3. Arguments regarding why the results did or did not support the hypotheses

4. Descriptions of possible sources of error in the results
5. A discussion of alternate explanations of the results
6. A discussion of additional experiments that could be done

REFERENCES

List any books, articles, or other materials used as a resource for your paper. Many methods for citing these resources can be used. Your instructor will decide which citation procedure you should use.

GUIDELINES FOR BETTER WRITING

There are a few simple steps you can take to ensure you communicate effectively in writing. They are described below.

1. Identify all prepositions used. Reword the passage to eliminate as many as possible.
2. Circle all forms of the verb "to be": am, is, are, was, were, be, being, been. Use a stronger verb whenever possible.
3. Figure out "who's kicking whom." That is, determine who is doing the action in the sentence. In very garbled writing, this actor/action connection is hard to identify.
4. Put that "kicking" action into a simple active verb. Avoid passive voice.
5. Get right to the point. Skip all mindless introductions.
6. Read each sentence aloud and mark off its basic rhythmic units with a "/". Bad sentences have no rhythm or very awkward rhythm.
7. Read the passage aloud with emphasis and feeling. If it sounds dumb, it probably is.
8. Compare the lengths of the sentences. The sentence lengths should be varied—not all long or all short, but a comfortable mixture.
9. As you write your paper, try to avoid the common errors listed below.

a. *Subject and verb disagree.* Example: "The bacter*ia is* grown on a starch-based med*ia*." The word *bacteria* is the plural of bacterium. The word media is also used incorrectly. It is the plural of medium.
b. *Missing sentence component.* Example: "Enzyme degrades starch." Is the sentence about one enzyme or all enzymes?
c. *Undefined pronoun.* Example: "I would scrape my mouth and put the remains on a Petri dish. I would let *it* cultivate." What is being cultivated, the remains or the Petri dish?
d. *Poor choice of words.* In the example given for (undefined pronouns) "teeth" is better than "mouth," and "sample" is better than "remains."
e. *Sentence does not say precisely what is meant.* In the example given for undefined pronouns, the organisms are grown on a "culture medium" contained within a Petri dish.
f. *Incorrect use of personal pronouns.* Example: "Take *your* culture medium and inoculate it with *your* bacteria." To correct this sentence, substitute "the" for the first "your" and delete the second "your." In general, it is best to write in the third person.
g. *Unneeded words.* Examples: now, well, so.
h. *Incorrect use of verbs.* Example: "A clear zone indicates the starch was *broke* down. We *seen* it."
i. *Lack of capitalization.*
j. *Use of symbols rather than words.* Examples: w/, w/o, &.
k. *Run-on sentences.* Example: Sentences with unrelated ideas combined into a single sentence, short, choppy sentences.
l. *Redundancy.* Example: "Later, after 2 days of incubation, we observed the results."
m. *Misplaced modifying phrase or word.* Example: "In the sewage sample, we observed many coliform bacteria." Were the bacteria in the sewage or was the writer?